# Community Medicine

# Practical Guide and Logbook

Name of Student: ..................................................................

Course of Student: ..................................................................

Name of College: ..................................................................

Name of University: ..................................................................

## Personal Details of Student

Name of Student: ----------------------------------------------------------------

Sex: M/F/T ----------------------------------------------------------------

Age (Date of Birth): ----------------------------------------------------------------

Mobile Number: ----------------------------------------------------------------

E-mail ID: ----------------------------------------------------------------

Local Address: ----------------------------------------------------------------
----------------------------------------------------------------

Permanent Address: ----------------------------------------------------------------
----------------------------------------------------------------

Course of Student: ----------------------------------------------------------------

Name of Teacher Guide: ----------------------------------------------------------------

Enrolment Number: ----------------------------------------------------------------

Date and Year of Registration: ----------------------------------------------------------------

Date of Joining: ----------------------------------------------------------------

Date of Examination: ----------------------------------------------------------------

Special Interest: ----------------------------------------------------------------

## Assessment of Student

| S. No. | Criteria | Marks Obtained (Out of Total 10 Marks) |
|---|---|---|
| 1 | Regularity | |
| 2 | Intelligence | |
| 3 | Diligence | |
| 4 | Academic Ability | |
| 5 | Practical Approach | |
| 6 | Initiation Ability | |
| 7 | Team work ability | |
| 8 | Leadership Quality | |
| 9 | Teaching Ability | |
| 10 | Research Aptitude | |
| 11 | Total Marks (Out of 100) | |

Signature of Teacher Guide                                        Signature of Professor and Head

## Summary of Student's Participation in Various Activities

| Type of Activities | Activities | No. Presented | No. Attended |
|---|---|---|---|
| **Departmental** | **Activities** | **No. Presented** | **No. Attended** |
| | Seminars Case Presentation | | |
| | Journal Club Presentation | | |
| | World Health Days/Special | | |
| | Activities Presentation | | |
| | Teaching | | |
| | Trainings | | |
| **Patient Care Activities** | **Places** | **Yes** | **No** |
| | UHTC | | |
| | RHTC | | |
| | IDH | | |
| | ARC | | |
| | Immunization Clinic | | |
| | Other Places (...............................) | | |
| **Community Care Activities** | **Activities** | **No. Participated** | **No. Attended** |
| | Community Surveys | | |
| | Health Education Camps | | |
| | World Health Days/Special Drives Celebration | | |
| **Field Visits** | | **Total No. Schedule** | **No. Attended** |
| | Field Visits | | |
| **Research Activities** | | **Yes** | **No** |
| | Research | | |
| **Other Activities** | | **Yes** | **No** |
| | Other Activities | | |

**Teacher Guide's Remark**                                        **Signature of Teacher Guide**

# Community Medicine

## Practical Guide and Logbook

**Kusum Lata Gaur**
MD (PSM) PGHFWM WHO Fellow for IEC
Professor, PSM

**SC Soni**
MD (PSM) PGHFWM WHO Fellow for IEC
Associate Professor, PSM

**Rajeev Yadav**
MD (PSM)
Assistant Professor, PSM

Department of Community Medicine
Sawai Man Singh Medical College
Jaipur, Rajasthan, India

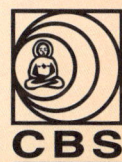

## CBS Publishers & Distributors Pvt Ltd

New Delhi • Bengaluru • Pune • Kochi • Chennai

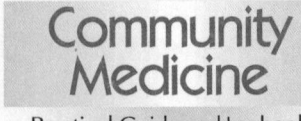

# Community Medicine

Practical Guide and Logbook

ISBN: 978-81-239-2394-9

Copyright © Authors and Publishers

First Edition: 2014

Published by Satish Kumar Jain for
**CBS Publishers & Distributors** Pvt Ltd
4819/XI Prahlad Street, 24 Ansari Road, Daryaganj, New Delhi 110 002, India.
Ph: 23289259, 23266861, 23266867          Website: www.cbspd.com
Fax: 011-23243014          e-mail: delhi@cbspd.com; cbspubs@airtelmail.in.
*Corporate Office:* 204 FIE, Industrial Area, Patparganj, Delhi 110 092
Ph: 4934 4934          Fax: 4934 4935          e-mail: publishing@cbspd.com; publicity@cbspd.com

*Branches*

- **Bengaluru:** Seema House 2975, 17th Cross, K.R. Road,
  Banasankari 2nd Stage, Bengaluru 560 070, Karnataka
  Ph: +91-80-26771678/79          Fax: +91-80-26771680          e-mail: bangalore@cbspd.com
- **Chennai:** 20, West Park Road, Shenoy Nagar, Chennai 600 030, Tamil Nadu
  Ph: +91-44-26260666, 26208620          Fax: +91-44-42032115          e-mail: chennai@cbspd.com
- **Kochi:** 36/14 Kalluvilakam, Lissie Hospital Road, Kochi 682 018, Kerala
  Ph: +91-484-4059061-65          Fax: +91-484-4059065          e-mail: kochi@cbspd.com
- **Mumbai:** 83-C, Dr E Moses Road, Worli, Mumbai-400018, Maharashtra
  Ph: +91-9833017933          e-mail: mumbai@cbspd.com
- **Pune:** Bhuruk Prestige, Sr. No. 52/12/2+1+3/2 Narhe, Haveli
  (Near Katraj-Dehu Road Bypass), Pune 411 041, Maharashtra
  Ph: +91-20-64704058, 64704059, 32392277 Fax: +91-20-24300160          e-mail: pune@cbspd.com

*Representatives*

- **Hyderabad** 0-9885175004
- **Nagpur** 0-9021734563
- **Kolkata** 0-9831437309, 0-9051152362
- **Patna** 0-9334159340
- **Vijayawada** 0-9000660880

*Printed at* HT Media Ltd., Noida

# Preface

This book is not only a guide on community medicine practical but it is also a manual, in which students can write down their observations and teachers can check and sign the work done by the students. In fact, this book is needed for each student which can serve the purpose of a Logbook.

Community medicine is called 'the father of medicine'. It is a very vast science as it includes the knowledge of other faculties also. It is difficult to concise the knowledge of community medicine as a whole. This book concentrates on the practical aspects of community medicine and is mainly designed for postgraduate students of this faculty of medicine but it also serves the purpose of undergraduates. As community medicine also covers the practical aspects of other faculties of medicine, this book may be useful to postgraduate students of other disciplines also along with undergraduate and postgraduate students of community medicine.

Community medicine practical, as per MCI, has sessionals, practical and viva voce. Sessionals will be assessed by daily performance of students which may be accessed through 'Logbook'. Practical has various activities at the time of practical examination which includes short cases, long cases, family presentation, water chemistry, spot exercises, exercises related to epidemiology and public health, statistical exercises, microbiological exercises, etc.

This book contains all the above referred contents of community medicine practical with some other important issues like investigation of an outbreak, thesis protocol, specimen sampling, water sampling, etc. It also contains visits to health-related places like hospital waste management facility, water treatment plant, sewage treatment plant, dairy plant, etc.

Hope this book on community medicine practical fulfills the aim which it is intended for.

Last, there is open invitation to the readers and users of this book to give suggestions which may help in further improvement. Good suggestions will be duly acknowledged.

**Kusum Lata Gaur**
**SC Soni**
**Rajeev Yadav**

## Activities Schedule Logbook

| S. No. | Date | Activity | Your Role | Teacher's Remark and Sign |
|---|---|---|---|---|
| 1 | | | | |
| 2 | | | | |
| 3 | | | | |
| 4 | | | | |
| 5 | | | | |
| 6 | | | | |
| 7 | | | | |
| 8 | | | | |
| 9 | | | | |
| 10 | | | | |
| 11 | | | | |
| 12 | | | | |
| 13 | | | | |
| 14 | | | | |
| 15 | | | | |
| 16 | | | | |
| 17 | | | | |
| 18 | | | | |
| 19 | | | | |
| 20 | | | | |
| 21 | | | | |
| 22 | | | | |
| 23 | | | | |
| 24 | | | | |
| 25 | | | | |
| 26 | | | | |
| 27 | | | | |
| 28 | | | | |
| 29 | | | | |
| 30 | | | | |
| 31 | | | | |
| 32 | | | | |
| 33 | | | | |
| 34 | | | | |
| 35 | | | | |
| 36 | | | | |
| 37 | | | | |
| 38 | | | | |
| 39 | | | | |
| 40 | | | | |
| 41 | | | | |
| 42 | | | | |
| 43 | | | | |
| 44 | | | | |

## Activities Schedule Logbook

| S. No. | Date | Activity | Your Role | Teacher's Remark and Sign |
|---|---|---|---|---|
| 41 | | | | |
| 42 | | | | |
| 43 | | | | |
| 44 | | | | |
| 45 | | | | |
| 46 | | | | |
| 47 | | | | |
| 48 | | | | |
| 49 | | | | |
| 50 | | | | |
| 51 | | | | |
| 52 | | | | |
| 53 | | | | |
| 54 | | | | |
| 55 | | | | |
| 56 | | | | |
| 57 | | | | |
| 58 | | | | |
| 59 | | | | |
| 50 | | | | |
| 61 | | | | |
| 62 | | | | |
| 63 | | | | |
| 64 | | | | |
| 65 | | | | |
| 66 | | | | |
| 67 | | | | |
| 68 | | | | |
| 69 | | | | |
| 60 | | | | |
| 61 | | | | |
| 62 | | | | |
| 63 | | | | |
| 64 | | | | |
| 65 | | | | |
| 66 | | | | |
| 67 | | | | |
| 68 | | | | |
| 69 | | | | |
| 70 | | | | |
| 71 | | | | |
| 72 | | | | |
| 73 | | | | |
| 74 | | | | |

## Activities Schedule Logbook

| S. No. | Date | Activity | Your Role | Teacher's Remark and Sign |
|--------|------|----------|-----------|----------------------------|
| 75 | | | | |
| 76 | | | | |
| 77 | | | | |
| 78 | | | | |
| 79 | | | | |
| 80 | | | | |
| 81 | | | | |
| 82 | | | | |
| 83 | | | | |
| 84 | | | | |
| 85 | | | | |
| 86 | | | | |
| 87 | | | | |
| 88 | | | | |
| 89 | | | | |
| 90 | | | | |
| 91 | | | | |
| 92 | | | | |
| 93 | | | | |
| 94 | | | | |
| 95 | | | | |
| 96 | | | | |
| 97 | | | | |
| 98 | | | | |
| 99 | | | | |
| 100 | | | | |
| 101 | | | | |
| 102 | | | | |
| 103 | | | | |
| 104 | | | | |
| 105 | | | | |
| 106 | | | | |
| 107 | | | | |
| 108 | | | | |
| 109 | | | | |
| 110 | | | | |
| 111 | | | | |
| 112 | | | | |
| 113 | | | | |
| 114 | | | | |
| 115 | | | | |

# Contents

Preface      v

1. **Case Study and Family Study**      1–42

2. **Microbiology**      43–48

3. **Water Chemistry**      49–59

4. **Spotting**      60–133
   - Food Stuffs Spots 60
   - Entomology 83
   - Insecticides 95
   - Disinfectants and Deodorants 98
   - Contraceptive Methods 101
   - Vaccines and Cold Chain Equipments 108
   - Cold Chain Equipments 114
   - Photographs and Miscellaneous Spots 118

5. **Field Visits**      134–160

6. **Water Sampling, Examination and Treatment**      161–173

7. **Specimen Sampling**      174–186

8. **Research Methodology and Biostatistics**      187–253
   - Research Methodology 187
   - Biostatistics 202
   - Computers in Statistics 233

9. **Thesis Protocol**      254–265

10. **Investigation and Management of an Epidemic**      266–275

## 11. Exercises                                            276–281

### *Appendix*                                              282–295

- India's Demography  282
- Important Days  283
- World Health Day Themes  289
- Chi-square Table  291
- 'Z' Score Test  292
- Table for 't' Test  293
- Random Number Table  294
- Hospital Waste Categories  294
- Final Treatment and Disposal  295

### *Index*                                                 297–298

# 1

# Case Study and Family Study

Cases should be examined thoroughly within the time allotted. Student should interpret following on the basis of history, examination and investigations done.

1. Provisional diagnosis (with reasons).
2. Investigations suggested for final diagnosis.
3. Preventive measures (including treatment/management).

Teacher's Remark .........................................
Teacher's Sign .........................................

## CASE STUDY

**Case no.** _____         **Date of Examination** —————

**Introductory Data**

Name of Patient _____*Age _____ Sex (Male/Female/Other)

Residence         _____    _____

_____

_____      _____

* Recorded in completed years, as on the last birthday

**Presenting Complaints** (In order of appearance of symptoms with their duration in chronological order).

1. _____

2. _____

3. _____

4. _____

5. _____

**History of Present Illness** (Describing all complaints in order of appearance with their nature)

_____

_____

_____

_____

_____

**History of Past Illness, if any**

_____

_____

**Previous Obstetric History (In case of Female)**

Gravid (G) ____ Para (P) ____ Stillbirth (S) ____ Abortion (A) ____ Live (L) ____

**No. of children with their nature of delivery**

| Order of delivery | Name of child | Sex | Date of birth | Nature of birth normal/LSCS/Inst | Status Sb/alive /dead if Sb/dead with reasons |
|---|---|---|---|---|---|
| | | | | | |
| | | | | | |
| | | | | | |

**Menstrual History**

Age at menarche: _____ with duration: _____ days cycle.

Regular/Irregular

Normal/Scanty/Heavy flow

**Family History of Illness**

_____

_____

**Social and Occupational History**

_____

_____

**Psychiatric History**

_____

_____

**Treatment History**

_____

_____

**Personal History**

Addiction-Yes / No          If, yes:

| S. no. | Type of Addiction | Quantity/day | Duration | |
|---|---|---|---|---|
| | | | From | To |
| | | | | |
| | | | | |
| | | | | |

Exercise:——————— Always/Often/Seldom/Rarely/Never

Any other: ——————— Always/Often/Seldom/Rarely/Never

**Personal Hygiene:** Poor/Fair/Good                                    Scores

| | | |
|---|---|---|
| Dressings: | Improper/Proper | 0/1 |
| | Unclean/Clean | 0/1 |
| | Un-ironed/Ironed | 0/1 |
| Skin: | Unclean/Clean | 0/1 |
| | Diseased/Non-diseased | 0/1 |
| Hairs: | Unclean/Clean | 0/1 |
| | With louse infestation/without louse infestation | 0/1 |
| | Un-combed/Combed | 0/1 |
| Eyes: | Unclean/Clean | 0/1 |
| Ears: | Unclean/Clean | 0/1 |
| Face: | Unclean/Clean | 0/1 |
| Teeth: | Un-brushed/Brushed | 0/1 |
| | Diseased/Non-diseased | 0/1 |
| Nails: | Unclean/Clean | 0/1 |
| Footwear: | No/Yes | 0/1 |

Total Score _____

**Personal Hygiene Status: Poor/Fair/Good**

**Poor:** Total score 5 and below

**Fair:** Total score between 6 and 10

**Good:** Total score more than 10

**General Examination**

Appearance: Conscious/Semiconscious/Unconscious

Weight _____ (kg) Height _____ cm   Built: Aesthetic/Athletic/Obese

Chest circumference (in case of child) _____        MAC (in case of child) _____

Skin-colour _____ Hair _____ Face _____              Mouth _____

Eyes _____ Ear _____ Neck _____ Upper limb _____ Abdomen _____

Lower limb _____ Any other _____

Temperature _____ Pulse _____ BP _____ Respiration rate _____

## Systemic Examination

| System | Observation | Palpation | Percussion | Auscultation | Diagnosis/Remark |
|---|---|---|---|---|---|
| GIT | | | | | |
| Respiratory | | | | | |
| CVS | | | | | |
| CNS | | | | | |
| Genitourinary | | | | | |
| Musculoskeletal | | | | | |
| Skin | | | | | |
| Other | | | | | |

## Investigations done with their Report

| Investigation | Normal value | Test value | Remark |
|---|---|---|---|
| | | | |
| | | | |
| | | | |
| | | | |

## Differential Diagnosis

| S. no. | D/D disease name | D/D variable | Points in favour | Points in against |
|---|---|---|---|---|
| 1. | | History | | |
| | | Examination | | |
| | | Investigation | | |
| 2. | | History | | |
| | | Examination | | |
| | | Investigation | | |
| 3. | | History | | |
| | | Examination | | |
| | | Investigation | | |

Probable diagnosis _____

## Suggestive Investigations for Diagnosis

1. _____

2. _____

## Treatment Advised

_____

_____

_____

## Preventive Measures Suggested

| Prevention level | Individual level | Family level | Community level |
|---|---|---|---|
| Primary | | | |
| Secondary | | | |
| Tertiary | | | |

## PROBLEM FAMILY

Find out psycho-socio-medical problems in the family.

```
Teacher's Remark .........................................
Teacher's Sign .........................................
```

## Family Presentation

Detailed history of the family should be taken on different aspects. Then every individual of the family should be examined thoroughly to find out any psycho-socio-medical problems in the family.

Family should be examined at the site, i.e. at its residence and within the time allotted. But before entering into any house, one should remember Hippocratic Oath. The Hippocratic Oath is an oath historically taken by physicians and other healthcare professionals swearing to practice medicine ethically and honestly.

**Hippocratic Oath:** I swear by *Apollo*, the *healer*, *Asclepius*, *Hygieia*, and *Panacea*, and I take to witness all the gods, all the goddesses, to keep according to my ability and my judgment, the following oath and agreement:

"Into whatever house I enter, I will go with the object of helping sick, holding aloof from all voluntary and all other hurtful wrong doing and from licentious practices and regarding the things I see or hear in the course of the treatment or even outside of the treatment in regard to the life of men, which on no account one must spread abroad, I will keep to myself holding such things shameful to be spoken about. In my intercourse with man which ought not to be divulged, I will keep silent regarding them as in violable secrets.

If I fulfill this path and do not violate it, may it be granted to me to enjoy life and art, being honored with fame among all men for all time to come; if I transgress it and swear falsely, may the opposite of all this be my lot."

To find out **psychosocio-medical problems** of the allotted family, one must strictly punctuate into following:

1. Environmental (external) status of family.
2. Socioeconomic status of family.
3. Psychosocial environment of family.
4. Medical examination of every individual of family.

## Module for Family Study
### Community Survey

Name of colony _____

Total population _____

Caste and origin _____

Community organizations _____

Principal modes of livelihood _____

Educational facilities _____

Health and health related facilities _____

    Health centres _____

      Government _____

      Private _____

    Water supply _____

    Excreta disposal _____

    Waste water disposal _____

    Refuse disposal _____

    Disposal of dead _____

Methods of recording birth and deaths _____

Channels of communication _____

Schools _____

## Spot Map of Colony Showing House

| **Housing Environment** | | **House No.** |
|---|---|---|
| Sketch of House | (Scale 1 cm = 1 meter) | N |

| **Housing Condition** | **Score** |
|---|---|
| Site: Bad/Fair/Good | 0/1/2 |
| Setback: No/Improper/Proper | 0/1/2 |
| Floor: Kacha/Pakka with crevices/Pakka without crevices | 0/1/2 |
| Walls: Kacha/Pakka with crevices/Pakka without crevices | 0/1/2 |
| Roof: Kacha/Pakka with crevices/Pakka without crevices | 0/1/2 |
| Height: Inadequate/Adequate | 0/1 |
| *Overcrowding: Present/Absent | 0/1 |
| **Light: Inadequate/Adequate | 0/1 |

Kitchen: Not separate/separate but without smoke

| | |
|---|---|
| Outlet/separate with smoke outlet | 0/1/2 |
| Storage facility: Improper/Proper | 0/1 |
| Drainage facility: Improper/Proper | 0/1 |
| Privy: Open air defaecation/Private service/Public sanitary/Private sanitary | 0/1/2/3 |
| Water supply: Surface/Well/Tape water/Tube well or treated tape water | 0/1/2/3 |
| Bath room: Not separate/Separate but Improper/Separate and proper | 0/1/2 |
| Domestic animals: Not separate/Separate | 0/1 |
| Refuse disposal: Improper/Proper | 0/1 |
| Drainage: Improper/Proper | 0/1 |

Environmental total score obtained _____

[*Overcrowding present if floor space/person is less than 50 feet$^2$ along with sex separation
** One can read newspaper in any corner of house is adequate lighting]

> **Criteria for housing environmental status of family**
> **Poor**: Score 10 or less
> **Fair**: Score 11 to 20
> **Good**: Score above 20

Housing environmental status of family:  Poor/Fair/Good

| **Living Status:** | **Scores** |
|---|---|
| *City: No/Category C/Category B/Category A | 0/1/2/3 |
| *Locality: No/Category C/Category B/Category A | 0/1/2/3 |
| Accommodation (BHK): 0/1/2/3/>3 | 0/1/2/3/4 |
| Conveyance: No/Cycle/Two wheeler/Four wheeler | 0/1/2/3/4 |
| Communication: No/News papers/Mobile | 0/1/2/3 |
| Audio-visual: No/Radio/Television/Computer/Laptop | 0/1/2/3/4 |
| Mechanical ventilation: No/Fan/Cooler/Air condition | 0/1/2/3 |
| **Modern amenities: 0/1/2/3/>3 | 0/1/2/3/4 |
| *Children's school: No/Category C/Category B/Category A | 0/1/2/3 |
| *Club membership: No/Category C/Category B/Category A | 0/1/2/3 |

Total scores gained _____

Living status:

> **Criteria for living status of family**
> **Poor**: Score 10 or less
> **Fair**: Score 11 to 21
> **Good**: Score above 21

[* Categories are as per criteria predefined by Government of India
**Number of other modern amenities]

## SOCIOECONOMIC SCHEDULE

Type of Family: Nuclear/Joint/3 Generation/Extended          **Religion:** _____

### Family Schedule

| S. no. | Name of family member | DOB | Sex | Relation to head of family | Education | Occupation | Income | Any chronic disease | Remark |
|--------|----------------------|-----|-----|---------------------------|-----------|------------|--------|--------------------|--------|
|        |                      |     |     |                           |           |            |        |                    |        |
|        |                      |     |     |                           |           |            |        |                    |        |
|        |                      |     |     |                           |           |            |        |                    |        |
|        |                      |     |     |                           |           |            |        |                    |        |

Total family income: ₹ _____/ Month   Per capita income: ₹ _____/Month

Expenditure: ₹_____/Month, i.e. _____% of income.

Mode of expenditure: Grocery _____ ,   Bills _____ ,   Any other_____

Debt/Loans = ₹ _____ Assets = ₹ _____

Debt to assets ratio = Debt: Assets = _____

*Socioeconomic status: Class: Upper/ Upper middle/Lower middle/Upper lower /Lower

(*Socioeconomic status is seen as per desired scale)

Births (during last year): Live _____ Stillbirths _____ Abortions _____

Deaths (during last year): Name _____ Age _____ Sex _____ Cause of death _____

## IMMUNIZATION RECORD

| S. no. | Name | Age (DOB) | Sex | Vaccines | | | | | | Remark |
|--------|------|-----------|-----|----------|--|--|--|--|--|--------|
|        |      |           |     | BCG | Hepatitis vaccine | OPV (1/2/3) | DPT (1/2/3) | Measles | Any other | |
|        |      |           |     |     |     |     |     |     |     |     |
|        |      |           |     |     |     |     |     |     |     |     |
|        |      |           |     |     |     |     |     |     |     |     |

### Immunization Status

Un-immunized/Incomplete immunization/Complete immunization for the age.

## DIET AND NUTRITIONAL STATUS SCHEDULE

**Diet–Survey:**                    **Type of Diet:** Vegetarian/Non-vegetarian/Eggeterian

| Food Stuffs | Quantity consumed | | | | |
|---|---|---|---|---|---|
| | 1st day | 2nd day | 3rd day | Total | Average/Day |
| Cereals (specify) | | | | | |
| Pulses (specify) | | | | | |
| Vegetable (specify) | | | | | |
| Meat (specify) | | | | | |
| Milk (specify) | | | | | |
| Sugar | | | | | |
| Oil | | | | | |
| Ghee | | | | | |
| Nuts (specify) | | | | | |
| Any other (specify) | | | | | |

### Average Daily Consumption of Family

| Food stuff | Quantity consumed | Nutrient consumed | | | | | | | |
|---|---|---|---|---|---|---|---|---|---|
| | | Calorie | Protein | Carbohydrate | Fat | Vit A | Vit B | Fe | Ca |
| | | | | | | | | | |
| | | | | | | | | | |
| | | | | | | | | | |
| | | | | | | | | | |
| | | | | | | | | | |
| | | | | | | | | | |
| | | | | | | | | | |

### Daily Nutrient Requirement of Family

| Name of family member | Age | Sex | Nutrient requirement | | | | | | | |
|---|---|---|---|---|---|---|---|---|---|---|
| | | | Calorie | Protein | Carbohydrate | Fat | Vit A | Vit B | Fe | Ca |
| | | | | | | | | | | |
| | | | | | | | | | | |
| | | | | | | | | | | |
| | | | | | | | | | | |
| | | | | | | | | | | |

### Nutritional Status of Family

| Nutritional status | Calorie | Protein | Carbohydrate | Fat | Vit A | Vit B | Fe | Ca |
|---|---|---|---|---|---|---|---|---|
| *Nutrient consumption | | | | | | | | |
| **Nutrient requirement | | | | | | | | |
| Nutrient deficit | | | | | | | | |
| Nutrient excess | | | | | | | | |

*Nutrient value of common foods given in Chapter Spots-Food Stuffs
**Daily requirement of nutrient given on pg. no. 39–41

## HEALTH KNOWLEDGE OF FAMILY

**Knowledge of Health Centre Available in Community: Yes/No**

| Vaccine | For which disease | At what age? | Rout of administration |
|---|---|---|---|
| BCG | | | |
| Hepatitis vaccine | | | |
| OPV | | | |
| DPT | | | |
| Measles | | | |
| DT | | | |
| TT | | | |
| Any other (specify) | | | |

**Feeding of babies/nutrition:** Knowledge about

Exclusive breastfeeding:  Yes/No   Weaning:   Yes/No

**Contraceptives /devices:** Knowledge about

Condom: Yes/No                 Oral pills (daily): Yes/No

Oral Pills (weekly): Yes/No        Emergency pills: Yes/No

IUD: Yes/No

Vasectomy: Yes/No               NSV: Yes/No

Tubectomy: Yes/No               Laparoscopic sterilization: Yes/No

Any other (specify): Yes/No

**Contraceptive Method in Use**

| Eligible couple no. | Names of EC | Type of CM in use | Duration of use |
|---|---|---|---|
| | | | |
| | | | |
| | | | |

**Unmet Need of Couple**

| Eligible couple no. | Names of EC | Desired family size | | | Family size in position | | | Unmet need | |
|---|---|---|---|---|---|---|---|---|---|
| | | Total | Male | Female | Total | Male | Female | Male | Female |
| | | | | | | | | | |
| | | | | | | | | | |
| | | | | | | | | | |

## SOCIAL PROBLEMS IN FAMILY

Any addiction in family _____

Any unemployment in family _____

Poverty (BPL) _____ (in SES Class V)

Any medical problem becoming social problem

    Physical _____

    Mental _____

    Social _____

Any criminal in family _____

Any unmarried mother in family _____

Any orphan in family _____

Any divorcee in family _____

Any child > 6 years not going to school _____

More than 2 old persons in family _____

Recreational facility not available in the house _____

More than 5 children per couple _____

Less than 2 years interval between two children _____

## ANTENATAL CASE RECORD

Name _____    Age _____    Reg. no. ( if reg.) _____

W/O _____

**Previous Obstetrical History**

Gravid (G) _____ Para (P) _____ Stillbirth (S) _____ Abortion (A) _____ Live (L) _____

**No. of children with their nature of delivery**

| Order of delivery | Name of child | Sex | Date of birth | Nature of birth | Place of birth | Status S/L/dead If dead with reasons |
|---|---|---|---|---|---|---|
| | | | | | | |
| | | | | | | |
| | | | | | | |
| | | | | | | |

**Present Pregnancy**

LMP EDD _____ Weeks of gestation _____

Complaints if any _____

H/O chronic illness _____

Family history of illness _____

Registration of pregnancy: Yes /No   If yes when _____    Where _____

**ANC Home Visit: Yes /No     If Yes:**

| ANC visit | Date | Visiting person | Gestational weeks | Findings | Advises |
|---|---|---|---|---|---|
| 1. | | | | | |
| 2. | | | | | |
| 3. | | | | | |
| 4. | | | | | |

**ANC Clinic Attended at Health Centre: Yes /No     If Yes,**

| ANC visit | Date | Visiting person | Gestational weeks | Findings | Advises |
|---|---|---|---|---|---|
| 1. | | | | | |
| 2. | | | | | |
| 3. | | | | | |
| 4. | | | | | |

**Laboratory Investigation done**

| ANC visit | Date | Investigation done | Test value | Normal value | Advises |
|---|---|---|---|---|---|
| 1. | | | | | |
| 2. | | | | | |
| 3. | | | | | |
| 4. | | | | | |

## POSTNATAL CASE

Name _____     Age _____     Reg. no. ( if reg.) _____

W/O _____

Delivered at (place) _____     Baby's birth weight _____

Date and time of admission _____     Date and time of delivery _____

Date and time of discharge _____ Result _____ Nature of delivery_____

### Mother's Component

Pulse _____ Temp. _____ Fundal Ht. _____ Lochia _____ Breast _____

Urine _____ Others _____

### Child's Component

Search for any congenital anomaly

Resuscitation

Care of cord

Care of eyes

Care of skin

Weight _____ Temperature _____ Stool _____ Feeding _____

### Advises given at time of discharge

Contraceptive

Vaccination

Related programmes like JSSY, IMNCI, etc.

Under five's clinics

Mother care in terms of observing for any complications, psycho-social support, encouraging for breastfeeding and health education specially for personal hygiene and baby care should be given.

## CHILD HEALTH RECORD (UP TO 2 MONTHS)

Name _____ Date of birth _____ Sex _____ Birth order _____

Birth place _____ Birth weight _____ Present weight _____

Name and relation of attendant: _____

### Ask Attendant about

Presenting complaints (in order of appearance)

_____

_____

_____

_____

Present history of illness _____
_____
_____

Past history of illness _____
_____
_____

Family history of illness _____
_____

| Check for feeding problem | Answers/observation | Assessed as |
|---|---|---|
| **Ask the mother**<br>• Have you started breastfeeding the baby?<br>• Do you have pain during breastfeeding?<br>• Is there any difficulty in feeding the baby? | | |
| **If yes, then look for**<br>• Flat or inverted nipples<br>• Sore nipples<br>• Engorged breast/breast abscess | | |
| **Ask the mother**<br>Have you given any other food or drink to baby: Yes/No | | |
| **If yes, what and how?**<br>Water/Dairy milk/Cow's milk/Buffalo milk/Any other | | |
| **And how?**<br>With bottle/with spoon/with any other | | |

| Check for feeding problem | Answers/observation | Assessed as |
|---|---|---|
| Count the breath in one minute _____ breaths per minute | | |
| Repeat if faster than normal _____ breaths per minute | | |
| Look for severe chest in drawing | | |
| Look at umbilicus: Is it red or draining pus? | | |
| Look for skin pustules: Are they 10 or more or a big boil | | |
| Measure auxiliary temperature: <br> • Normal: 36.5 to 37.4°C <br> • Mild hypothermia: 36 to 36.5°C <br> • Moderate hypothermia: 32 to 36°C <br> • Sever hypothermia: < 32°C <br> • Fever hyperthermia: 37.5°C and more <br> Is young infant lethargic or unconscious? | | |
| Look at young infant's movement, if normal or less | | |
| Look for jaundice | | |
| Look for anaemia | | |
| Has the infant have convulsions? | | |
| **Has the child receive** <br> • BCG: Yes/No <br> • OPV: Yes/No <br> • DPT: Yes/No <br> • Any other: Yes/No, If Yes what _____ When _____ | | |
| **Assess any other problem** | | |
| **Assess breastfeeding** | **Answers/observation** | **Assessed as** |
| Has the infant breastfeed in the previous one hour? If the infant has not breastfeed in the previous one hour, ask the mother to breastfeed her infant and observe | | |
| **Attachment to breast** <br> Is the infant able to attached <br> • Chin touching breast: Yes/No <br> • Mouth wide open: Yes/No <br> • Lower lip turned outwards: Yes/No <br> • More areola above than below the mouth: Yes/No | **Classify:** <br> 1. No attachment at all <br> 2. Poorly attached <br> 3. Well attached | |
| **Suckling** | **Classify** | |
| Is the infant suckling effectively, i.e. slow deep sucks: Yes/No | 1. Not suckling at all <br> 2. Not suckling efficiently <br> 3. Suckling efficiently | |
| **If not suckling efficiently** <br> • Look for ulcers in mouth: Yes/No <br> • Look for ulcers white patches in mouth: Yes/No | | |

## Systemic Examination

| System | Observation | Palpation | Percussion | Auscultation | Diagnosis/Remark |
|---|---|---|---|---|---|
| GIT | | | | | |
| Respiratory | | | | | |
| CVS | | | | | |
| CNS | | | | | |
| Genitourinary | | | | | |
| Muskuloskeletal | | | | | |
| Skin | | | | | |
| Other | | | | | |

## Investigations done with their report

| Investigation | Normal value | Test value | Remark |
|---|---|---|---|
| | | | |
| | | | |
| | | | |

## Differential Diagnosis

| S. no. | D/D disease name | D/D variable | Points in favour | Points in against |
|---|---|---|---|---|
| 1. | | History | | |
| | | Examination | | |
| | | Investigation | | |
| 2. | | History | | |
| | | Examination | | |
| | | Investigation | | |
| 3. | | History | | |
| | | Examination | | |
| | | Investigation | | |

Probable diagnosis _____

## Suggestive Investigations for Diagnosis

1. _____

2. _____

## Treatment Advised

1. _____

2. _____

## Preventive Measures Suggested

| Prevention level | Individual level | Family level | Community level |
|---|---|---|---|
| Primary | | | |
| Secondary | | | |
| Tertiary | | | |

## CHILD HEALTH RECORD (2 months to 5 years)

Name _____     Age _____     Sex _____     Birth order _____

Birth place _____     Birth weight _____     Present weight _____

### Development

Teething                           Date _____

Sitting with support               Date _____

Sitting without support            Date _____

Talking 1st word                   Date _____

Walking                            Date _____

**Immunization status:** (No. of doses)

BCG _____ OPV _____ DPT _____ Measles _____ Any other _____

Present history of illness _____

_____

_____

Past history of illness _____

_____

_____

Family history of illness _____

_____

### Examination

Signs of malnutrition:   Yes/No   Tick if any of the following present

| Signs of malnutrition | If yes, tick(√) | Signs of malnutrition | If yes, tick (√) |
|---|---|---|---|
| Xerosis: | | Flage sign | |
| Glossitis: | | Rickety rosary | |
| Angular stomatitis: | | Bleeding gums | |
| Keratomalacia | | Harrison's sulcus | |
| Bitot's spot | | Bowing of legs | |
| Oedema | | Night blindness | |
| Any other (specify) | | | |

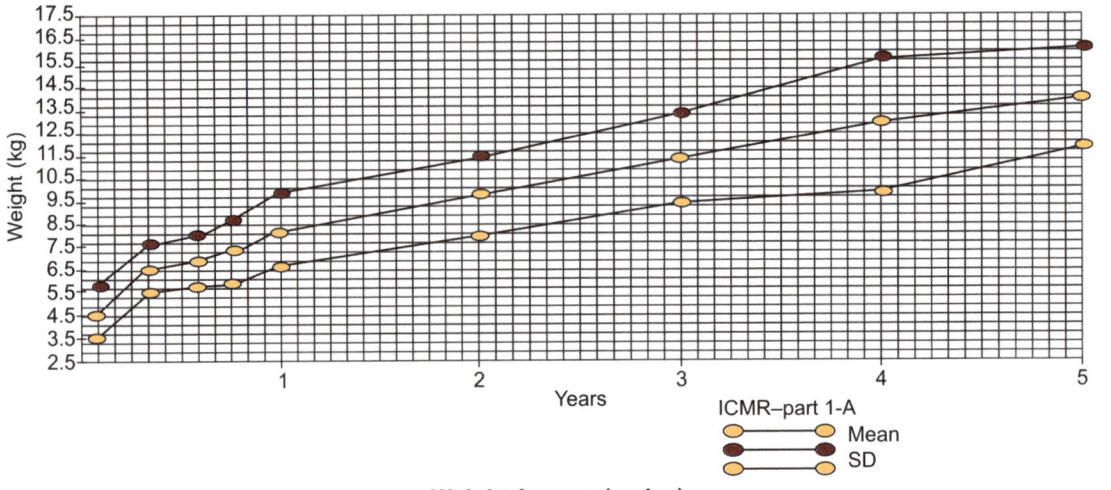

**Weight for age (males)**

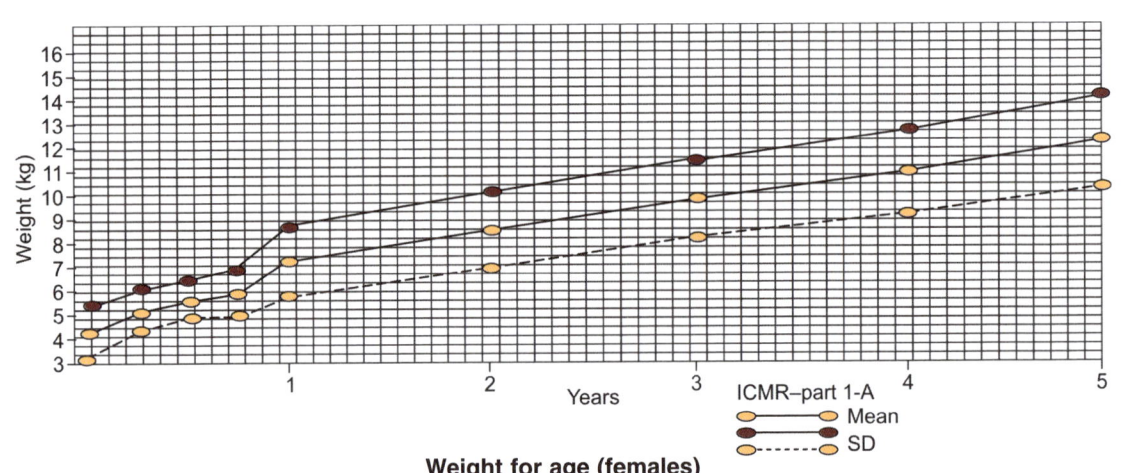

**Weight for age (females)**

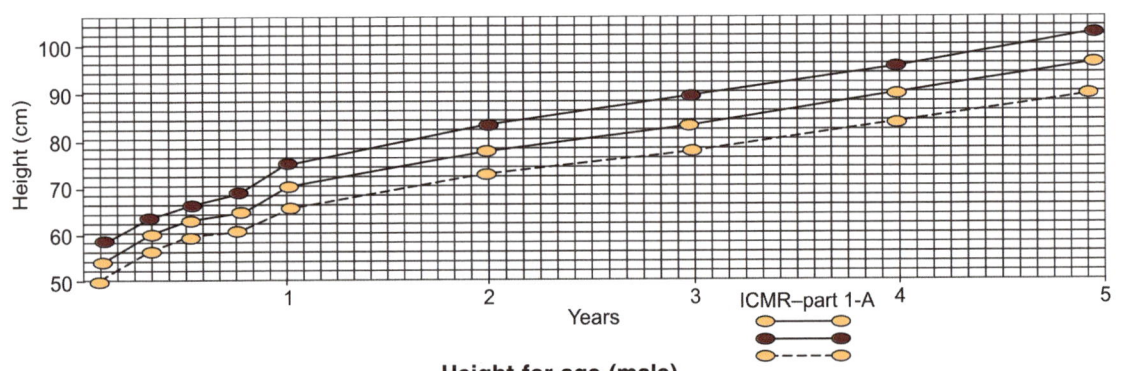

**Height for age (male)**

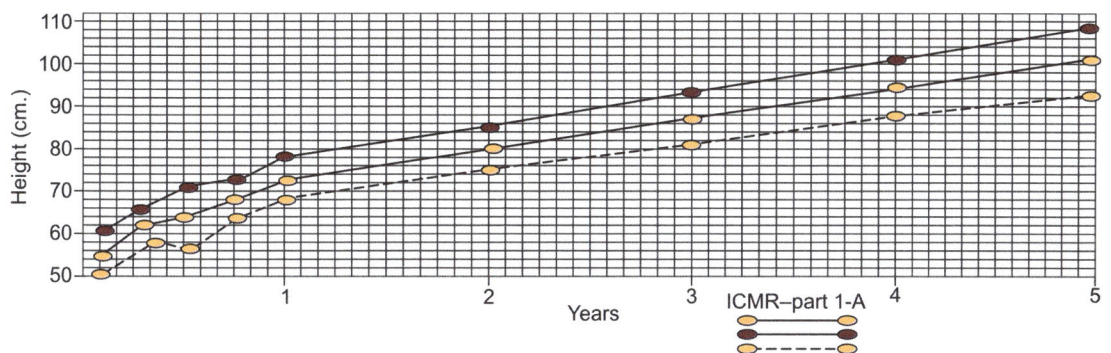

**Height for age (females)**

| Personal Hygiene: Poor/Fair/Good | | Scores |
|---|---|---|
| Dressings: | Improper/Proper | 0/1 |
| | Unclean/Clean | 0/1 |
| | Un-ironed/Ironed | 0/1 |
| Skin: | Unclean/Clean | 0/1 |
| | Diseased/Non-diseased | 0/1 |
| Hairs: | Unclean/Clean | 0/1 |
| | With louse infestation/without louse infestation | 0/1 |
| | Un-combed/Combed | 0/1 |
| Eyes: | Unclean/Clean | 0/1 |
| Ears: | Unclean/Clean | 0/1 |
| Face: | Unclean/Clean | 0/1 |
| Teeth: | Un-brushed/Brushed | 0/1 |
| | Diseased/Non-diseased | 0/1 |
| Nails: | Unclean/Clean | 0/1 |
| Footwear: | No/Yes | 0/1 |
| | Total score | _____ |

**Personal hygiene status: Poor/Fair/Good**

> **Poor:** Total score 5 and below
> **Fair:** Total score between 6 and 10
> **Good:** Total score more than 10

### General Examination

Appearance: Conscious/Semiconscious/Unconscious

Weight _____ (kg) Height _____ cm   Built: Aesthetic/Athletic/Obese

Chest circumference (in case of child) _____          MAC (in case of child) _____

Skin-colour _____ Hair _____ Face _____          Mouth _____ Eyes _____

Ear _____ Neck _____ Upper limb _____ Abdomen _____ Lower limb _____

Any other _____

Temperature _____ Pulse _____ BP _____ Respiration rate _____

## Systemic Examination

| System | Observation | Palpation | Percussion | Auscultation | Diagnosis/Remark |
|--------|-------------|-----------|------------|--------------|------------------|
| GIT | | | | | |
| Respiratory | | | | | |
| CVS | | | | | |
| CNS | | | | | |
| Genitourinary | | | | | |
| Musculoskeletal | | | | | |
| Skin | | | | | |
| Other | | | | | |

## Investigations done with their report

| Investigation | Normal value | Test value | Remark |
|---------------|--------------|------------|--------|
| | | | |
| | | | |
| | | | |
| | | | |

## Differential Diagnosis

| S. no. | D/D disease name | D/D variable | Points in favour | Points in against |
|--------|------------------|--------------|------------------|-------------------|
| 1. | | History | | |
| | | Examination | | |
| | | Investigation | | |
| 2. | | History | | |
| | | Examination | | |
| | | Investigation | | |
| 3. | | History | | |
| | | Examination | | |
| | | Investigation | | |

Probable diagnosis _____

## Suggestive Investigations for Diagnosis

1. _____

2. _____

## Treatment Advised

_____

_____

_____

**Preventive Measures Suggested**

| Prevention level | Individual level | Family level | Community level |
|---|---|---|---|
| Primary | | | |
| Secondary | | | |
| Tertiary | | | |

## INDIVIDUAL HEALTH RECORD

**Family member no.** _____      **Date of examination** _____

**Introductory Data**

Name of patient _____ *Age _____ Sex (Male/Female/Other) _____

Residence _____

_____

     _____           _____

\* Recorded in completed years as on the last birthday.

**Presenting Complaints** (In order of appearance of symptoms with their duration in chronological order).

1. _____

2. _____

3. _____

4. _____

5. _____

**History of Present Illness** (Describing all complaints in order of appearance with their nature)

_____

_____

_____

_____

_____

**History of Past Illness**

_____

_____

**Previous Obstetric History (in case of female)**

Gravid (G) ____ Para (P) ____ Stillbirth (S) ____ Abortion (A) ____ Live (L) ____

**No. of children with their nature of delivery**

| Order of delivery | Name of child | Sex | Date of birth | Nature of birth Normal/LSCS/Inst | Status Sb/Alive/Dead If Sb/Dead with reasons |
|---|---|---|---|---|---|
| | | | | | |
| | | | | | |
| | | | | | |

**Menstrual History (in case of females)**

Age at menarche: _____ with duration: _____ days cycle.

Regular/Irregular

Normal/Scanty/Heavy flow

**Family History of Illness**

_____

_____

**Social and Occupational History**

_____

_____

**Psychiatric History**

_____

_____

**Treatment History**

_____

_____

**Personal History**

Addiction: Yes/No          If yes:

| S. no. | Type of addiction | Quantity/day | Duration | |
|--------|-------------------|--------------|----------|----|
| | | | From | To |
| | | | | |
| | | | | |
| | | | | |

Exercise: Always/Often/Seldom/Rarely/Never

Any other: Always/Often/Seldom/Rarely/Never

**Personal Hygiene:** Poor/Fair/Good                                         Scores

| | | |
|---|---|---|
| Dressings: | Improper/Proper | 0/1 |
| | Unclean/Clean | 0/1 |
| | Un-ironed/Ironed | 0/1 |
| Skin: | Unclean/Clean | 0/1 |
| | Diseased/Non-diseased | 0/1 |
| Hairs: | Unclean/Clean | 0/1 |
| | With louse infestation/without louse infestation | 0/1 |
| | Un-combed/Combed | 0/1 |
| Eyes: | Unclean/Clean | 0/1 |
| Ears: | Unclean/Clean | 0/1 |
| Face: | Unclean/Clean | 0/1 |
| Teeth: | Un-brushed/Brushed | 0/1 |
| | Diseased/Non-diseased | 0/1 |
| Nails: | Unclean/Clean | 0/1 |
| Footwear: | No/Yes | 0/1 |

Total Score _____

**Personal hygiene status:** Poor/Fair/Good

**Poor:** Total score 5 and below
**Fair:** Total score between 6 and 10
**Good:** Total score more than 10

## General Examination

Appearance: Conscious/Semiconscious/unconscious

Weight ____ (kg) Height _____ cm   Built: Aesthetic/Athletic/Obese

Chest circumference (in case of child) _____        MAC (in case of child) _____

Skin-colour _____ Hair _____   Face _____                    Mouth _____ Eyes _____

Ear _____   Neck _____   Upper limb _____   Abdomen _____ Lower limb _____

Any other _____

Temperature _____   Pulse _____   BP _____   Respiration rate _____

## Systemic Examination

| System | Observation | Palpation | Percussion | Auscultation | Diagnosis/Remark |
|---|---|---|---|---|---|
| GIT | | | | | |
| Respiratory | | | | | |
| CVS | | | | | |
| CNS | | | | | |
| Genitourinary | | | | | |
| Musculoskeletal | | | | | |
| Skin | | | | | |
| Other | | | | | |

## Investigations done with their Report

| Investigation | Normal value | Test value | Remark |
|---|---|---|---|
| | | | |
| | | | |
| | | | |
| | | | |

## Differential Diagnosis

| S. no. | D/D disease name | D/D variable | Points in favour | Points in against |
|---|---|---|---|---|
| 1. | | History | | |
| | | Examination | | |
| | | Investigation | | |
| 2. | | History | | |
| | | Examination | | |
| | | Investigation | | |
| 3. | | History | | |
| | | Examination | | |
| | | Investigation | | |

Probable diagnosis _____

## Suggestive Investigations for Diagnosis

1. _____

2. _____

## Treatment Advised

_____

_____

_____

## Preventive measures suggested

| Prevention level | Individual level | Family level | Community level |
|---|---|---|---|
| Primary | | | |
| Secondary | | | |
| Tertiary | | | |

## PROBLEMS IN FAMILY

### Social Problems

1. _____

2. _____

### Psychiatric Problems

1. _____

2. _____

### Environment Problems

1. _____

2. _____

### Socioeconomic Status _____

### Immunization Status

Child no. 1. _____

Child no. 2. _____

### Nutritional Status

| Nutritional status | Calorie | Protein | Carbohydrate | Fat | Vit A | Vit B | Fe | Ca |
|---|---|---|---|---|---|---|---|---|
| Nutrient deficit | | | | | | | | |
| Nutrient excess | | | | | | | | |

### Diseased Person in Family

| S. no. | Name of family member | Type of disease | Duration |
|---|---|---|---|
| | | | |
| | | | |
| | | | |

## MANAGEMENT OF FAMILY

**Socio-therapy Advised**

_____

_____

_____

**Psychotherapy Advised**

_____

_____

**Medical Therapy with Treatment**

_____

_____

_____

## Operational Definitions of Various Variables

**Family:** A family is a group of individuals, who are related by blood or by marriage, living under same shelter and share a common kitchen.

**Nuclear family:** A group of person comprising numbers of a single or at most two generations united by blood or adoptive or marital or equivalent ties, e.g. wife, husband and their children.

**Joint family:** This type of family is merger of several nuclear families or as a vertical extension of a nuclear family and having more than one couple.

**Three generation family:** When three generations are living together and sharing from one kitchen, e.g. children, parents and grandparents.

**Extended family:** When some unrelated or in distinctly related members live together besides the wife, husband and their children.

## Religion

Religion is simply defined as belief in interaction of man with supernatural (since no universally accepted definition exists). On the basis of their beliefs, usual religions are like Hindu, Muslim, Christian, Sikh, etc.

## Education

Literacy measures the incorporation of knowledge and values in individuals. It is recorded as follows.

**Illiterate:** Person who could neither read nor write or those who could merely read but could not write in any of language with understanding considered as illiterate.

**Just literate:** Person who could read and write a short statement on everyday life in any of language with understanding but either never attended a school or not cleared V standard called just literate.

**Primary:** Person who has studied but not beyond V standard.

**Middle:** Person who has studied beyond V standard but not beyond eighth standard.

**Secondary:** Person who has 8th standard but not beyond matriculation, i.e. 10th standard.

**Graduation:** Person who has studied beyond matriculation or post-matriculation diplomas but not beyond bachelor degree.

**Postgraduation:** Those who studied beyond graduation or had been awarded masters degree.

**Professional:** Those who had been awarded some prsofessional degre, e.g. MBBS/BE/ BTech/MD/MS/BBA/MBA/BCA/MCA/B.Ed/M.Ed.

## Occupation

Occupation is a trade, profession or type of work performed by an individual for his/her livelihood. These occupations are of the following types:

1. Unemployment: Not earning at all but dependent on others for their livelihood.
2. Unskilled worker: Doing work which does not require any type of skill, e.g. peon.
3. Semi-skilled worker: Doing work which requires some skill, e.g. helpers.
4. Skilled worker: Doing work which requires specific type of skill, e.g. mason, lab and technician.
5. Clerk/farmers/shopkeepers: Office clerk or person having their own farms/shops.
6. Semiprofessionals: Doing work which requires some knowledge of a specific profession, e.g. nurses, ophthalmic assistant, building contractors.
7. Professionals: Doing work which requires knowledge of a specific profession, e.g. doctors and engineers.
8. Corporate CMD/Chairman: Either having own limited company or is director or chairman of some limited company or organization.

## Socioeconomic Status

Socioeconomic status (SES) assessment is an important aspect in community based studies. SES assessment will categorize the socioeconomic position of families in respect of defined variables such as education, occupation, economic status, physical assets, etc.

## Socioeconomic Status Scales

Several methods or scales for socioeconomic status assessment were proposed time to time like:

P. Prasad's scale (1960)

Kuppuswamy scale (1962, 1976)

Rahudkar scale 1960

Udai Pareek scale 1964,

Jalota scale 1970

Kulshrestha scale 1972

Shrivastava scale 1978, and

Bharadwaj scale 2001 (1–7).

Gaur's classification (1996, 2004 and 2012)

Some of the widely accepted SES assessment scales are detailed here for practical purpose.

## P. Prasad's Scale (1960)

This classification was first proposed in 1961. It is based on the per capita income of the family. Incidentally base year for All India Consumer Price Index (AICPI) was also proposed in 1960–61. AICPI in April 2012 was 4678 (as per base year 1960), i.e. ₹ 100 of year 1960 = ₹ 4678 of April 2012, i.e. ₹ 4680 (rounded off to nearest ten rupees).

So ₹ one of year 1960 will equals to 4680 × 1/100 of April 2012.

Following table is updated (April 2012) B.G. Prasad's socioeconomic classification:

| Socioeconomic class | Original Prasad's classification Per capita family income, 1960 (₹) | Per capita family income (₹) for 2012 |
|---|---|---|
| Class I | 100 and above | 4680 and above |
| Class II | 50–99 | 2340–4679 |
| Class III | 30–49 | 1400–2339 |
| Class IV | 15–29 | 700–1399 |
| Class V | <15 | <700 |

**Note:** Updating of B.G. Prasad's classification by Kumar P (1993) method.

## Advantages

It is easy for calculation and considers major criteria of SES.

## Drawbacks

This scale considers only one criterion of SES, i.e. income.

Further, steady inflation and consequent fall in the value of currency make the economic criteria in the scale less relevant.

## Kuppuswamy SES Scale (1962, 1976)—By B. Kuppuswamy

It was introduced in 1962 and is developed mainly for subjects of urban areas and of nuclear families. This scale is based on three main variables, education, occupation and income. For each factor, there are seven plausible alternatives. Range of scores which can be obtained is from 3 to 29.

**Scoring:** The information is collected about education, occupation and income of head of family. Scores are given as per the information collected. On the basis of the total score, categorization of SES will be done.

## Kuppuswamy's Classification

It is based on education, occupation and income of family head.

### A. Education

| | |
|---|---|
| Professional degree, PG and above | 7 |
| Graduate | 6 |
| Intermediate or past high school diploma | 5 |
| High school certificate | 4 |
| Middle school completion | 3 |
| Primary school or literate | 2 |
| Illiterate | 1 |

### C. Per capita income (₹ per month)

| | |
|---|---|
| 1500 or above | 12 |
| 750–1499 | 10 |
| 555–749 | 6 |
| 375–564 | 4 |
| 225–374 | 3 |
| 75–224 | 2 |
| Below 75 | 1 |

### B. Occupation

| | |
|---|---|
| Profession | 10 |
| Semiprofession | 6 |
| Clerk, shop owner, farm owner | 5 |
| Skilled worker | 4 |
| Semi-skilled worker | 3 |
| Unskilled | 2 |
| Unemployed | 1 |

### The total score is graded as follows

| | |
|---|---|
| Upper | 26–29 |
| Upper middle | 16–25 |
| Lower middle | 11–15 |
| Upper lower | 5–10 |

## Advantages

This scale considers major three criteria of SES.

## Drawbacks

The norms which were established can only be applicable for urban population and may become irrelevant to rural population.

In addition to this, the highest level of income which is shown by Kuppuswamy is also inconsistent across various economic groups in the present time.

Information about the person-concerned cannot be observed.

## Udai Pareek's SES Scale: By Udai Pareek and G. Trivedi (1964)

This scale has nine variables which assessed to assess the socioeconomic status of the individual:

1. Caste
2. Occupation
3. Education
4. Social participation
5. Land
6. House
7. Farm powers
8. Material possession
9. Family

**Scoring:** Scoring is done for each of the nine variables then cumulative score will be assessed. SES will be finally assessed as per the total score gained as follows:

| Socioeconomic class | Pareek's classification (Total scores) |
|---|---|
| Upper class (class I) | 43 and above |
| Upper middle class (class II) | 33–42 |
| Middle class (class III) | 24–32 |
| Lower middle class (class IV) | 13–23 |
| Lower class (class V) | <13 |

This scale does not emphasize the economic aspect and is more suitable for rural subjects.

### Gaur's SES Classification (2012)

This scale was first introduced in year 1996 and then revised in year 2004. In year 2012, it is again revised with inflation of time.

**Gaur's SES classification (2012)** is having seven variables are to assess the socioeconomic status, these variables are:

1. Education
2. Occupation
3. @Income per capita
4. Expenditure
5. Housing condition
6. Living status
7. Debt to assets ratio

@To make it compatible in measuring the SES over the years with fast growing economy; Income is linked with All India Consumer Price Index (AICPI). Values in present SES is as per AICPI April 2012, i.e. 4680 (AICPIIW base year 1960)/949 (base year 1982)/205 (base year 2001)

It is having **rule of seven**, i.e. seven variables with '0' to '7' scoring of each variable. Scoring is done for each of these seven variables from 0 to 7, where '0' is the lowest category whereas '7' is the highest category. So, the equal weightage is given to all the seven variables related to socioeconomic status.

In case of living status and housing condition, scoring is done for different variables related respectively. To find out the final scoring of living status and housing condition, total scoring is divided into eight equal parts to get further scoring '0' to '7'.

Socioeconomic group is divided into five classes as per total score gained as follows:

| Socioeconomic class | Total scores gained |
|---|---|
| Class I | 40 and above |
| Class II | 30–39 |
| Class III | 20–29 |
| Class IV | 10–19 |
| Class V | < 10 |

The reliability of the scale was found to be very high ($r = 0.93$).

### Advantages

- This scale considers majority of criteria for SES.
- More relevant in modern ages.

### Drawback

This scale requires much more information in comparison to 'P' Prasad's and Kuppuswamy to find out SES.

## Gaur's Socioeconomic Classification

| Education | Scores |
|---|---|
| Illiterate | 0 |
| Primary | 1 |
| Middle | 2 |
| High school | 3 |
| Intermediate | 4 |
| B.A./B.Sc/B.com/Equivalent | 5 |
| M.A/M.Sc/M.com/Equivalent | 6 |
| Professional | 7 |

| Occupation: | Scores |
|---|---|
| Unemployment | 0 |
| Unskilled worker | 2 |
| Semi-skilled worker | 3 |
| Skilled worker | 3 |
| Clerk/farmers/shopkeepers | 4 |
| Semiprofessionals | 5 |
| Professionals | 6 |
| Corporate CMD/chairman | 7 |

| ©Income per capita per month: (In rupees as per CPI April 2012) | Scores |
|---|---|
| < 1000 | 0 |
| 1,000 to 4,999 | 1 |
| 5,000 to 9,999 | 2 |
| 10,000 to 14,999 | 3 |
| 15,000 to 19,999 | 4 |
| 20,000 to 24,999 | 5 |
| 25,000 to 29,999 | 6 |
| 30,0000 and above | 7 |

| Expenditure | Scores |
|---|---|
| <10% of income | 0 |
| 10 to 19% of income | 1 |
| 20 to 29% of income | 2 |
| 30 to 39% of income | 3 |
| 40 to 49% of income | 4 |
| 50 to 59% of income | 5 |
| 60 to 69% of income | 6 |
| 70 and above | 7 |

| Housing enviornmental status | Scores |
|---|---|
| Score < 4 | 0 |
| Score 4 to 7 | 1 |
| Score 8 to 11 | 2 |
| Score 12 to 15 | 3 |
| Score 16 to 19 | 4 |
| Score 20 to 23 | 5 |
| Score 24 to 27 | 6 |
| Score 28 and above | 7 |

| *Living status | Scores |
|---|---|
| Score < 4 | 0 |
| Score 4 to 7 | 1 |
| Score 8 to 11 | 2 |
| Score 12 to 15 | 3 |
| Score 16 to 19 | 4 |
| Score 20 to 23 | 5 |
| Score 24 to 27 | 6 |
| Score 28 and above | 7 |

| Debt to assets ratio | Scores |
|---|---|
| < 2 | 0 |
| 1 to 2 | 1 |
| 0.5 to 0.99 | 2 |
| 0.25 to 0.24 | 3 |
| 0.12 to 0.24 | 4 |
| 0.06 to 0.11 | 5 |
| 0.03 to 0.059 | 6 |
| < 0.059 | 7 |

### Gaur's socioeconomic classification

| Socioeconomic status | Total scores |
|---|---|
| Upper class (I) | Score 40 and above |
| Upper middle class (II) | Score between 30 and 39 |
| Lower middle class (III) | Score between 20 and 29 |
| Upper lower class (IV) | Score between 10 and 19 |
| Lower class (V) | Score < 10 |

©Income per capita is linked with AICPI (April 2012 AICPI IW is ₹. 205 (base year 2001).

*Scoring for living status and housing condition is as follows.

| Housing condition | Score |
|---|---|
| Site: Bad/Fair/Good | 0/1/2 |
| Setback: No/Improper/Proper | 0/1/2 |
| Floor: Kacha/Pakka with crevices/Pakka without crevices | 0/1/2 |
| Walls: Kacha/Pakka with crevices/Pakka without crevices | 0/1/2 |
| Roof: Kacha/Pakka with crevices/Pakka without crevices | 0/1/2 |
| Height: Inadequate/Adequate | 0/1 |
| *Overcrowding: Present/Absent | 0/1 |
| **Light: Inadequate/Adequate | 0/1 |
| Kitchen: Not separate/separate but without smoke outlet/separate with smoke outlet | 0/1/2 |
| Storage facility: Improper/Proper | 0/1 |
| Drainage facility: Improper/Proper | 0/1 |
| Privy: Open air defaecation/Private service/Public sanitary/Private sanitary | 0/1/2/3 |
| Water supply: Surface/Well/Tape water/Tube well or treated Tape water | 0/1/2/3 |
| Bathroom: Improper/Proper | 0/1 |
| Domestic animals: Not separate/Separate | 0/1 |
| Refuse disposal: Improper/Proper | 0/1 |
| Drainage: Improper/Proper | 0/1 |
| Environmental total score obtained | |

*Overcrowding present if floor space/person is less than 50 feet$^2$ along with sex separation.

** One can read newspaper in any corner of house is adequate lighting.

| Living Status | Scores |
|---|---|
| *City: No/Category C/Category B/Category A | 0/1/2/3 |
| *Locality: No/Category C/Category B/Category A | 0/1/2/3 |
| Accommodation (BHK): 0/1/2/3/>3 | 0/1/2/3/4 |
| Conveyance: No/Cycle/Two wheeler/Four wheeler | 0/1/2/3/4 |
| Communication: No/News papers/Mobile | 0/1/2/3 |
| Audiovisual: No/Radio/Television/Computer/Laptop | 0/1/2/3/4 |
| Mechanical ventilation: No/Fan/Cooler/Air condition | 0/1/2/3 |
| **Modern amenities: 0/1/2/3/>3 | 0/1/2/3/4 |
| *Children's school: No/Category C/Category B/Category A | 0/1/2/3 |
| *Club membership: No/Category C/Category B/Category A | 0/1/2/3 |

Total scores gained _____

*Categories as per predefined criteria by the government.

**Number of modern amenities other than included already.

## All India Consumer Price Index (AICPI)

Before AICPI, Wholesale Price Index (WPI), which was first published in 1902, was only economic indicator. WPI has measure impact of inflation more on business than consumers whereas CPI actually measure increase in price that a consumer will ultimately have to pay. So WPI was replaced by most developed countries by the Consumer Price Index (CPI) in the 1970s.

All India Consumer Price Index (AICPI) was proposed in 1960, i.e. ₹ 100 of year 1960 = ₹ AICPI of that specific time (base year 1960). AICPI was again revised in year 1982 with linking factor of 4.93. AICPI was further revised in year 2001 with linking factor of 4.63 to link with base year 1982.

AICPI of base year 2001 × 4.63 = AICPI of base year 1982 of that specific point of time.

AICPI of base year 1982 × 4.93 = AICPI of base year 1960 of that specific point of time.

AICPI of base year 1960 = ₹ 100 of that specific point of time.

Consumer Price Index (CPI) in India comprises multiple series classified based on different economic groups. There are four series, viz. the CPI UNME (urban non-manual employee), CPI AL (agricultural labourer), CPI RL (rural labourer) and CPI IW (industrial worker). While the CPI UNME series is published by the Central Statistical Organisation within the *Ministry of Statistics and Programme Implementation* while the other three are published by the Labour Bureau in the *Ministry of Labour*. From February 2011, the CPI (UNME) released by CSO is replaced as CPI (urban), CPI (rural) and CPI (combined). CPI published by Reserve Bank of India (RBI) can be found at URL link "bulletin.rbi.org.in" (under the head Price Sl. No.36 onwards). It is published on monthly basis and quarterly basis.

**All India Consumer Price Index (Base 1960) for industrial workers** (Quarterly Average)

| Year | Jan–March | April–June | July–Sept | Oct–Dec |
|------|-----------|-----------|-----------|---------|
| 2006 | 2716 | 2770 | 2838 | 2899 |
| 2007 | 2907 | 2945 | 3028 | 3059 |
| 2008 | 2907 | 2945 | 3028 | 3059 |
| 2009 | 3089 | 3173 | 3302 | 3371 |
| 2010 | 3378 | 3454 | 3690 | 3820 |
| 2011 | 4246 | 4276 | 4443 | 4520 |
| 2012 | 4550 | | | |

**All India Consumer Price Index (Base 1982) for industrial workers (monthly)**

| Year | Jan | Feb | March | April | May | June | July | Aug | Sep | Oct | Nov | Dec |
|------|-----|-----|-------|-------|-----|------|------|-----|-----|-----|-----|-----|
| 2006 | 551 | 551 | 551 | 557 | 560 | 570 | 574 | 574 | 579 | 588 | 588 | 588 |
| 2007 | 588 | 593 | 588 | 593 | 597 | 602 | 611 | 616 | 616 | 620 | 620 | 620 |
| 2008 | 620 | 625 | 634 | 639 | 644 | 648 | 662 | 671 | 676 | 685 | 685 | 681 |
| 2009 | 685 | 685 | 685 | 695 | 699 | 708 | 741 | 750 | 755 | 764 | 778 | 782 |
| 2010 | 796 | 787 | 787 | 787 | 796 | 806 | 824 | 824 | 829 | 838 | 843 | 857 |
| 2011 | 870 | 857 | 857 | 861 | 866 | 875 | 894 | 898 | 912 | 917 | 921 | 912 |
| 2012 | 917 | 921 | 931 | 949 | | | | | | | | |

## Consumer Price Index numbers for industrial workers on base year 2001

| State | S. no. | Centre | April 2012 | State | S. no. | Centre | April 2012 |
|-------|--------|--------|-----------|-------|--------|--------|-----------|
| AP | 1. | Godavarikhani | 212 | MP | 40. | Bhopal | 213 |
| | 2. | Guntur | 208 | | 41. | Chhindwara | 207 |
| | 3. | Hyderabad | 185 | | 42. | Indore | 196 |
| | 4. | Vijayawada | 201 | | 43. | Jabalpur | 206 |
| | 5. | Vishakhapatnam | 207 | MHR | 44. | Mumbai | 208 |
| | 6. | Warrangal | 214 | | 45. | Nagpur | 234 |
| ASM | 7. | Doom Dooma Tinsukia | 177 | | 46. | Nasik | 215 |
| | 8. | Guwahati | 178 | | 47. | Pune | 212 |
| | 9. | Silchar | 191 | | 48. | Sholapur | 214 |
| | 10. | Mariani Jorhat | 183 | ORI | 49. | Angul Talcher | 217 |
| | 11. | Rangapara Tezpur | 166 | | 50. | Rourkela | 216 |
| BIH | 12. | Munger Jamalpur | 210 | PUD | 51. | Puducherry | 201 |
| CHD | 13. | Chandigarh | 208 | PUN | 52. | Amritsar | 225 |
| CHS | 14. | Bhilai | 235 | | 53. | Jalandhar | 203 |
| DLI | 15. | Delhi | 214 | | 54. | Ludhiana | 202 |
| GOA | 16. | Goa | | RJN | 55. | Ajmer | 215 |
| GUJ | 17. | Ahmedabad | 202 | | 56. | Bhilwara | 217 |
| | 18. | Bhavnagar | 203 | | 57. | Jaipur | 212 |
| | 19. | Rajkot | 212 | TN | 58. | Chennai | 190 |
| | 20. | Surat | 190 | | 59. | Coimbatore | 188 |
| | 21. | Vadodara | 197 | | 60. | Coonoor | 198 |
| HRY | 22. | Faridabad | 206 | | 61. | Madurai | 190 |
| | 23. | Yamunanagar | 213 | | 62. | Salem | 191 |
| HP | 24. | Himachal Pradesh | 185 | | 63. | Tiruchirapally | 203 |
| J and K | 25. | Srinagar | 186 | TRP | 64. | Tripura | 173 |
| JRK | 26. | Bokaro | 205 | UP | 65. | Agra | 216 |
| | 27. | Giridih | 243 | | 66. | Ghaziabad | 207 |
| | 28. | Jamshedpur | 227 | | 67. | Kanpur | 210 |
| | 29. | Jharia | 214 | | 68. | Lucknow | 200 |
| | 30. | Kodarma | 231 | | 69. | Varanasi | 203 |
| | 31. | Ranchi Hatia | 225 | WB | 70. | Asansol | 226 |
| KNT | 32. | Bangalore | 209 | | 71. | Darjeeling | 192 |
| | 33. | Belgaum | 213 | | 72. | Durgapur | 203 |
| | 34. | Hubli Dharwar | 213 | | 73. | Haldia | 206 |
| | 35. | Mercara | 198 | | 74. | Howrah | 194 |
| | 36. | Mysore | 203 | | 75. | Jalpaiguri | 186 |
| KRL | 37. | Ernakulam | 194 | | 76. | Kolkata | 196 |
| | 38. | Mundakkayam | 209 | | 77. | Raniganj | 190 |
| | 39. | Quilon | 200 | | 78. | Siliguri | 191 |
| **All India Index** | | | **205** | | | | |

1. The CPI-IW for the month of May, 2012 will be released on 29th June, 2012.
2. E-Mail Address: dglbsm@dataone.in, dglb@nic.in
3. Website : http://www.labourbureau.gov.in

## Type of Food

Vegetarian: Those who take only vegetarian diet.

Mixed: Those who take vegetarian as well as non-vegetarian diet.

Eggeterian: Those who do not take non-vegetarian diet but take eggs.

**Body Mass Index (BMI):** BMI is calculated by many means, out of that one as follows:

  *BMI (kg/sq.m) = Weight/Height square.

 *As per BMI, individuals are classified in to three categories that are as follows:

| BMI (kg/M$^2$) | Person as per BMI |
|---|---|
| < 18.5 | Underweight |
| 18.5–24.9 | Normal weight |
| 25–30 | Overweight |
| > 30 | Obese |

*Source-ICMR

## 'At Risk' Mothers

'At Risk' mothers are those whose:

1. Pre-pregnancy weight is 36 kg or less.

2. Weight is 40 kg or less at 20th week.

3. Weight increase less than 1 kg/month to 40 kg weight after 20th week of pregnancy.

4. Height 145 cm or below.

5. Primipara.

6. Heavy weight in pregnancies.

7. Previous history of stillbirths/abortions/antepartum haemorrhage/postpartum haemorrhage/eclampsia/early neonatal deaths/caesarian or forceps deliveries.

8. Age above 35 years or below 18 years.

9. Suffering from tuberculosis/severe anaemia/heart diseases/diabetes.

10. Has conceived after treatment for infertility.

11. Has had 4 or more pregnancies.

## 'At Risk' Children

1. Twins or low birth weight singletons.

2. Where breastfeeding has not been established or is insufficient.

3. One parent.

4. Working mother.

5. Fails to gain weight during 3 successive months.

6. Loses weight during 2 successive months.

7. History of death or more than 2 siblings during the 2 years of life.

8. Develops acute episodes of acute gastroenteritis/measles/whooping cough.

9. Weight below 70% of the reference (2nd degree of malnutrition).

10. Birth order 5 or more.

11. Spacing less than 2 years.

12. Illness of parents.

## Pregnant Women Vaccination

| Vaccine | When to give |
|---------|-------------|
| TT 1 | Early pregnancy |
| TT2 | 4 wks after TT1 |
| TT Booster | If received TT1 and TT2 in previous pregnancy is within 3 years |

## Children Vaccination

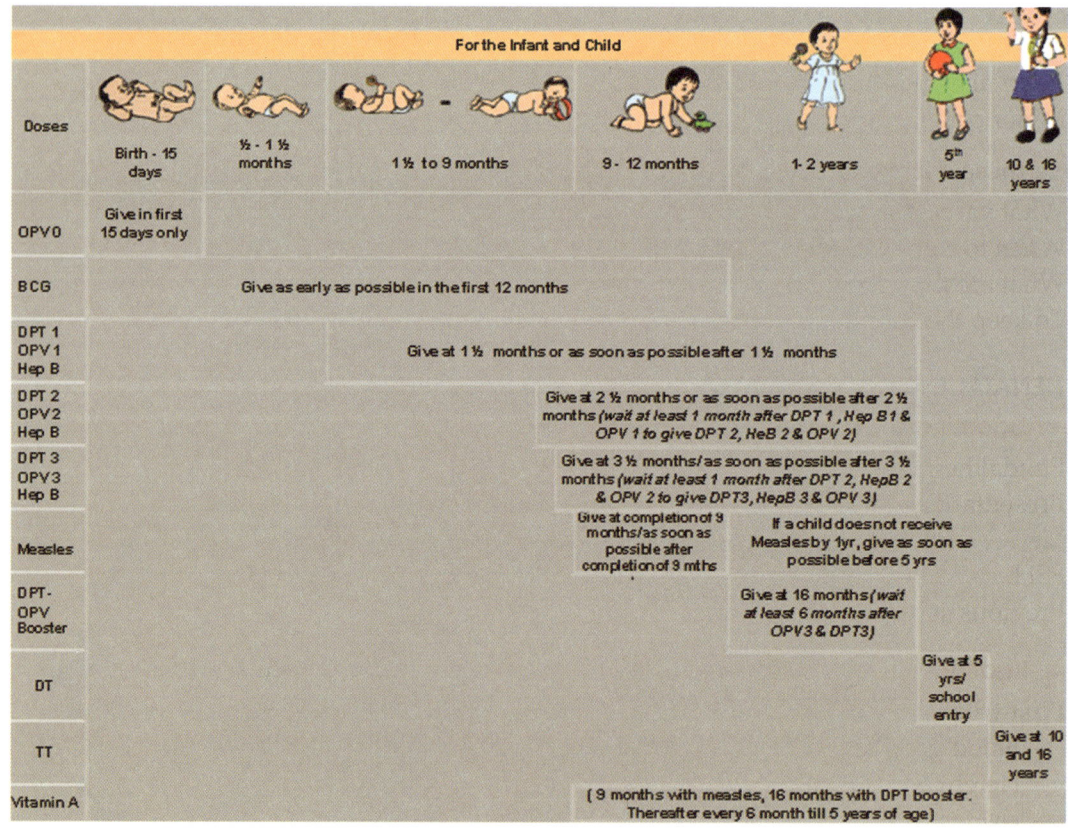

Vaccination schedule of children

## Remember

- All due vaccines can be given at same time but in different limbs (sites).
- Even if the child is suffering from diarrhoea, mild fever or malnutrition, it should be vaccinated.
- Unless a child is so sick that it has to be taken to hospital, do not stop its vaccination.

  The goal is to fully immunise each child before its first birthday.

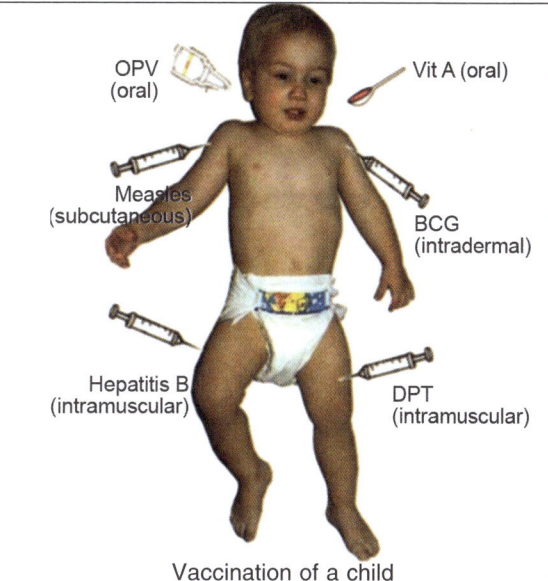

OPV (oral)

Vit A (oral)

Measles (subcutaneous)

BCG (intradermal)

Hepatitis B (intramuscular)

DPT (intramuscular)

Vaccination of a child

## Note

- Interval between two doses should be 4–6 weeks and should not be less than one month.
- Minor cough colds and mild fever are not a contraindication for vaccination.

### Give these 4 Key Messages to the Caregiver

1. What vaccine was given and what disease it prevents (e.g. BCG for preventing TB)
2. When to come for the next dose.
3. What are the minor side-effects and how to deal with them?
4. To keep the vaccination card safe and to bring it along for the next visit.

## ANTENATAL CASE

### Per Abdominal Examination of Antenatal Case

- Fundal height
- Presentation
- Lie
- FSH
- Previous surgery scare

### Investigations Recommended in Antenatal Case

- **First trimester**
  - Blood pressure
  - Height and weight
  - Urine test
  - Routine urine examination and microscopy: Includes test for sugar and protein
  - Blood tests:
    - Complete blood count
    - Includes haemoglobin, red blood cell counts to rule out anaemia

♦ Blood type and Rh type testing (A, B, AB, O and Rh +ve or Rh −ve need to be determined)

♦ HIV/Hepatitis B tests

♦ Syphilis (by VDRL test)

♦ If you have a high risk of developing diabetes, you may need other special tests like the GTT (glucose tolerance test). If you have a strong family history of diabetes you should talk to your treating doctor about it.

♦ The serology for TORCHES is done based on the history, risk factors and physical examination by the treating doctor.

– Ultrasound scans: This will determine how well your baby is growing. It is also the most reliable in determining the EDD when done in the first trimester (ideally at around the 10th week of pregnancy).

- **Second and third trimester:** Along with regular physical check-up, followings are required:
  - Weight: Weight gain monitoring
  - Regular BP check-up
  - Blood glucose around 24th week of pregnancy as is the time to detect gestational diabetes
  - Urine culture at 28th week
  - Urine routine examination including for sugar and protein.
  - Ultrasound as anomaly scan at 18 to 20 weeks and subsequently final scan at 28 to 32 weeks
  - There are a few more investigations that are not routine but based on the conditions and the risk factors such as chorionic villous sampling done at 10 to 12 weeks, amniocentesis done around 18 weeks.

## Treatment/Prophylaxis given to ANC

- IFA (at least 100 )
- Inj. TT
- Pregnancy preparedness counselling

## Pregnancy Preparedness and Counselling

1. **Be aware of the changes in your body:** As the child in your womb grows from its first to third trimester, your body will undergo specific changes. You should be prepared for:
   a. **During first trimester:** You can experience morning sickness, vomiting and a feeling of being ill. This is usually a result of the hormonal changes that your body is undergoing so it's normal.
   b. **During second trimester:** You should be prepared for weight gain.
   c. **During third trimester:** You will feel most uncomfortable as the weight in your belly grows bigger and bigger until the time that you will actually give birth.
2. **Do away with any unwanted habit like smooking and alcoholism.** Smoking while pregnant may lead to miscarriage, bleeding or if you successfully carry your baby onto its third trimester, it might be premature or underweight.
3. **Be physically prepared:** Eating right and balanced diet.

4. **Be prepared financially:** additional finance needed for the costs of giving birth in the hospital and cost of addition of one more member to your family.

5. **Plan for the birth and the delivery details:** Plan about the medical aspect of things, i.e. place of delivery and doctor from whom you want your delivery conducted. About a week before expected date of delivery, you should make sure that you already packed the essentials like your clothes, the toiletries and some clothes that you bought for your baby.

6. **Be prepared for pregnancy backup plan**: Although you may be preparing for a vaginal birth, you should still have a backup plan in case of emergency C-section may be needed.

7. **Prepare your home in welcoming a new member of the family**: It's not just the nursery that you need to prepare when welcoming a new member of your family, it's the entire household which should be child-proof.

8. **Practice multitasking**: You will have to do multitask with a little baby, so as early as possible, you can practice multitasking.

9. **Decide on the parenting style**: This is an especially crucial decision for both parents. Which parenting style will you take? If both parents are working, should one give up his or her job in order to personally care for the baby, or is hiring a full-time baby sitter an option that you are considering?

10. **Enjoy the experience to the fullest:** By following these pregnancy tips, you can rest assured that you are prepared for your pregnancy, the labour phase and the post-natal care of that new member of your family which everyone is eagerly awaiting with open arms.

## NUTRITION

### Recommended Daily Allowances (RDA) of Major Nutrients for Indians

| Group | Energy kcal/D | Carbohydrate gm/D | Protein gm/D | Fat gm/D | Calcium mg/D | Iron mg/D | Folic acid µg/D |
|---|---|---|---|---|---|---|---|
| Man (R) | 2875 | 60 | 60 | 20 | 400 | 28 | 100 |
| Woman (R) | 2225 | 50 | 50 | 20 | 400 | 30 | 100 |
| Infant < 6 mth | 108/kg | 5.4 | 2.05/kg | 20 | 500 | 5 | |
| Infant > 6 mth | 98/kg | 8.6 | 1.65/kg | 20 | 500 | 5 | 25 |
| Children 1–3 yrs | 1240 | 12.2 | 22 | 25 | 400 | 12 | 30 |
| Children 4–6 yrs | 1690 | 19 | 30 | 25 | 400 | 18 | 40 |
| Children 7–9 yrs | 1950 | 26.9 | 41 | 22 | 400 | 26 | 60 |
| Boys 10–12 yrs | 2190 | 35.4 | 54 | 22 | 600 | 34 | 70 |
| Girls 10–12 yrs | 1970 | 31.5 | 57 | 22 | 600 | 19 | 70 |
| Boys 13–15 yrs | 2450 | 47.8 | 70 | 22 | 600 | 41 | 100 |
| Girls 13–15 yrs | 2060 | 46.7 | 65 | 22 | 600 | 28 | 100 |
| Boys 16–18 yrs | 2640 | 57.1 | 78 | 22 | 500 | 50 | 100 |
| Girls 16–18 yrs | 2060 | 49.9 | 63 | 22 | 500 | 30 | 100 |

## Recommended Daily Allowances (RDA) of Micronutrients for Indians _____

| Group | Vitamin A (µg/D) Reti. β Carotene | | Thiamine mg/D | Riboflavin mg/D | Niacin mg/D | Pyridoxine mg/D | Vitamin B$_{12}$(µg/D) | Vitamin C (mg/D) |
|---|---|---|---|---|---|---|---|---|
| Man (reference) | 600 | 2400 | 1.4 | 1.6 | 18 | 2 | 1 | 40 |
| Woman (reference) | 600 | 2400 | 1.1 | 1.3 | 14 | 2 | 1 | // |
| Infant < 6 months | 350 | 1200 | 55 µg/kg | 65 µg/kg | 710 µg/kg | 0.1 | 0.2 | 25 |
| Infant > 6 months | 350 | 1200 | 50 µg/kg | 60 µg/kg | 650 µg/kg | 0.4 | 0.2 | 25 |
| Children 1–3 yrs | 400 | 1600 | 0.6 | 0.7 | 8 | 0.9 | 0.2–1 | 40 |
| Children 4–6 yrs | 400 | 1600 | 0.9 | 1 | 11 | 0.9 | 0.2–1 | // |
| Children 7–9 yrs | 600 | 2400 | 1 | 1.2 | 13 | 1.6 | 0.2–1 | 40 |
| Boys 10–12 yrs | 600 | 2400 | 1.1 | 1.3 | 15 | 1.6 | 0.2–1 | // |
| Girls 10–12 yrs | 600 | 2400 | 1 | 1.2 | 13 | 1.6 | 0.2–1 | // |
| Boys 13–15 yrs | 600 | 2400 | 1.2 | 1.5 | 16 | 2 | 0.2–1 | // |
| Girls 13–15 yrs | 600 | 2400 | 1 | 1.2 | 14 | 2 | 0.2–1 | // |
| Boys 16–18 yrs | 600 | 2400 | 1.3 | 1.6 | 17 | 2 | 0.2–1 | // |
| Girls 16–18 yrs | 600 | 2400 | 1 | 1.2 | 14 | 2 | 0.2–1 | // |

## Recommended Daily Allowances (RDA) of Major Nutrients for Indians Special Groups

| Group | Status | Energy kcal/D | Carbohydrate gm/D | Protein gm/D | Fat gm/D | Calcium mg/D | Iron mg/D | Folic acid µg/D |
|---|---|---|---|---|---|---|---|---|
| Man | Sedentary worker | 2425 | 60 | 60 | 20 | 400 | 28 | 100 |
| | Moderate worker | 2875 | // | // | // | // | // | // |
| | Heavy worker | 3800 | // | // | // | // | // | // |
| Woman | Sedentary worker | 1875 | 50 | 50 | 20 | // | 30 | 100 |
| | Moderate worker | 2225 | // | // | // | // | // | // |
| | Heavy worker | 2925 | // | // | // | // | // | // |
| | Pregnant | + 300 | +15 | + 15 | 30 | 1000 | 38 | 400 |
| | Lactating < 6 months | + 550 | +25 | + 25 | 45 | 1000 | 30 | 150 |
| | Lactating > 6 months | + 400 | +18 | + 18 | 45 | 1000 | 30 | 150 |

## Recommended Daily Allowances (RDA) of Micronutrients for Indians Special Groups_____

| Group | Status | Vitamin A (µg/D) Retin.β Car. | | Thiamine Mg/D | Riboflavin Mg/D | Niacin mg/D | Pyridoxine mg/D | Vit. B$_{12}$ (µg/D) | Vit. C mg/D |
|---|---|---|---|---|---|---|---|---|---|
| Man | Sedentary worker | 600 | 2400 | 1.2 | 1.4 | 16 | 2 | 1 | 40 |
| | Moderate worker | " | " | 1.4 | 1.6 | 18 | " | " | " |
| | Heavy worker | " | " | 1.6 | 1.9 | 21 | " | " | " |
| Woman | Sedentary worker | " | " | 0.9 | 1.1 | 12 | " | " | " |
| | Moderate worker | " | " | 1.1 | 1.3 | 14 | " | " | " |
| | Heavy worker | " | " | 1.2 | 1.5 | 16 | " | " | " |
| | Pregnant | " | " | +0.2 | +0.2 | + 2 | 2.5 | " | " |
| | Lactating < 6 months | +350 | +1400 | +0.3 | +0.3 | + 4 | " | 1.5 | 80 |
| | Lactating > 6 months | " | " | +0.2 | +0.2 | + 3 | " | " | " |

**Sedentary worker:** Doctors, nurses, managers, clerk, teacher, tailor, barber, goldsmith, priest, shoapkeepers, maid, peon, retiered personnel, etc.

**Moderate worker:** Site supervisor, mason, carpenter, electrician, welder, fitterman, fisherman, postman, potter, driver, colie, etc.

**Heavy worker:** Army soldiers, stone cutter, wood cutter, blacksmith, mine workers, farm labourer, etc.

## Energy Requirements of Adults in terms of BMR Units

| Activities | Duration (Hrs) | Rate of energy expenditure in terms of *BMR Units | | |
|---|---|---|---|---|
| | | Sedentary activity | Moderate activity | Heavy activity |
| Sleep | 8 | 1 | 1 | 1 |
| Occupational activity | 8 | 1.7 | 2.8 | 4.5 |
| Non-occupational activity | 8 | 2.2 | 2 | 1.5 |
| Average for 24 hrs | | 1.6 | 1.9 | 2.5 |
| Energy expenditure for reference man in 24 hrs | | 2425 | 2882 | 3788 |
| Energy expenditure for Reference woman in 24 hrs | | 1872 | 2223 | 2925 |
| **Break-up of non-occupational energy requirement** | | | | |
| Resting, moving around, etc. average rate of 1.7 BMR units | | 4 Hrs 30 Mts | 5 Hrs 30 Mts | 5 Hrs 30 Mts |
| Household, physical exercise, etc. average rate of 2.8 BMR units | | 3 Hrs 30 Mts | 2 Hrs 30 Mts | 2 Hrs 30 Mts |

## Energy Cost of Common Activities in Terms of *BMR Units

| Activities | Energy cost in terms of BMR units |
|---|---|
| Sleep quietly | 1.2 |
| Standing quietly | 1.4 |
| Sitting doing light work | 1.3 |
| Sitting doing moderate work | 1.6 |
| Standing doing light work | 2 |
| Standing doing moderate work | 3.6 |
| Standing doing heavy work | 7.4 |
| Walking 3 km/hr | 3.7 |
| Walking 6 km/hr | 7.4 |
| Dancing | 6.8 |

* One BMR unit is energy required for a reference person to maintain basal metabolic rate at sleep, i.e. 25.25 kcal/kg/day for males and 23.4 kcal/kg/day for females

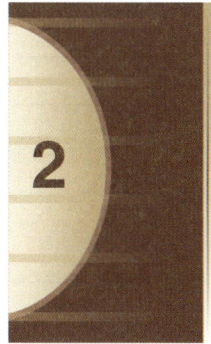

# 2

# Microbiology

## Microbiology

Exercise: Identify the bacteria in a given specimen.

Teacher's Remark .........................................

Teacher's Sign .........................................

## MICROBIOLOGY

**Exercise: Identify the bacteria in a given specimen**.

Solution through following steps:

Step 1: Observe type of specimen

Step 2: Observe culture media

Step 3: Gram staining

Step 4: Hanging drop preparation

Step 5: Sugar set reaction

### STEP (1)—TYPES OF SPECIMEN

**Blood sample:** Streptococci, staphylococci, *E. coli*, *Klabsiella*, *Pseudomonas*, meningococci, pneumococci, gonococci and *Vibrio cholerae* are found in blood samples.

**Urine sample:** Coliform and enterococci are found in urine samples.

**Stool sample:** *E. coli*, staphylococci, *Vibrio*, *Salmonella* and *Shigella* are found in stool samples.

**CSF sample:** Meningococci and pneumococci are found in CSF samples.

**Throat swabs:** Streptococci, staphylococci and diphtheroids are found in throat swabs.

**Sputum:** Staphylococci, *Tubercular bacilli*, pneumococci and *Klebsiella* are found in sputum sample.

**Nasopharyngeal and middle ear swab:** Pneumococci and haemolytic streptococci are found in nasopharyngeal and middle ear swabs.

**Genital sample:** Gonococci and syphilis are found in genital samples.

### STEP (2)—TYPES OF MEDIA

**Mac Conkey's:**

a. Pink colony of lactose fermenting bacteria, e.g. *E. coli*, *Klebsiella*.

b. Pale yellow colony of non-lactose fermenting bacteria, e.g. *Shigella*, *Salmonella*, *Proteus*, *Pseudomonas*.

**Blood agar:** All most all bacteria easily grow on blood agar.

**Nutrient agar:** All most all bacteria easily grow on nutrient agar.

**Peptone water:** Usually *E. coli*, *Salmonella*, *Shigella*, etc.

### STEP (3)—GRAM'S STAINING

**Aims of Gram Staining**

**To classify bacteria into two groups:**

Gram-positive (stain violet)

Gram-negative (stain pink)

**Bacteria can also be identified morphologically:**

Bacilli (rod-shaped)

Cocci (dot-shaped)

Cocobacilli.

**Bacteria can also be identified as per arrangements:**

Strept (in chains)

Staph (in group)

Diplo (in group of two)

## Principle

- Crystal violet stains all bacteria as violet.
- Iodine fixes violet colour of stain in bacteria more or less strongly.
- 95% alcohol/ethanol decolorize certain bacteria which stain less strongly (i.e. Gram-negative).
- Whereas it has no effect on strongly stained bacteria (i.e. on Gram-positive)
- Decolourized bacteria (i.e. Gram-negative) can be stained with carbol fuchsin/safranin stains as pink.

## Technique

Step 1: Prepare thin smear, if specimen is liquid, direct smear can be used and if it is thick then add a few drops of normal saline till it becomes liquid as required, emulsify it in a test tube and then it is used.

Step 2: Sterilize the loop (wire loop) on flame.

Step 3: Prepare thin smear on a clear wax free glass slide.

Step 4: Dry smear in air.

Step 5: Fix it on flame passing 3–4 times.

Step 6: Pour crystal violet on slide.

Step 7: Wait for one minute.

Step 8: Wash with water.

Step 9: Pour iodine solution on slide.

Step 10: Wait for one minute.

Step 11: Wash with water.

Step 12: Pour 95% alcohol/ethanol.

Step 13: Wait for one minute.

Step 14: Wash with water.

Step 15: Pour carbol fuchsin mixture/safranin on slide.

Step 16: Wait for one minute.

Step 17: Wash with water.

Step 18: Dry it in air.

Step 19: Pour one drop of oil.

Step 20: See in oil immersion lens and identify the type of bacteria.

## Result of Gram Staining

Bacteria in given specimen are Gram _____ cocci/bacilli.

### Sources of Error in Gram Staining

| False  Gram + ve | False Gram – ve |
|---|---|
| 1. Smear too thick. | 1. Smear too thin. |
| 2. Smear fixed before it  was dry. | |
| 3. Sediment in crystal violet. | |
| 4. Iodine not drained properly. | |
| 5. Less strong alcohol/ethanol. | |
| 6. Safranin/carbol fuchsin mix is too strong. | |
| 7. Safranin/carbol fuchsin mix is left for more time. | |

## STEP (4)—HANGING DROP PREPARATION
### Aims of Hanging Drop
- To see motility of bacteria and differentiate between motile and non-motile bacteria.
- To observe type of motility of bacteria.

### Technique: Steps
1. Dissolve specimen in peptone water.
2. Leave it for an hour or two to activate bacteria.
3. Form a ring of plasticine and put it on clean glass slide.
4. Put a drop or two of dissolved specimen on clean cover-slip in middle.
5. Put the slide on the cover-slip in such a way that drops of dissolved specimen should come in the middle of ring of plasticine of the slide and turn it upside down.
6. Focus the edge of drop in low power lens (10x).
7. Then focus the same place in high power (45x) lens and see motility.

**Result:** Bacteria in given specimen are motile/non-motile.

(Motility can be best observed at the edges of the drop.)

**False motility:** Basically bacteria are non-motile but look motile.

| Reason for false motility | Type of motility | Solution |
|---|---|---|
| 1 Due to wave of water | >>>>>>>> | See motility at the edge of drop |
| 2. Due to forces on bacteria | < > > > < < | By observing motility thoroughly and usually it is not regular. |

## STEP (5)—SUGAR REACTIONS
### Aims of Sugar Set Reactions
To differentiate bacteria on the basis of production of acid and/or gas on reaction with different sugars.

### Observations
**Sugar set:** There (usually 7) are test tubes for sugar set reaction containing peptone water with 1 % of specific sugar of which reaction is to be observed. One small tube called Durham's tube is also suspended inverted in all the test tubes containing sugar.
1. Test tube (1): Lactose
2. Test tube (2): Glucose
3. Test tube (3): Maltose
4. Test tube (4): Mannitol
5. Test tube (5): Sucrose
6. Test tube (6): Glactose
7. Test tube (7): Xylose

**Observation:** Reaction of bacteria with specific sugar is observed as follows:
1. If there is no change, i.e. no reaction of bacteria with sugar.
2. If there is air bubbles in top of 'D'tube, i.e. bacteria produce **gas** with sugar.
3. If peptone water became pink, i.e. bacteria produce **acid** with sugar.

4. If peptone water became pink with air bubbles on top of 'D' tube, i.e. bacteria produce **acid** and **gas** with sugar.

**Result:**  Bacteria in given sample are producing _____ with lactose

Bacteria in given sample are producing _____ with glucose

Bacteria in given sample are producing _____ with maltose

Bacteria in given sample are producing _____ with mannitol

Bacteria in given sample are producing _____ with sucrose

Bacteria in given sample are producing _____ with galactose

Bacteria in given sample are producing _____ with xylose

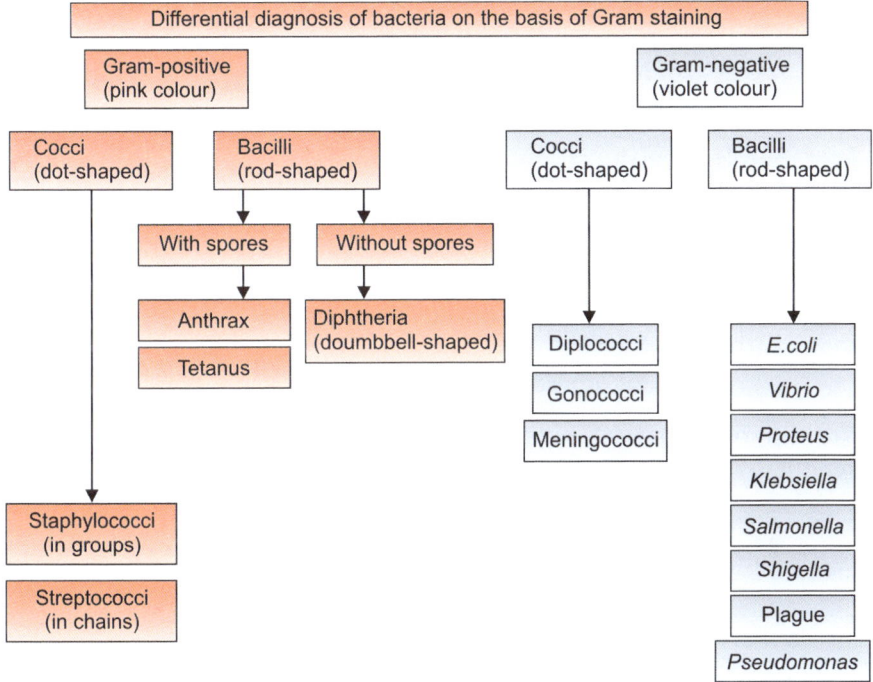

D/D of bacteria on Gram's staining

## D/D of Bacteria on the Basis of Reaction with Sugar

| S. no. | Sugar | E. coli | Vibrio | Proteus | Klebsiella | Salmonella | Shigella | Pseudomonas |
|--------|----------|---------|--------|---------|------------|------------|----------|-------------|
| 1 | Lactose | A + G | – | – | A + G | – | – | – |
| 2 | Glucose | A + G | A | A + G | A + G | A/A +G | A | A |
| 3 | Maltose | A + G | A | – | A + G | A | – | Variable |
| 4 | Mannitol | A + G | A | – | A + G | A | – | Variable |
| 5 | Sucrose | A + G | A | – | A + G | – | – | – |
| 6 | Glactose | A + G | – | – | A + G | – | – | – |
| 7 | Xylose | A + G | – | A | A + G | – | – | – |

## D/D of Bacteria on the Basis of Hanging Drop Preparation

| Motile | Non-motile |
|---|---|
| *Vibrio cholerae* | *Shigella* |
| *Salmonella typhi* | *Salmonella dysentery* |
| *E. coli* | *Klebsiella* |

## Result of Microbiology Exercise

Bacterium in given specimen is _____ (Name of bacterium)

Because (reasons)

1. Specimen is of stool/urine/vaginal/CSF/oropharyngeal/ _____
2. Bacteria are grown on _____ medium.
3. Bacteria colonies grown are _____ type.
4. Bacteria are Gram _____ positive/negative cocci/bacilli.
5. Bacteria are morphologically _____
6. Bacteria are having following reaction with specific sugar in sugar set reactions:

    1. With lactose produce _____
    2. With glucose produce _____
    3. With maltose produce _____
    4. With mannitol produce _____
    5. With sucrose produce _____
    6. With galactose produce _____
    7. With xylose produce _____

7. Bacteria are motile/non-motile.

# 3

# Water Chemistry

## Water Chemistry

Exercise 1: Find out the chlorine demand of a given sample of water with given bleaching powder

Exercise 2: Estimate the total hardness of given sample of water.

Exercise 3: Estimation of Ca hardness of given sample of water.

Exercise 4: Estimation of Mg hardness of water.

Exercise 5: Estimation of chlorides in given sample of water.

Exercise 6: Estimate sulphates in given sample of water.

Exercise 7: Estimate available chlorine in bleaching powder.

Teacher's Remark .............................................

Teacher's Sign .............................................

### Exercise 1: Find out the chlorine demand of a given sample of water with given bleaching powder

**Objective:** To find out the chlorine demand of given water sample.

## Apparatus

Horrock's apparatus containing:
1. 6 white cup measuring 200 ml capacity each
2. One black cup, 200 ml capacity
3. 2 metallic spoons measuring 2 gm each
4. 7 glass stirring rods
5. One special pipette
6. 2 droppers
7. One starch iodide/potassium iodide bottle

## Principle

$H_2O + Cl_2 = HOCl + HCl$

$HOCl = H^+ + OCl^-$

$OCl^- + 2H^+ + 2I = I_2 + H_2O + Cl^-$,   $I_2 + Starch = Starch$ iodide (blue colour)

## Procedure

Step 1:  Prepare stock solution of bleaching powder with following steps:
      a.  Take one level full of spoon (2 gm) of bleaching powder in black cup.
      b.  Add some sample water to it to make a paste.
      c.  Now fill the cup up to circular mark and stir it with a rod. Now stock solution is ready.

Step 2:  Fill six white cups with sample water up to 1 cm below the rim, i.e. 200 ml.

Step 3:  With the help of special pipette add one drop of stock solution in cup no. '1', two drops in cup no. '2', three drops in cup no. '3', four drops in cup no. '4', five drops in cup no. '5', and six drops in cup no. '6' after arranging cups in sequence.

Step 4:  Stir each cup using separate rod for each cup.

Step 5:  Wait for contact period (half hour for treated water and 1 hour for untreated water)

Step 6:  Add 3 drops of starch iodide/potassium iodide solution to each white cup.

Step 7:  Note the 1st cup showing blue colour in the series of 6 cups.

Step 8:  Repeat the whole procedure (step 1 – 7) at least 2 times more.

Step 9:  Take mode of observations.

Step 10: Calculate amount of bleaching powder for given sample water with formula.

## Observations

| S. no. | No. of 1st cup showing blue colour | Mean of no. of 1st cup |
|--------|------------------------------------|------------------------|
| 1.     |                                    |                        |
| 2.     |                                    |                        |
| 3.     |                                    |                        |

## Calculations

Amount of bleaching powder $= \dfrac{\text{No. of 1st cup showing blue colour}}{455} \times 2 \text{ gm/litre of water}$

Amount of bleaching powder required (BP) = _____ gm/l of water

If, bleaching powder is having 25% strength, then

Amount of chlorine in _____ gm bleaching powder is = BP × 25/100

**Result:** Chlorine demand of water is _____ l

For super-chlorination, calculation is as follow:

Amont of bleaching powder for super-chlorination

$= \dfrac{\text{No. of 2nd cup showing blue colour}}{455} \times 2 \text{gm/l of water}$

## Exercise 2: Estimate the total hardness in given sample of water

**Objective:** To estimate the total hardness in given sample of water.

## Apparatus

1. Beaker
2. Pipette capacity 25 ml
3. Small pipette
4. Burette
5. EDTA (ethylenediaminetetra-acetic acid)
6. Chrome black-T
7. Ammonium buffer ($NH_4OH$) to make pH 8.5 to 11.5).

## *Principle

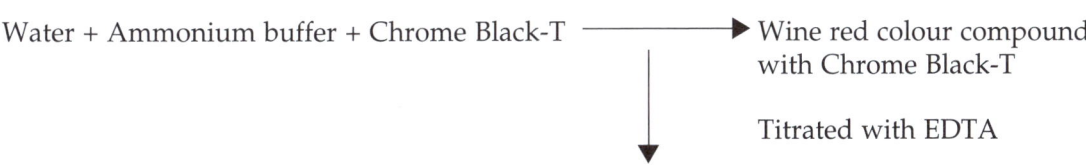

Water + Ammonium buffer + Chrome Black-T ⟶ Wine red colour compound with Chrome Black-T

Titrated with EDTA

Pinkish blue colour (original colour of dye)
Colourless compounds with EDTA

## Procedure

Step 1: With the help of a pipette, take 25 ml of sample water in a beaker.

Step 2: Add 1 ml of $NH_4OH$ (ammonium buffer) in it.

Step 3: Add a pinch (5 ml) of Chrome Black-T to it.

Step 4: After observing wine red colour (due to chrome complexes with Ca and Mg), start titrating it with EDTA.

Step 5: Stop titration on appearing pinkish blue colour and note the reading.

Step 6: Repeat the whole exercise (step 1–5) at least two times more or uptill two reading coincides.

Step 7: Take mode of reading.
Step 8: Calculate the EDTA used for 25 ml sample water.
Step 9: Now calculate total hardness of sample water.

## Observations

| S. no. | Sample water + $NH_4OH$ + Chrome Black-T | EDTA used | Final reading |
|--------|------------------------------------------|-----------|---------------|
| 1. | 25 ml | | |
| 2. | 25 ml | | |
| 3. | 25 ml | | |

## **Calculations

Total hardness of water = EDTA used × 40 mg/l of water
**Result:** Total hardness of given sample, water is _____ (mg/l)

## *Principle

1. $NH_4OH$ is used to make pH suitable (8.5 to 11.5) for reaction of Ca, Mg, etc. with Chrome Black-T.
2. Chrome Black-T forms wine red colour complexes, Ca, Mg, etc. as hardness.
3. EDTA forms more durable colourless complexes of Ca and Mg, etc. for which EDTA extracts Ca and Mg from Ca, Mg complexes of Chrome Black-T, then wine red colour slowly gets converted to pinkish blue, which is the original colour of dye itself.

## **Calculations

25 ml of water needs = E ml of EDTA to utilize Ca and Mg present in water.

$$1 \text{ ml of water needs} = \frac{E \text{ ml of EDTA to utilize Ca and Mg present in water}}{25}$$

$$1000 \text{ ml of water needs} = \frac{E \text{ (EDTA used)} \times 1000 \text{ mg}}{25}$$

1 Liter of water needs = E (EDTA used) × 40 mg
Total hardness = E (EDTA used) × 40 mg/l of water

## Exercise 3: Estimation of Ca hardness in given sample of water

**Objective:** To estimate the Ca hardness of given sample of water.

## Apparatus

1. Beaker
2. Pipette capacity 25 ml
3. Small pipette
4. Burette
5. EDTA
6. Murexide
7. NaOH (2 ml)

## *Principle

Water + Sodium buffer (NaOH) + Murexide ⟶ Pink-coloured complex with murexide

↓ Titrated with EDTA

Purple colour (original colour of dye)
Colourless complex with EDTA

## Procedure

Step 1: Take 25 ml of sample water in beaker with the help of pipette.
Step 2: Add 1 ml of sodium buffer to it to make pH about 12.
Step 3: Add a pinch of murexide to it.
Step 4: After observing pink colour of complex, titrate it with EDTA.
Step 5: Stop titration on appearing purple colour and note the reading.
Step 6: Repeat whole process two times more.
Step 7: Take mode of reading of EDTA.
Step 8: Calculate Ca hardness with the help of formula.

## Observations

| S. no. | Sample water + NaOH + Murexide | EDTA used | Final reading |
|--------|-------------------------------|-----------|---------------|
| 1. | 25 ml | | |
| 2. | 25 ml | | |
| 3. | 25 ml | | |

## **Calculations

Calcium hardness of water = EDTA use × 40 mg/l of water

**Result:** Calcium hardness of given sample water is _____ (mg/l)

## *Principle

1. Murexide makes complexes with Ca not with Mg.
2. NaOH is used to make pH suitable (12) for reaction of Ca with murexide.
3. Murexide makes pink colour complexes with calcium as hardness.
4. EDTA form more durable colourless complexes of Ca for which EDTA extract Ca from calcium complexes of murexide.
5. Then pink colour slowly is converted to purple which is the original colour of dye itself.

## **Calculations

25 ml of water need × ml of EDTA to use Ca present in given sample of water

$$1 \text{ ml of water need} = \frac{E \text{ ml of EDTA to use}}{25}$$

$$1000 \text{ ml of water need} = \frac{E \times 1000}{25} = E40 \text{ mg of Ca hardness}$$

## Exercise 4: Estimation of Mg hardness in given sample of water

**Objective:** To estimate the Mg hardness in given sample of water.

### Apparatus

1. Beaker
2. Pipette capacity 25 ml
3. Small pipette
4. Burette
5. EDTA
6. Chrome Black-T
7. Murexide
8. NaOH
9. Ammonia buffer ($NH_4OH$)

### *Principle

Total hardness – Ca hardness = Mg hardness
**Procedure:** Same as that of exercise '2' and '3'

### Observations

**For Total Hardness 'A'**

| S. no. | Sample water + $NH_4OH$ + Chrome Black-T | EDTA used | Final reading |
|--------|------------------------------------------|-----------|---------------|
| 1. | 25 ml | | |
| 2. | 25 ml | | |
| 3. | 25 ml | | |

**For Calcium Hardness 'B'**

| S. no. | Sample water + NaOH + Murexide | EDTA used | Final reading |
|--------|--------------------------------|-----------|---------------|
| 1. | 25 ml | | |
| 2. | 25 ml | | |
| 3. | 25 ml | | |

### **Calculations

Total hardness of water = EDTA used in exercise 'A' × 40 mg/l

Calcium hardness of water = EDTA used in exercise 'B' × 40 mg/l

Total hardness – Ca hardness = Mg hardness

or Mg hardness = (EDTA used 'A' – 'B') × 40 mg/l of water

**Result:** Magnesium hardness of given sample of water is _____ (mg/l)

*Principle: Same as that of exercise '2' and '3'.
**Calculations: Same as that of exercise '2' and '3'.

### Exercise 5: Estimation of chlorides in given sample of water

**Objective:** To estimate the chlorides in given sample of water.

## Apparatus

1. Beaker
2. Pipette capacity 25 ml
3. Small pipette
4. Burette
5. $AgNO_3$
6. Potassium chromate ($K_2CrO_4$)

## *Principle

Chlorides of water + Potassium chromate ($K_2Cr\ O_4$) $\longrightarrow$ Silver chlorides (colourless complex)

Titrated with $AgNO_3$

Silver Chromate (brick red colour complex)

$CaCl_2 + 2\ AgNO_3 = 2\ AgCl$ (colourless complex) $+ Ca(NO_3)_2$

$MgCl_2 + 2\ AgNO_3 = 2\ AgCl$ (colourless complex) $+ Ca(NO_3)_2$

$K_2CrO_4$ (yellow colour) $+ 2\ AgNO_3 = 2\ KNO_3 + Ag_2CrO_4$ (brick red colour)

## Procedure

Step 1: Take 25 ml of water in a beaker with the help of pipette.
Step 2: Add a few drops of potassium chromate into it.
Step 3: Titrate it with $AgNO_3$ after a few minutes.
Step 4: Titrate it until the whole chlorides of water converted to $AgCl_2$
Step 5: Stop titration on appearance of brick red colour of silver chromate.
Step 6: Note the reading.
Step 7: Repeat the whole process (steps 1 to 5) at least for two times more.
Step 8: Take mode of reading of $AgNO_3$.
Step 9: Calculate amount of chloride in water with the help of formula.

## Observations

| S. no. | Sample water + $K_2CrO_4$ | $AgNO_3$ used | Final reading |
|--------|---------------------------|---------------|---------------|
| 1. | 25 ml | | |
| 2. | 25 ml | | |
| 3. | 25 ml | | |

## **Calculations

Chlorides in sample water = Amount of $AgNO_3$ used × 40 mg/l
**Result:** Chlorides in given sample water is _____ (mg/l)

### *Principle

1. Potassium chromate ($K_2CrO_4$) is yellow coloured compound.
2. When $AgNO_3$ titrates it makes AgCl (colourless complexes) with chlorides present in water.
3. As soon as whole chloride in water is used by $AgNO_3$ (forming AgCl), potassium chromate ($K_2CrO_4$) titrated with $AgNO_3$ it makes red colour complexes of silver chromate.

### **Calculations

25 ml of water need 'A' ml of $AgNO_3$ use chlorides present in given sample of water

$$1 \text{ ml of water need} = \frac{\text{'A'ml of} AgNO_3}{25}$$

$$1000 \text{ ml of water need} = \frac{A \times 1000}{25} = A \text{ 40 mg of chlorides}$$

### Exercise 6: Estimate sulphates in given sample of water

**Objective:** To estimate sulphates in given sample of water.

### Apparatus

1. Beaker
2. Pipette capacity 25 ml
3. Small pipette
4. Burette
5. $BaCl_2$
6. Ammonium buffer
7. Chrome Black-T
8. EDTA

*Principle: Principle for total hardness is given in exercise no '2'.
**Calculations: Total hardness–hardness except $SO_4$ = $SO_4$ hardness

### Principle for Hardness Except $SO_4$

Water + $BaCl_2$ + Ammonium buffer + Chrome Black-T ⟶ Wine red colour complex with Chrome Black-T

$BaSO_4$ PPT | Titrated with EDTA

Blue colour (original colour of Chrome Black-T)

$$CaSO_4 \text{ (in water)} + BaCl_2 = BaSO_4 \text{ (wine red colour)} + CaCl_2$$
$$MgSO_4 \text{ (in water)} + BaCl_2 = BaSO_4 \text{ (wine red colour)} + MgCl_2$$

**Procedure:** Procedure for total hardness is given in exercise '2'.

### For Hardness Except $SO_4$

Step 1: Take 25 ml water in a beaker with the help of burette.
Step 2: Add 10 ml $BaCl_2$ to it and keep it for a few minutes.
Step 3: Add 1 ml ammonium buffer and a pinch of Chrome Black-T to it.
Step 4: Titrate it with EDTA after observing wine red colour of $BaSO_4$.

Step 5: Stop titration when wine red colour disappears and blue colour of dye starts appearing.

Step 6: Note the reading of EDTA used.

Step 7: Repeat the whole process (steps 1–6) at least for two times more.

Step 8: Take final (mode) reading.

Step 9: Calculate $SO_4$ hardness as per principle with the help of formula.

## Observations

**For Total Hardness 'A'**

| S. no. | Sample water + $NH_4OH$ + Chrome Black-T | EDTA used | Final reading |
|--------|------------------------------------------|-----------|---------------|
| 1.     | 25 ml                                    |           |               |
| 2.     | 25 ml                                    |           |               |
| 3.     | 25 ml                                    |           |               |

**For Hardness other than Sulphate 'B'**

| S. no. | Sample water + $BaCl_2$ + $NH_4OH$ + Chrome Black-T | EDTA used | Final reading |
|--------|-----------------------------------------------------|-----------|---------------|
| 1.     | 25 ml                                               |           |               |
| 2.     | 25 ml                                               |           |               |
| 3.     | 25 ml                                               |           |               |

## **Calculations

**Total** hardness of water = EDTA used in exercise 'A' × 40 mg/l

Hardness without sulphate ($SO_4$) of water = EDTA used in exercise 'B' × 40 mg/l

Total hardness – Hardness without sulphate ($SO_4$) = Sulphate ($SO_4$) hardness

**Result:** Sulphate ($SO_4$) hardness of given sample water is _____ (mg/l)

*Principle: Same as that of exercise '2'. Here $BaCl_2$ makes complexes with '$SO_4$' which precipitates colourless.

**Calculations: Same as that of exercise '2'.

## Exercise 7: Estimate available chlorine in bleaching powder

**Objective:** To estimate available chlorine in bleaching powder.

## Apparatus

1. Beaker
2. Pipette capacity 25 ml
3. Small pipette
4. Burette
5. Flask
6. Bleaching powder (sample)
7. Potassium iodide
8. Acetic acid
9. Starch solution
10. Sodium thiosulphate

## *Principle

Bleaching P.Soln + Pot. iodide +Acetic acid ──────────▶ Blue colour of starch iodide
+ Starch solution

Titrated with sodium thiosulphate

▼

Sodium thiosulphate complex (colourless)

## Procedure

Step 1: Take 5 gm of bleaching powder in a flask.

Step 2: Dissolve it in 250 ml of distilled water.

Step 3: Take 25 ml of water in a beaker.

Step 4: Add 10 ml of 10% potassium iodide.

Step 5: Add 5 ml of acetic acid.

Step 6: Add a few drops of starch solution.

Step 7: Titrate it with sodium thiosulphate.

Step 8: Stop titration when blue colour disappears and note the reading.

Step 9: Repeat the whole process (steps 1–8) for at least two more times.

Step 10: Take final reading (mode of 3 readings).

Step 11: Calculate amount of chlorine available in given sample of bleaching powder with the help of given calculation.

## Observations

| S. no. | Bleaching soln. + Pot. iodide + Acetic acid +Starch solution | Sodium thiosulphate | Final reading |
|--------|------------------------------------------------------------|---------------------|---------------|
| 1. | 25 ml | | |
| 2. | 25 ml | | |
| 3. | 25 ml | | |

## **Calculations

% of chlorine available in bleaching powder = Sodium thiosulphate used × 200 × 0.00346

**Result:** Amount of chlorine in bleaching powder is _____%.

## *Principle

*Chlorine in bleaching powder react with KI and starch as follows:

$(R_1)$ $Cl_2$ + 2 KI + Starch = 2 KCl + Starch iodide (blue colour)

When $Cl_2$ consumed with KI and starch then starch react with sodium thiosulphate and makes colourless complex.

$(R_2)$ $Na_2S_2O_3$ + Starch iodide = Colourless complex

## **Calculations

250 ml of water contains 5 gm of bleaching powder

1 ml of water contains $\dfrac{5}{250}$ gm bleaching powder

25 ml of water contains $= \dfrac{5 \times 25}{250}$ gm $= 0.5$ gm of bleaching powder

0.5 gm bleaching powder requires '$S$' ml of sodium thiosulphate

1 gm of bleaching powder requires $= \dfrac{'S'}{0.5}$ ml  ml of sodium thiosulphate.

100 gm of bleaching powder requires $= \dfrac{'S' \times 100}{0.5}$ ml of sodium thiosulphate

$= 200 \times$ '$S$' ml of sodium thosulphate.

(1 ml of thiosulphate $= 0.003546$ gm chlorine) (0.003546 is mol. wt. of chlorine)

$= 200 \times 0.003546$ gm of chlorine.

# 4

# Spotting

➢ 10 to 20 spots are kept for examination
➢ With every spot 2/3 questions are asked
➢ Questions usually asked are given with the type of spots
➢ Time allotted is 2 to 3 minutes for answering questions given with the spot.

## Food Stuffs Spots

Question 1: Indentify the spot with reasons.

Question 2: Write down nutrient value of given spot.

Question 3: Enumerate the diseases, its deficiency can cause?

Question 4: Write down the public health importance of given spot.

Teacher's Remark ..........................................

Teacher's Sign ..........................................

# CEREALS

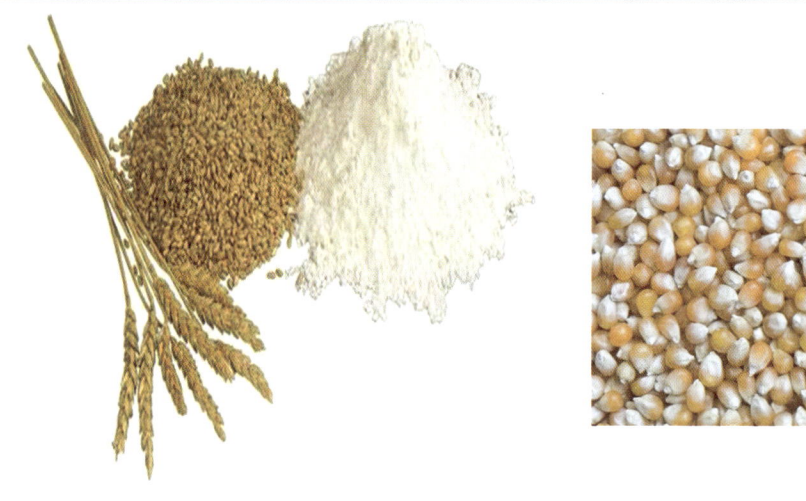

| Wheat | Maize |
|---|---|

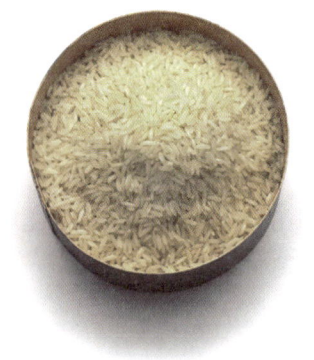 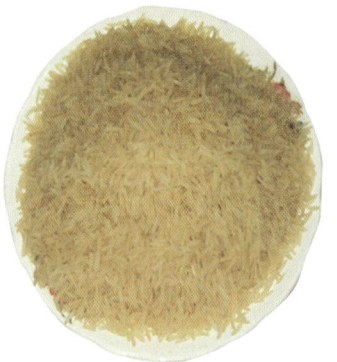 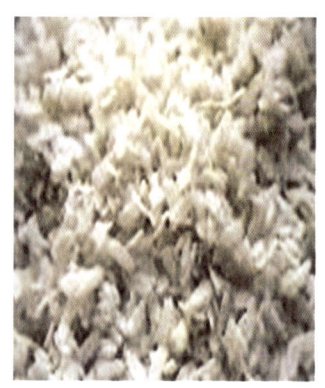

| Rice | Parboiled rice | Rice flakes |
|---|---|---|

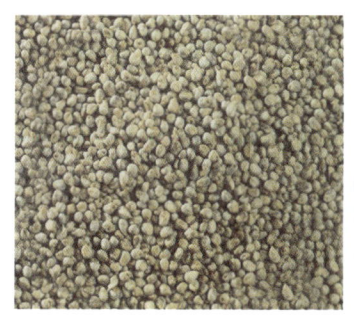 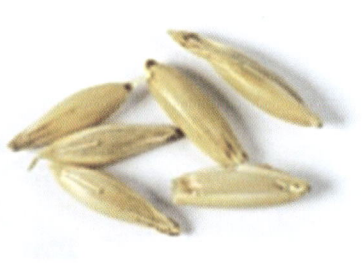 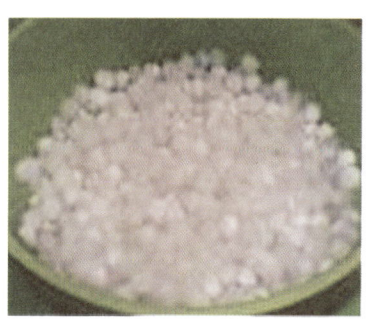

| Bajara | Oat | Sago (Sabudana) |
|---|---|---|

## Nutrient value of cereals (per 100 g)

| Nutrient | Carbohydrate (g) | Protein (g) | Fat (g) | Fibre (g) | Iron (mg) | Vit B comp (μg) | Energy (kcal) |
|---|---|---|---|---|---|---|---|
| Wheat | 69.4 | 12.1 | 1.7 | 1.9 | 4.9 | 5.62 | 341 |
| Maize | 66.2 | 11.1 | 3.6 | 2.7 | 2.3 | 2.3 | 342 |
| Rice | 78.2 | 6.8 | 0.5 | 0.2 | 0.7 | 3.1 | 345 |
| Parboiled rice | 79 | 6.4 | 0.4 | 0.2 | 1 | 5.1 | 346 |
| Bajara | 67.5 | 11.6 | 5 | 1.2 | 8 | 2.1 | 361 |
| Oat | 21 | 9 | 10 | 3.1 | 28 | 3.7 | 240 |
| Sago | 87.1 | 0.2 | 0.2 | 0.5 | 1.2 | 0.21 | 351 |

### General Features of Cereals
- Consumed in large bulk in Indian diet.
- Main sources of energy (carbohydrates)—350 kcal/100 gm.
- Contain proteins (6 to 12 %) minerals and B group vitamins
- Provide 70–80% of total energy intake and >50% of protein intake.

### Proteins of Cereals
- Poor in nutritive quality deficient in essential amino acid (EAA) lysine.
- Maize deficient lysine and tryptophan (precursor of niacin).

### Supplementary Action of the Proteins
- When cereals are taken with pulses, cereals and pulse proteins complement each other and provide a complete protein intake.

### Wheat
- Limiting amino acids lysine and threonine.
- Wheat protein (gluten) may cause allergy.
- In India, wheat is consumed as wheat flour, whiter the flour greater the loss of vitamins and minerals.

### Maize
- Yellow variety is rich in carotenoid pigments.
- Proteins are deficient in lysine and tryptophan
- High leucine contents interfere in conversion of tryptophan into niacin. Hence, excess of consumption causes 'pellagra'.

**Rice:** It is a grain consis of 3 parts:
1. Germ (embryo) – nutrients
2. Endosperm – starch
3. Pericarp layer – nutrients

## Nutritive Value of Rice

- Rich—thiamine, niacin, pyridoxine and riboflavin (B group vitamins).
- Poor—vitamins A, C, D, calcium and iron.
- Richer in lysine than other cereals.

**Effect of milling on rice:** Loss of 15% of protein, 75% of thiamine, 60% of riboflavin and niacin.

Looks clean and attractive and becomes more digestable but highly polished rice predisposes to beriberi.

## Effect of Washing and Cooking on Rice

- Washing in large quantity of water removes 60% of vitamins and minerals.
- Cooking in large quantity of water and draining of excess water at the end leads to loss of group B vitamins.

**Parboiling:** Recommended by "Central Food Technological Research Institute, Mysore"

- Soak the paddy (unhusked rice) in hot water (65 to 70°F) for 3 to 4 hrs.
- Drain the water and apply the steam to the soaked paddy for 5 to 10 miniutes
- Paddy is dried now.
- During steaming process, greater part of vitamins and minerals present in the inner layer of rice enter into endosperm layer of rice grain, so during milling process nutrients are not removed.

## PULSES

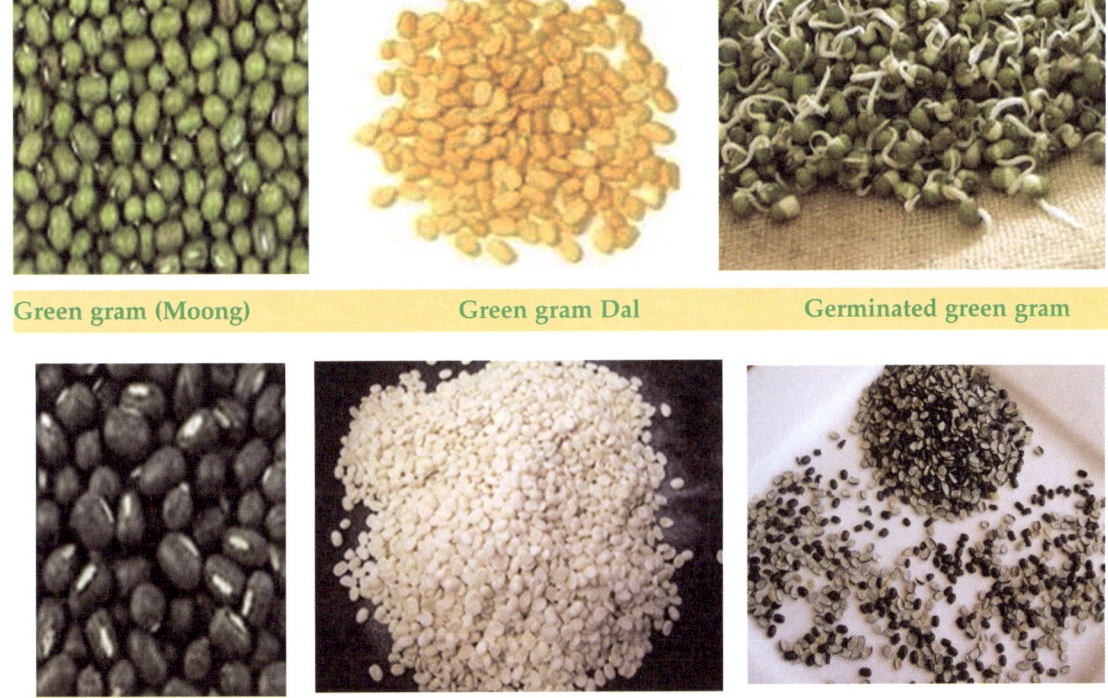

| Green gram (Moong) | Green gram Dal | Germinated green gram |

| Black gram (Urad) whole | Black gram Dal without skin | Black gram Dal with skin |

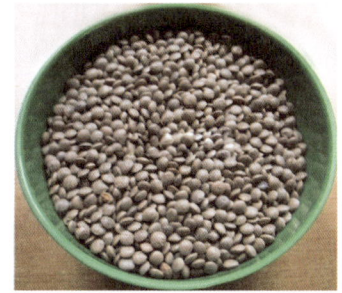
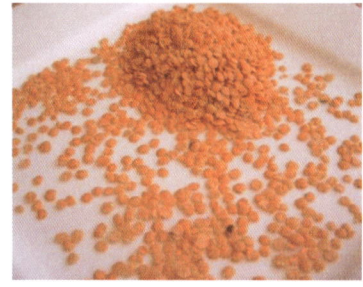
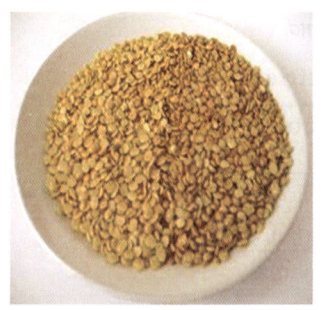

| Red gram lentil (Masoor) | Yellow gram (Arhar) Dal |

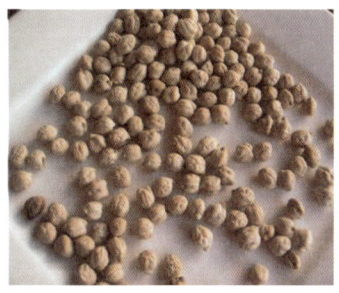
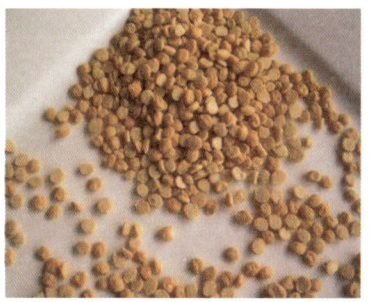

| Bangal gram whole (Chhole) | Bangal gram Dal (Chana Dal) |

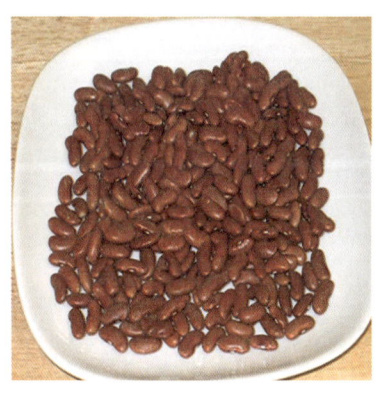
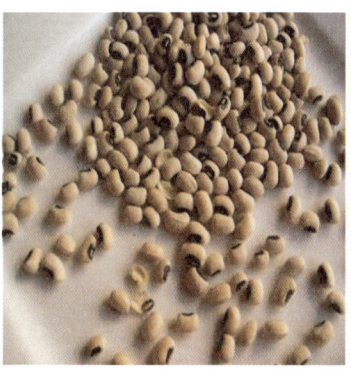
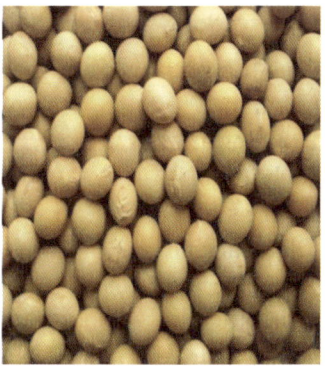

| Kidney beans (Rajma) | Black eye beans | Soyabean |

## Nutrient value of legumes (per 100 g)

| Nutrient | Carbohydrate (g) | Protein (g) | Fat (g) | Fibre (g) | Energy (kcal) |
|---|---|---|---|---|---|
| Green gram | 59.9 | 24.5 | 1.2 | 2.8 | 348 |
| Red gram | 57.6 | 22.3 | 1.7 | 2.1 | 335 |
| Black gram | 59.6 | 24.0 | 1.4 | 2.3 | 347 |

Contd.

*Contd.*

## Nutrient value of legumes (per 100 g)

| Nutrient | Carbohydrate (g) | Protein (g) | Fat (g) | Fibre (g) | Energy (kcal) |
|---|---|---|---|---|---|
| Yellow gram | 57.6 | 28.2 | 0.6 | 3.2 | 345 |
| Bangal gram | 58.1 | 22.5 | 5.2 | 3.9 | 369 |
| Rajama | 60.6 | 22.9 | 1.3 | 4.8 | 432 |
| Soyabean | 20.9 | 43.2 | 19.2 | 3.7 | 432 |
| Beans dry | 24.5 | 19.7 | 1.1 | 1.8 | 315 |

## Micronutrient value of legumes (per 100 g)

| Nutrient | | Mineral (mg) | | | Vitamins (µg) | |
|---|---|---|---|---|---|---|
| | Ca | Iron | Vit B$_1$ | Vit B$_2$ | Vit B$_4$ | Vit C |
| Green gram | 75 | 3.9 | 0.47 | 0.21 | 2.4 | 0 |
| Red gram | 73 | 2.7 | 0.45 | 0.19 | 2.9 | 0 |
| Black gram | 154 | 3.8 | 0.42 | 0.2 | 2 | 0 |
| Yellow gram | 202 | 4.6 | 0.42 | 0.2 | 1.5 | 1 |
| Bangal gram | 202 | 4.6 | 0.3 | 0.15 | 2.9 | 3 |
| Rajma | 260 | 5 | 0.5 | 0.3 | 2.4 | 0 |
| Soyabean | 240 | 10.4 | 0.73 | 0.39 | 3.2 | 0 |
| Beans dry | 75 | 7.05 | 0.47 | 0.19 | 3.4 | 0 |

**Pulses (Legumes):** Most commonly known as 'dals'.
- Contain 20% to 25% of proteins but they are poor in the quality of protein.
- Proteins are rich in lysine but poor in methionine and cysteine.
- Rich in minerals and group B vitamins like thiamine and riboflavin.
- In dry state, no vitamin C but germinating pulses contain vitamins C and B.
- Oligosaccharides of pulses cause flatulence.
- Anti-nutritional factors: In raw states, pulses have phytates and tannins which adversely affect the bioavailability of some nutrients in the body but can be destroyed by heat.

**Soyabeans:** It is 'Queen' of pulses.
- Contains high protein (43 gm/100 gm) and fat (19 gm/100 gm)
- Nutritive value of proteins is equivalent to milk proteins.
- Good source of iron, folic acid, niacin and carotene.
- Blend taste is made suitable by cooking or processing it.
- Cooked as dal or prepared with other legumes as mixed dal.
- Mixed in wheat flour to be more nutritious.
- Soya milk or curd is also popular.
- Nutrinugetts are also one of the preparation of soyabeans.
- As it contains high amount of fats, its oil is extracted and used as cooking oil.
- This oil is one of the very few oils rich in alpha-linolenic acid (>5%) besides high linolenic acid (53%).

## Effect of Sprouting

- It increases riboflavin, niacin, choline, biotin and vitamin C.
- It destroys anti-nutrients and toxic factors.

## VEGETABLES

### GREEN LEAFY VEGETABLES

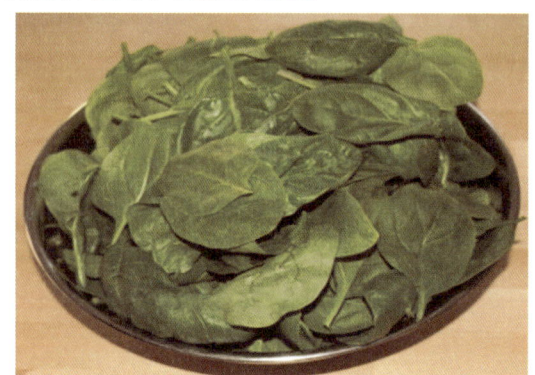

Spinach

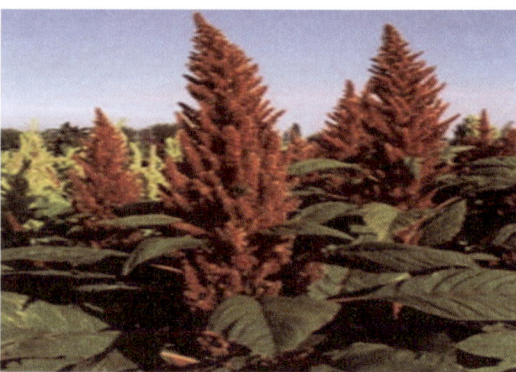

Amaranth

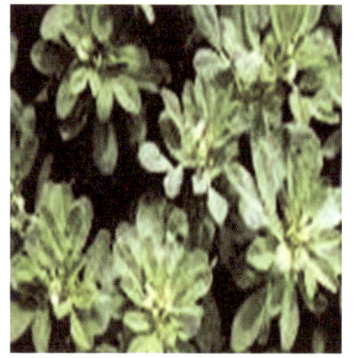

Fenugreek (Methi) leaves

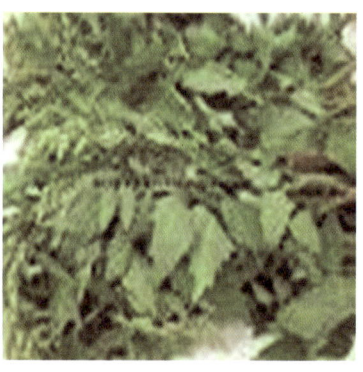

Bathua leaves

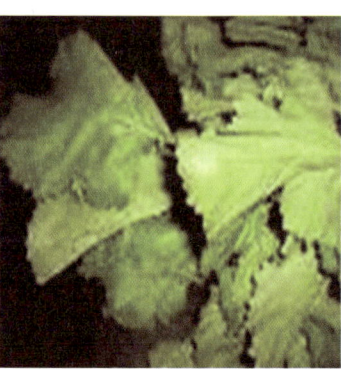

Sarso leaves

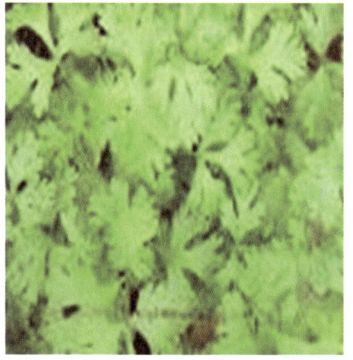

Coriander (Dhania) leaves

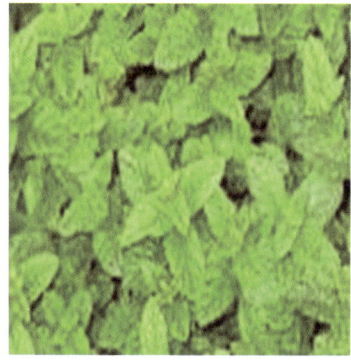

Mint (Podina) leaves

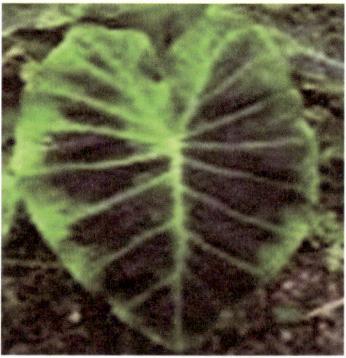

Colocasia (Arbi) leaves

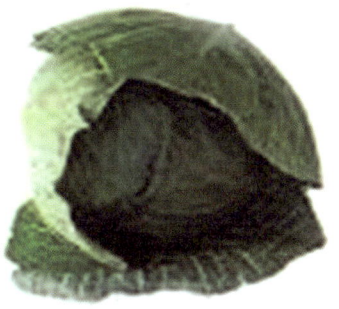 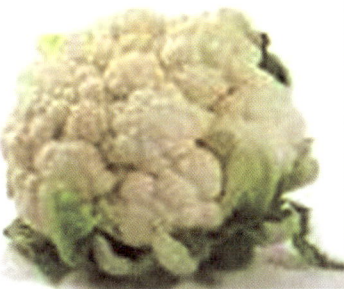 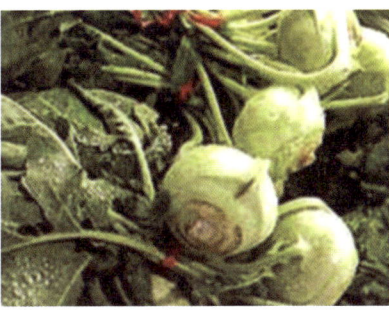

**Cabbage (Band Gobhi)**      **Cauliflower (Fool Gobhi)**      **Ganth Gobhi**

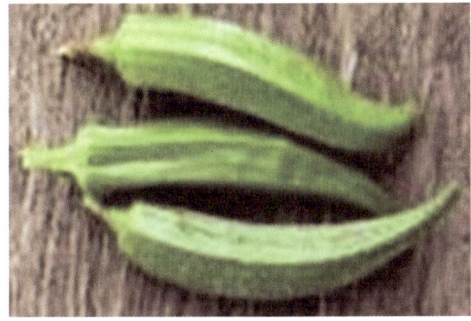 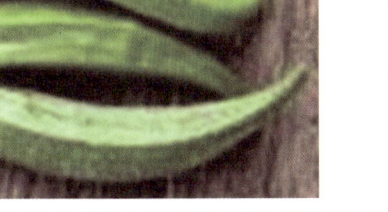 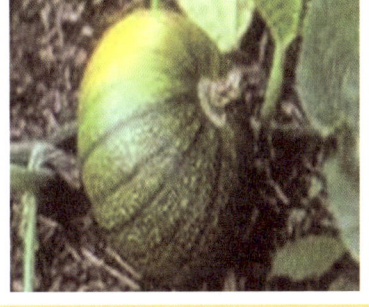

**Ladies finger (Bhindi)**      **Pumpkin (Kashiphal)**

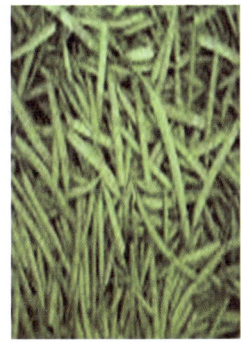 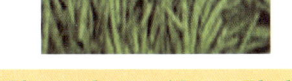 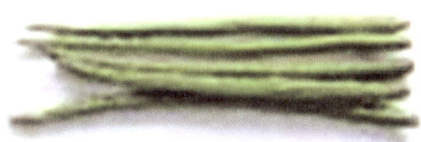

**Cluster beans (Gwar Phali)**      **Drumstick**

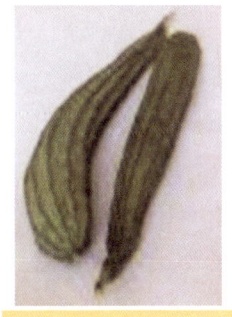 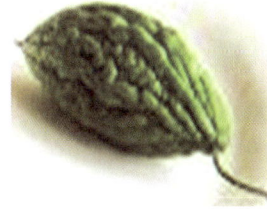 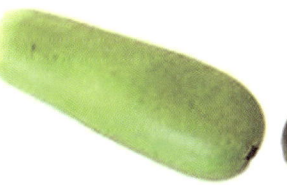 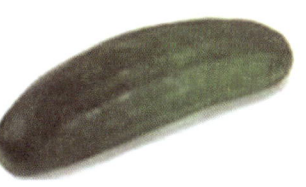

**Ridge guard (Turai)**      **Bitter guard (Karela)**      **Bottle guard (Loki)**      **Cucumber**

## ROOTS AND TUBERS

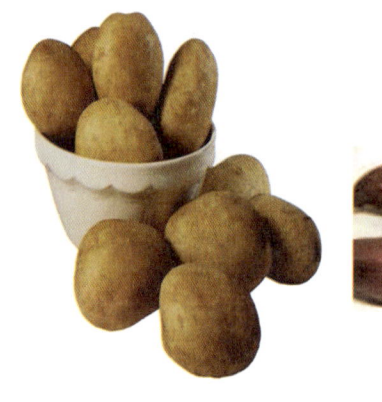 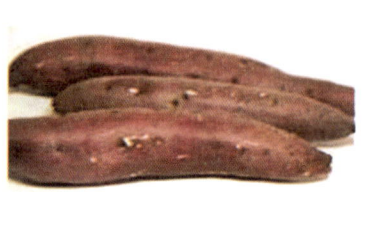 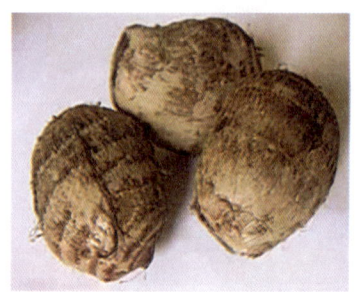

| Potato | Sweet potato | Colocasia (Arbi) |

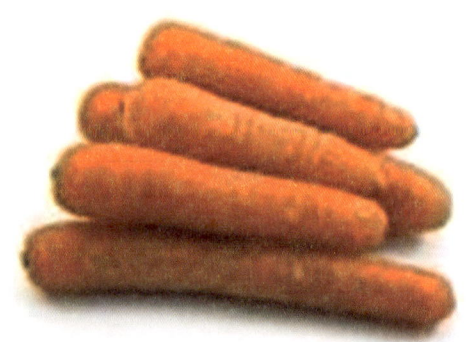 

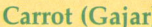

| Carrot (Gajar) | Raddish (Muli) |

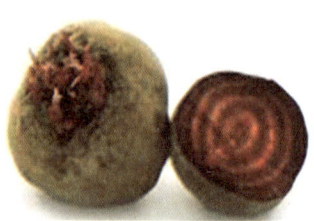 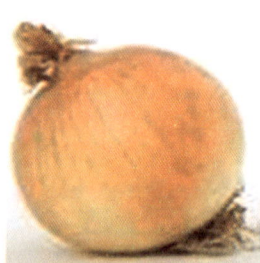 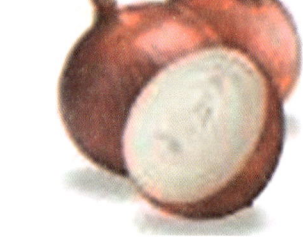

| Beet root (Chukander) | Onion (Pyaj) |

## OTHER VEGETABLES

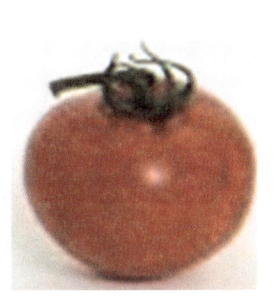 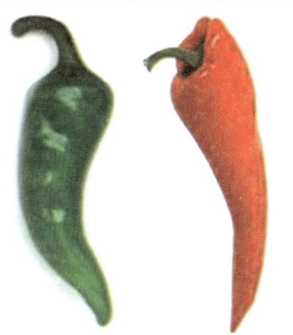 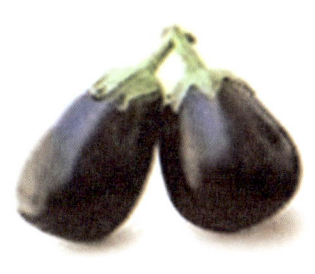

| Tomato | Chilies | Brinjal (Baingan) |

### Nutrient value of vegetables (per 100 g)

| Nutrient | Energy (kcal) | Carbo-hydrate (g) | Protein (g) | Fat (g) | Calcium (mg) | Iron (mg) | Vit. C (µg) | Carotene (µg) |
|---|---|---|---|---|---|---|---|---|
| Amaranth | 45 | 6.3 | 4 | 0.5 | 397 | 3.49 | 99 | 5620 |
| Spinach | 26 | 2.9 | 2 | 0.7 | 73 | 1.14 | 28 | 5580 |
| Fenugreek (methi) | 49 | 6 | 4.4 | 0.9 | 335 | 1.99 | 52 | 2340 |
| Sarso leaves | 45 | 6 | 4 | 0.5 | 205 | 1 | 50 | |
| Coriander L | 44 | 6.3 | 3.3 | 0.6 | 184 | 18.5 | 27 | 337 |
| Mint L | 48 | 5.8 | 4.8 | 0.6 | 200 | 16 | 27 | 1620 |
| Colocasia L | 56 | 7 | 4 | 1 | 227 | 10 | 25 | 324 |
| Cabbage | 27 | 4.6 | 1.8 | 0.1 | 39 | 0.8 | 124 | 120 |
| Cauliflower | 30 | 4 | 2.6 | 0.4 | 33 | 1.5 | 56 | 30 |
| Ladies finger | 35 | 6.7 | 1.9 | 0.2 | 66 | 0.35 | 13 | 52 |
| Pumpkin | 25 | 4.6 | 1.4 | 0.1 | 10 | 0.7 | 21 | 368 |
| Cluster beans | 16 | 11 | 3 | 0 | 130 | 1 | 23 | 86 |
| Drumstick | 92 | 12.5 | 6.7 | 1.7 | 440 | 0.85 | 220 | 6780 |
| Ridge gourd | 17 | 3.4 | 0.5 | 0.1 | 40 | 1.6 | 95 | 120 |
| Bitter gourd | 25 | 4.2 | 1.6 | 0.2 | 20 | 0.61 | 96 | 126 |
| Bottle gourd | 18 | 3.3 | 0.5 | 0.3 | 50 | 1.1 | 95 | 120 |
| Cucumber | 13 | 2.5 | 0.4 | 0.1 | 10 | 1.5 | 96 | 120 |
| Chilies G | 35 | 6.7 | 1.9 | 0.2 | 66 | 0.35 | 95 | 4545 |
| Mango green | 44 | 10.1 | 0.7 | 0.1 | 10 | 5.4 | 137 | 312 |
| Tomato | 20 | 3.6 | 0.9 | 0.2 | 34 | 0.64 | 131 | 276 |
| Brinjal | 24 | 4 | 1.4 | 0.3 | 18 | 0.9 | 23 | 68 |
| Potato | 97 | 22.6 | 1.6 | 0.1 | 10 | 0.48 | 17 | 24 |
| Sweet potato | 120 | 28.2 | 1.2 | 0.3 | 46 | 0.21 | 24 | 6 |
| Beet root | 43 | 8.8 | 1.7 | 0.1 | 18.3 | 1.19 | 10 | – |
| Colocasia | 97 | 21.1 | 3 | 0.1 | 40 | 0 | 16 | – |
| Carrots | 48 | 10.6 | 0.9 | 0.2 | 80 | 1.3 | 3 | 1840 |
| Radish | 17 | 3.4 | 0.7 | 0.1 | 35 | 0.4 | 15 | 3 |
| Onion | 49 | 11 | 1.2 | 0.1 | 40 | 1.2 | 2 | 25 |

## Vegetables

- Classified as a "protective food".
- High vitamin and mineral content.
- Usually have a large water content, low energy and protein content and varying amount of dietary fibre.
- Some vegetables are good source of protein, e.g. green peas and beat.

## Vegetables are Divided into three Groups

1. Green leaves
2. Roots and tubers
3. Others

## Green Leefy

- Rich sources of carotene, calcium, iron and vitamin C.
- Fairly good sources of riboflavin, folic acid and many other micronutrients.
- Leaf proteins are good sources of lysine, although deficient in sulphur containing amino acid.
- Bioavailability of calcium and iron from green leaves is rather poor due to presence of high amount of oxalates and phylates.
- Because of their low caloric value and high bulk, they have an important place in diet of obese persons, who want to cut down their calorie intake.
- RDA of leafy vegetables is about 40 g for an adult.

## Roots and Tubers

- They are good source of carbohydrates such as potatoes.
- In general, roots and tubers are poor in proteins, vitamins and minerals.
- Vegetables like cluster beans, drumsticks and green mango contain fair amount of iron.
- Carrots contain high amount of beta carotene.
- RDA is about 50 to 60 g for adult.

### FRUITS

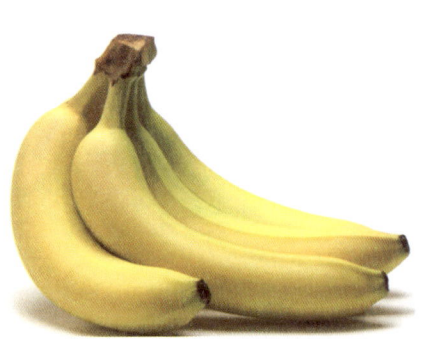

Banana

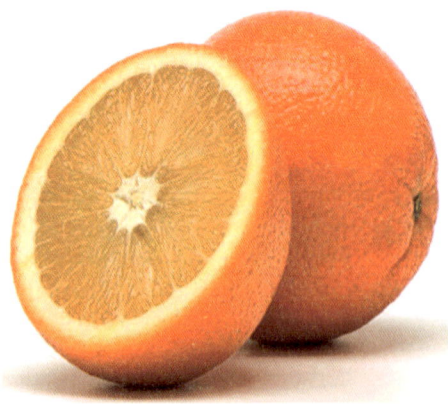

Orange

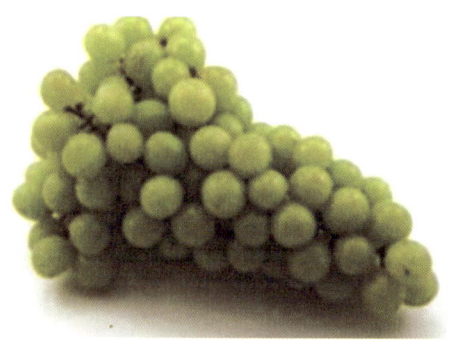

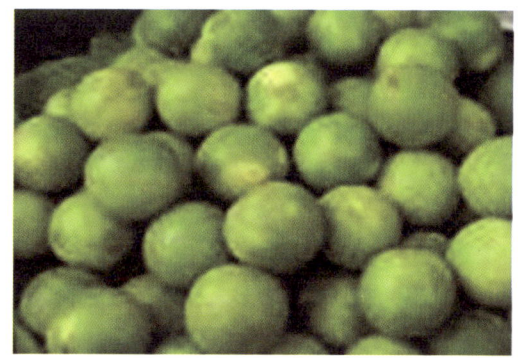

Grapes

Mausami

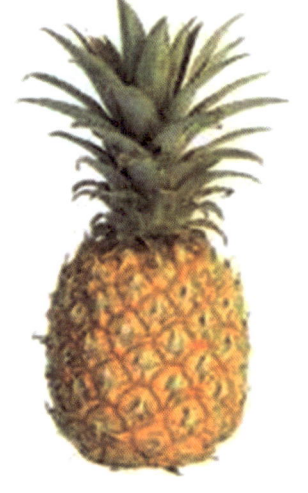

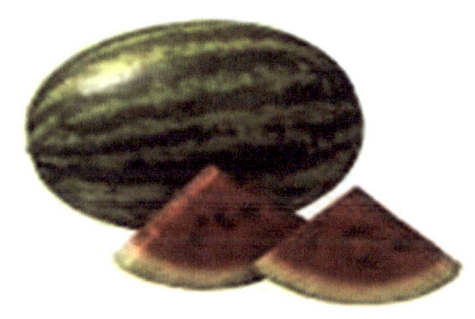

Pineapple

Watermellon

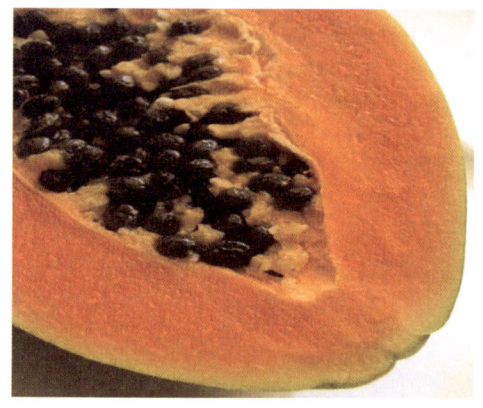

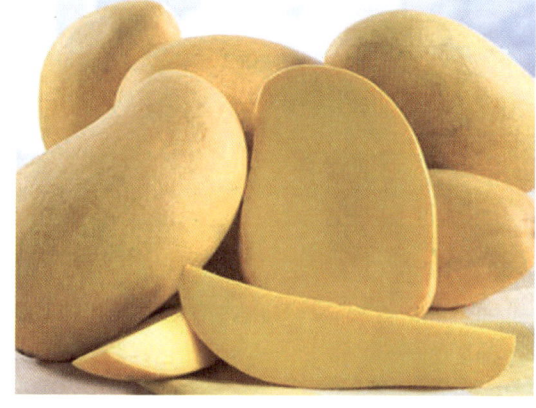

Papaya

Mango

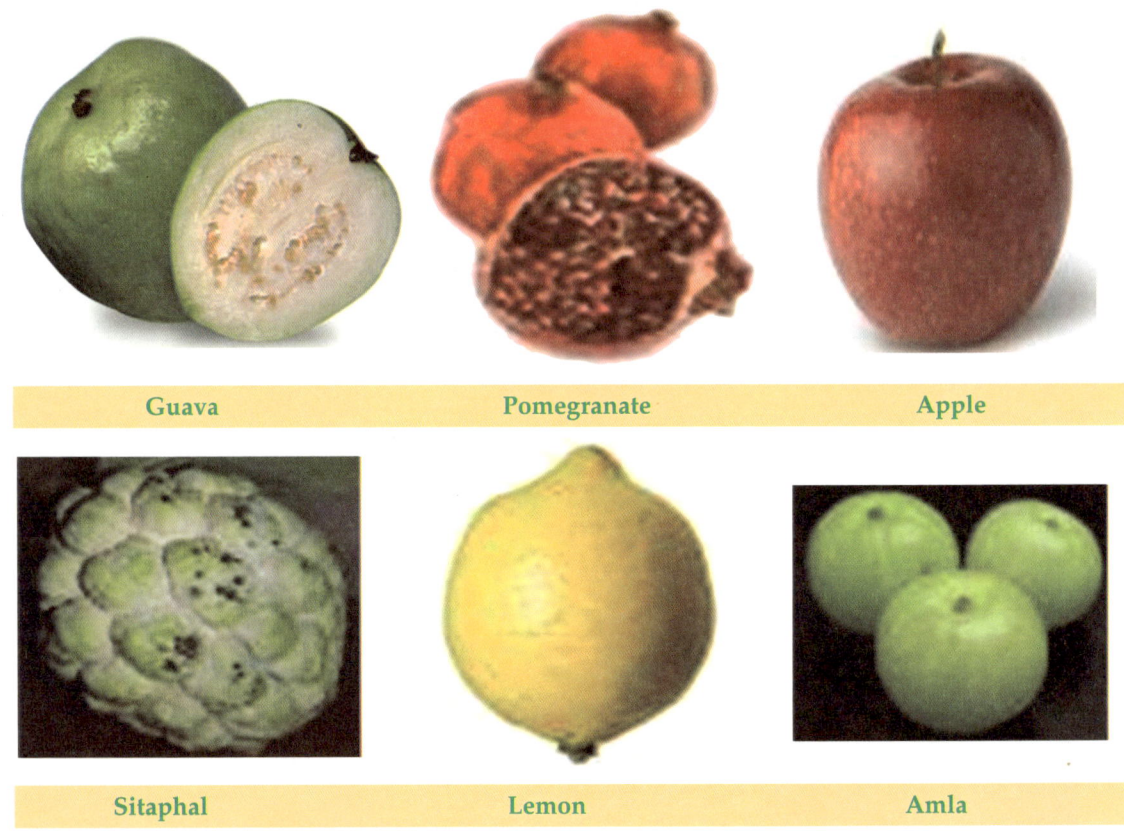

| Guava | Pomegranate | Apple |

| Sitaphal | Lemon | Amla |

## Nutrient value of fruits (per 100 g)

| Nutrient | Energy (kcal) | Carbo-hydrate (g) | Protein (g) | Fat (g) | Calcium (mg) | Fibre (g) | Iron (g) | Carotene (µg) | Vit. C (µg) |
|---|---|---|---|---|---|---|---|---|---|
| Banana | 116 | 27.2 | 1.2 | 0.3 | 10 | 0.4 | 0.36 | 124 | 7 |
| Orange | 40 | 8.9 | 0.6 | 0.2 | 20 | 0.3 | 0.5 | 2240 | 68 |
| Grapes | 71 | 18.1 | 0.72 | 0 | 20 | 0.4 | 0.36 | 0.45 | 10.8 |
| Mausami | 52 | 8 | 0.72 | 0 | 24 | 0.8 | 0.30 | 0.45 | 48.8 |
| Pineapple | 46 | 10.8 | 0.4 | 0.1 | 20 | 0.8 | 1.2 | 228 | 36.2 |
| Watermelon | 16 | 3.3 | 0.2 | 0.2 | 11 | 5.1 | 7.9 | 28 | 8.1 |
| Papaya | 32 | 7.2 | 0.6 | 0.1 | 17 | 0.8 | 0.5 | 2740 | 57 |
| Mango | 82 | 17.8 | 0.8 | 0.8 | 10 | 0.9 | 1.3 | 2210 | 16 |
| Guava | 51 | 11.2 | 0.9 | 0.3 | 10 | 5.20 | 0.27 | 527 | 212 |
| Pomegranate | 65 | 14.5 | 1.6 | 0.1 | 10 | 4.8 | 0.3 | 453 | 32 |
| Apple | 55 | 13.3 | 0.3 | 0.1 | 9 | 5.20 | 1 | 138 | 10 |
| Tamato | 20 | 3.6 | 0.9 | 0.2 | 0.8 | 4.7 | 0.64 | 26 | 51 |
| Sitaphal | 104 | 23.5 | 0 | 3.7 | 17 | 0.3 | – | 0 | 37 |
| Lemon | 57 | 11.1 | 1.0 | 0.9 | 70 | 0.4 | 2.3 | 0 | 53 |
| Amla | 58 | 14 | 0 | 0 | 50 | 0.8 | 1 | 9 | 600 |

**Fruits:** They are the edible envelope containing the seeds of plant or tree.

- They are classified as protective foods and are good sources of vitamins and minerals.
- Raw fruits contain varying proportion of starch.
- Process of ripening imparts a sweet taste and makes it readily absorbable.
- Flavour of fruit is due to presence of various organic acids.
- Most fruits contain significant amount of ascorbic acid, e.g. orange, guava, Indian gooseberry.
- Several fruits also contain good amount of carotene, e.g. papaya and mango.
- Fruits like sitaphal are rich in calcium.
- Intake of fruits leads to alkaline urine.
- In general low energy value.
- Some fruits like banana and mango contain good amount of carbohydrate.
- Pectin, present in fruits like guava is helpful in preparation of fruit jellies.
- Fruit sugars are easily digestible and completely absorbed.
- Cellulose: Contain cellulose which assists in normal bowel movement.

## NON-VEGETARIAN FOOD STUFFS

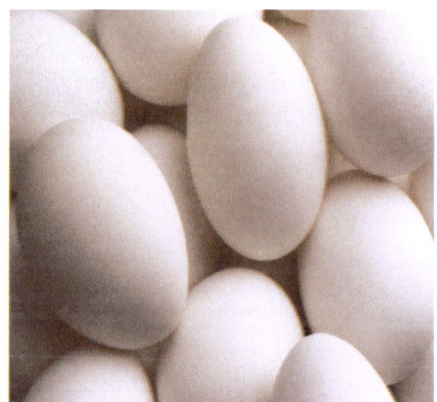

Eggs

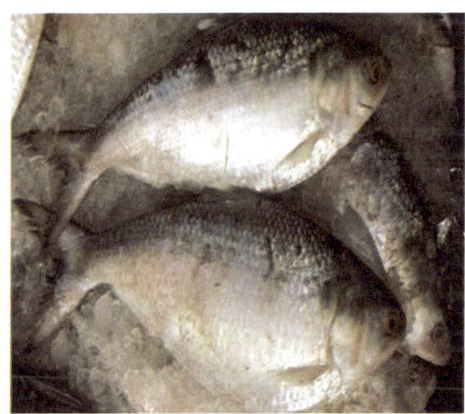

Fishes

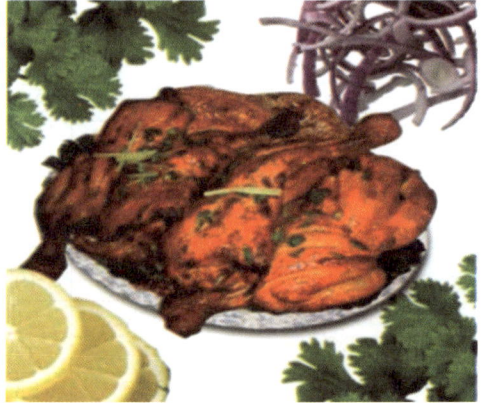

Chicken

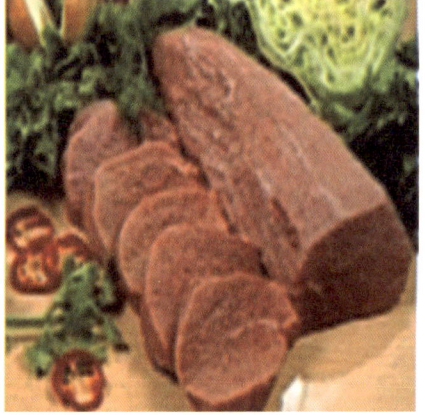

Meat pieces

**Nutrient value of non-vegetarian food stuffs (per 100 gm)**

| Nutrient | Carbohydrate (g) | Protein (g) | Fat (g) | Fibre (g) | Calcium (mg) | Iron | Energy (kcal) |
|----------|------------------|-------------|---------|-----------|--------------|------|---------------|
| Egg | – | 13.3 | 13.3 | – | 60 | 2.1 | 173 |
| Fishes | 1.8 | 17 | 1.3 | – | 200 | 0.9 | 87 |
| Chicken | – | 25.9 | 0.6 | – | 25 | – | 109 |
| Meat | – | 18.7 | 4.4 | – | 30 | 2.2 | 114 |

## Eggs

- Contain all nutrients except carbohydrate and vitamin C.
- About 12% of the egg is made of shell, 58% of egg white and 30% of egg yolk.
- An egg weighing 60 g contains 6 g of proteins, 6 g of fat, 30 mg of calcium and 1.5 mg of iron and supplies about 70 kcal of energy.
- Egg protein contains all nine essential amino acids (EAA) needed by the body in right proportions.
- Except for vitamin C, contains all fat-soluble and water-soluble vitamins in appreciable amounts.
- Also contains important minerals like calcium, phosphorus, iron, zinc and others.
- Boiling of egg destroys 'avidin', a substance which prevents the body from obtaining biotin (one of B complex). Boiled egg is, therefore, nutritionally superior to raw egg.
- NPU is same as its biological value, i.e. 100 for egg which is 80 for meat and 75 for milk.

## Fish

- Food rich in protein with good biological value and satisfactory amino acid balance.
- Fat of fish is rich in unsaturated fatty acid and vitamins A and D.
- Fish liver oil is the richest source of vitamins A and D.
- Fish bones when eaten are good source of calcium, phosphorus and fluoride.
- Lesser rich in iron than meat.
- Fresh water fishes do not contain iodine, but sea fishes do.

## Meat

- Term meat is applied to the flesh of cattle, sheep and goat.
- Contains 15–20 % of protein and is good source of (EAA).
- Contains varying amount of fat, which is composed of saturated fat.
- Poor in iron and calcium but rich in phosphorus.

# MILK AND MILK PRODUCTS

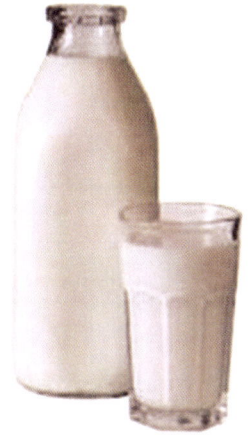
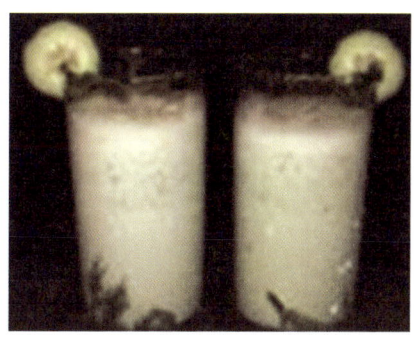
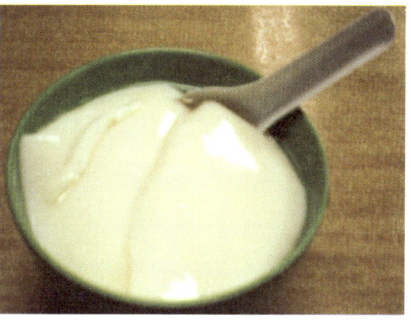

| Milk | Butter milk (Chhachh) | Curd |

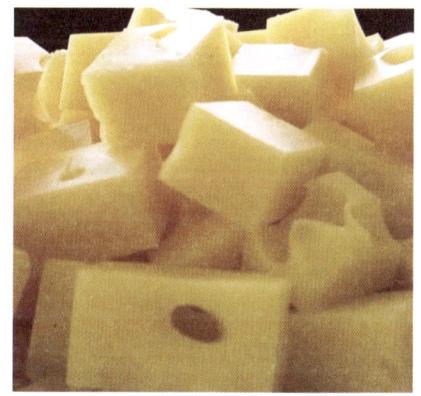
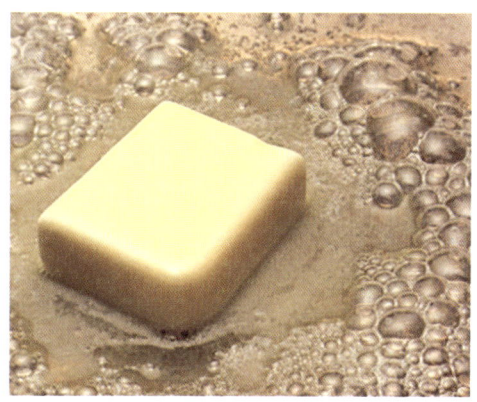

| Cheese | Butter |

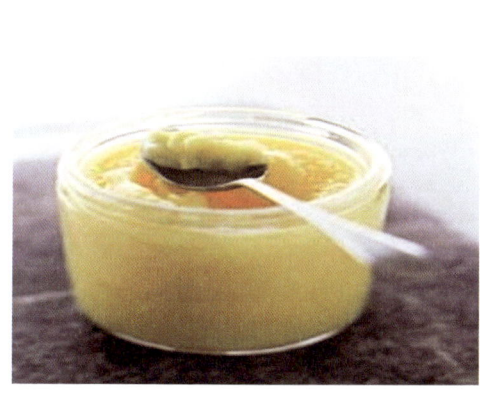
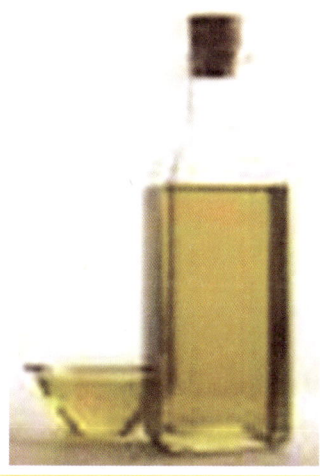

| Ghee | Oil |

**Nutrient value of milk and milk products (per 100 g)**

| Nutrient | Energy (kcal) | Carbohydrate (g) | Protein (g) | Fat (g) | Calcium | Iron (g) | Vit A (g) | Vit C (µg) | Water (mg) |
|---|---|---|---|---|---|---|---|---|---|
| Human milk | 65 | 7.4 | 1.1 | 3.4 | 28 | 0.1 | 50 | 3 | 88 |
| Cow's milk | 67 | 4.4 | 3.2 | 4.1 | 120 | 0.2 | 50 | 2 | 87 |
| Buffalo's milk | 117 | 5.1 | 4.3 | 8.8 | 210 | 0.2 | 50 | 1 | 81 |
| Goat's milk | 72 | 4.6 | 3.3 | 4.5 | 170 | 0.3 | 50 | 1 | 86.8 |
| Curd | 60 | 3 | 3.1 | 4 | 149 | 0.2 | 31 | 1 | 85 |
| Butter milk | 38 | 1.7 | 2.1 | 1 | 59 | 0.1 | 21 | 1 | 90 |
| Cheese | 348 | 6.3 | 25.1 | 25.1 | | 2.1 | | | 11 |
| Butter | 729 | – | – | 81 | – | – | 960 | – | – |
| Ghee | 900 | – | – | 100 | – | – | 600 | – | – |
| Oil | 900 | – | – | 100 | – | – | – | – | – |

**Milk:** It is secreted by the mammals to serve as a wholesome food for their suckling young ones.
- Complete food, i.e. good source of proteins, fats, sugars, vitamins and minerals.
- It is a fine blend of all the nutrients necessary for growth and development of young ones.

## Proteins
- Chief protein of milk is casein that is combined with calcium as calcium caseinogenate. Other proteins are lactalbumin and lactoglobulin.
- Animal milk contains three times more protein than human milk.
- Contains all the essential amino acids.
- Human milk protein contains greater amount of tryptophan and sulphur containing amino acids especially cysteine than the animal milk proteins.

## Fats
- Fat content of milk varies from 3.4% in human milk to 8.8 % in buffalo milk.
- Human milk contains high percentage of linoleic acid and oleic acid than animal milk.
- Milk fat is good source of retinol and vitamin D.

## Sugars
- Carbohydrate in all milk is lactose or milk sugar.
- It is less sweet than cane sugar and is readily fermented by lactic acid bacilli.
- It is found nowhere else in nature.
- Human milk contains more sugar than animal milk.

**Minerals:** Contain almost all minerals needed by the body, poor source of iron.

**Vitamins:** Good source of all vitamins except vitamin C.

**Milk products:** Consumed in a variety of forms — as whole milk, curd, butter, ghee, cheese, dried and condensed milk, khoa, ice-cream.

**Skimmed milk:** Milk from which fat has been removed is known as a skimmed milk.
- Devoid of fat and fat-soluble vitamins, but good source of protein and calcium.

**Toned milk:** It is a blend of natural milk and made up milk.
- It contains one part of water, one part of natural milk and 1/8 part of skimed milk powder.
- Mixture is stirred, pasteurized and supplied in bottles.
- Composition nearly equivalent to cow's milk.
- Cheaper and yet a wholesome product.

### Fermentation of Milk (Making Curd)
- Starting point for products like curd, buttermilk and ghee.
- 40 % of the lactose in milk is changed into lactic acid by lactobacilli.

### Advantages
- Fermented products are better tolerated by some people than unfermented milk, which produces flatulence.
- More nutritious than fresh milk with higher riboflavin and thiamine content.
- Reported to partially inhibit the growth of *B. dysenteriae* and *V. cholerae* .

## NUTS

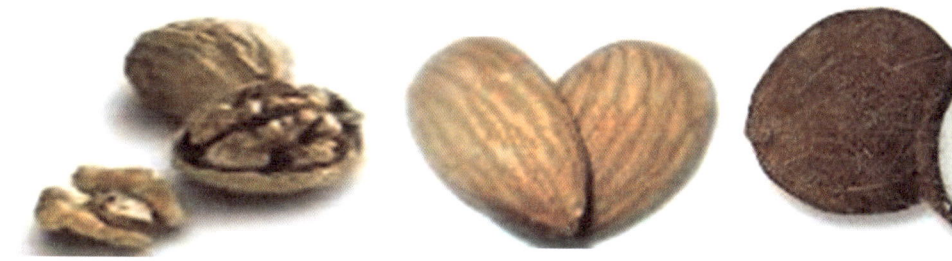

| Walnut (Akhrot) | Almond (Badam) | Coconut |

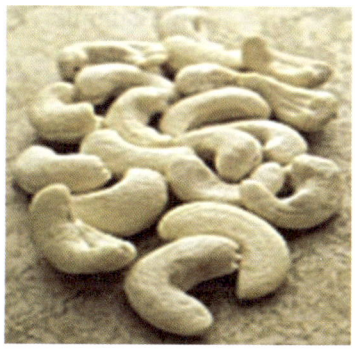 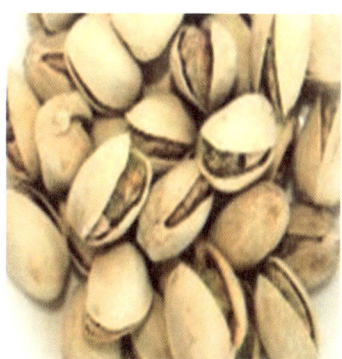 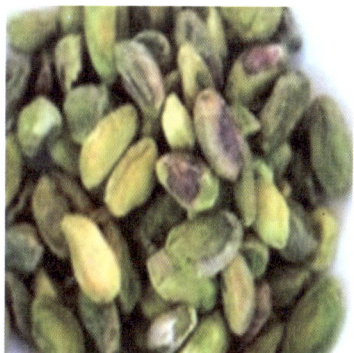

Cashew nut (Kaju)       Pistachio (Pista)

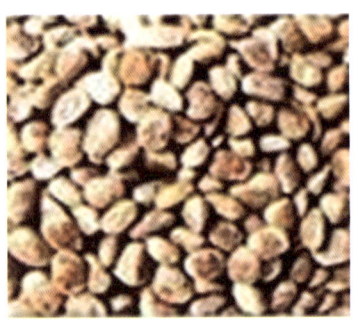
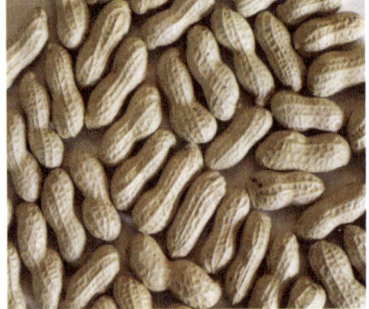
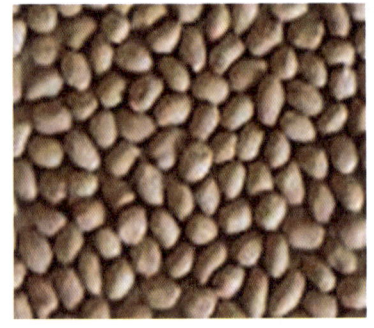

**Cudpohunut (Chirongi)**          **Groundnut (Mungphali)**

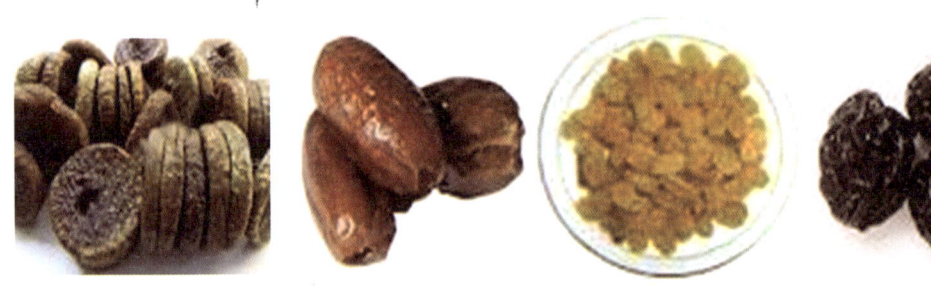

**Fig (Anjeer)**          **Dates**          **Raisins (Kishmish)**          **(Dakh)**

## Nutrient value of nuts and oil  (per 100 g)

| Nutrient | Energy (kcal) | Carbohydrate (g) | Protein (g) | Fat (g) | Calcium (mg) | Iron (mg) | Phosphorus (mg) |
|---|---|---|---|---|---|---|---|
| Walnut | 687 | 11 | 15.6 | 64.5 | 100 | 4.8 | 380 |
| Almond | 655 | 10 | 21 | 59 | 230 | 5 | 489 |
| Coconut | 662 | 18 | 7 | 62 | 400 | 8 | 340 |
| Cashew nut | 596 | 22 | 21 | 47 | 50 | 6 | 450 |
| Pistachio | 626 | 16.2 | 20 | 53.5 | 140 | 8 | 430 |
| Cudpohunut | 636 | 21 | 19.8 | 51 | 125 | 8 | 435 |
| Ground nut | 567 | 26.1 | 25.3 | 40.1 | 90 | 2.5 | 350 |
| Anjeer | 676 | 31.3 | – | 23 | 75 | 24 | 465 |
| Dates | 317 | 20.4 | 15.2 | 15.6 | 120 | 6 | 342 |
| Raisins | 308 | 67.8 | – | 18 | 87 | 52 | 651 |
| Oil | 900 | – | – | 100 | – | – | – |

Dry fruits like raisins, dates and apricots are good source of calcium and iron.

## SWEETNERS

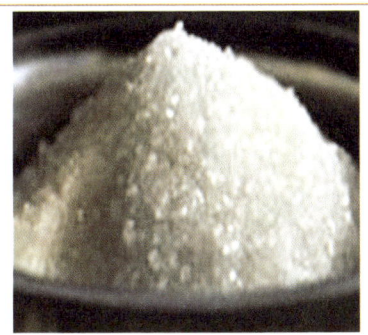 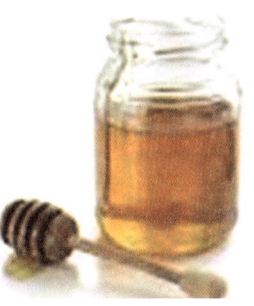 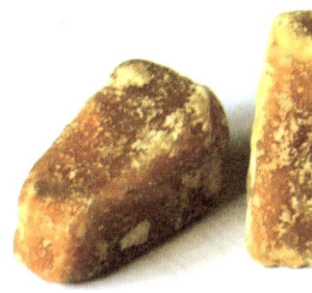 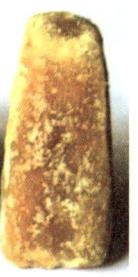

| Sugar | Honey | Jaggery |

### Nutrient value of sugar and jaggery (per 100 g)

| Nutrient | Carbohydrate (g) | Protein (g) | Fat (g) | Calcium (mg) | Iron (µg) | Vit A (µg) | Vit B (µg) | Vit C (µg) | Energy (kcal) |
|---|---|---|---|---|---|---|---|---|---|
| Sugar | 99.4 | 0.1 | 0 | 12 | 0 | – | 0 | – | 400 |
| Honey | 79.5 | 0.3 | 0 | 5 | 0.9 | – | 0.24 | 4 | 319 |
| Jaggery | 95 | 0.4 | 0.1 | 80 | 11.4 | 168 | 0.56 | – | 383 |

## MISCELLANEOUS FOODS

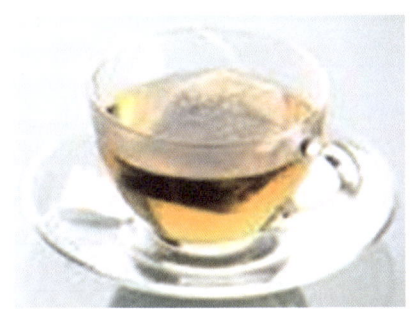 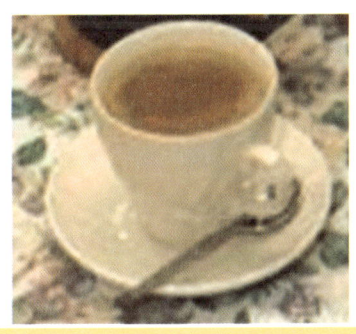 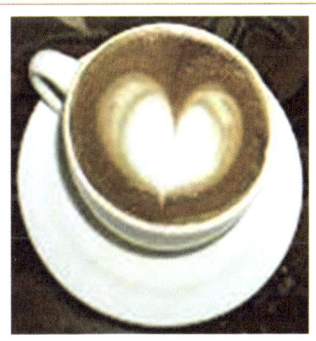

| Green tea | Tea | Coffee |

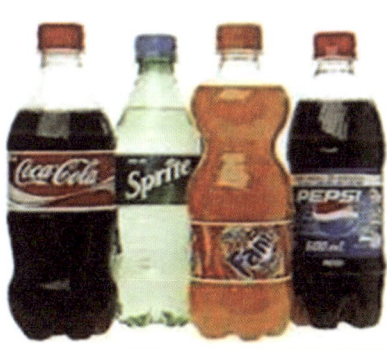

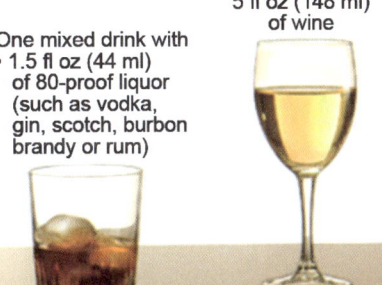

One mixed drink with
• 1.5 fl oz (44 ml) of 80-proof liquor (such as vodka, gin, scotch, burbon brandy or rum)

5 fl oz (148 ml) of wine

12 fl oz (355 ml) of beer or wine cooler

**Soft drinks**          **Hard drinks**

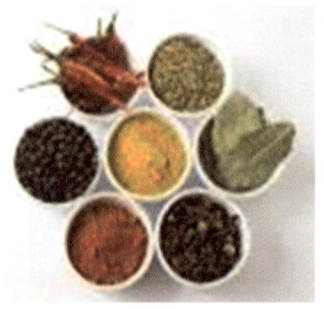
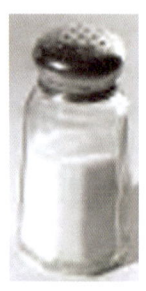
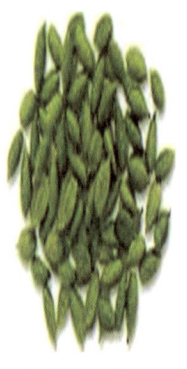
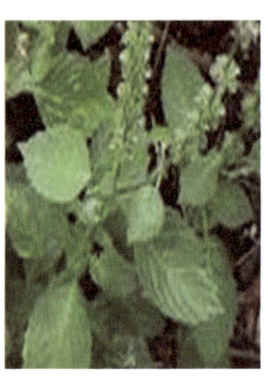

| Spices | Salt | Cardamom | Tulsi leaves |

## Nutrient value of miscellaneous food items (per 100 g/100 ml)

| Nutrient | Carbohydrate (g) | Protein (g) | Fat (g) | Calcium (mg) | Iron (mg) | Vit A (µg) | Vit B (µg) | Vit C (µg) | Energy (kcal) |
|---|---|---|---|---|---|---|---|---|---|
| *Tea | 19 | 0.3 | 0.2 | 0.6 | 0 | 24 | 0 | 0 | 70 |
| G. Tea | 0.2 | 3 | 0.2 | 6 | 0 | 1 | 0 | 0 | 14 |
| *Coffee | 0.2 | 0 | 0 | 0 | 0 | 0 | 0 | 0 | 13 |
| Cold drink (soft) | 28 | 0 | – | 28 | – | – | – | –, | 100 |
| Cold drink (hard) | – | – | – | – | – | – | – | – | 90 |
| Spices | 40.6 | 9.8 | 6.6 | 410.3 | 14.5 | 241.2 | 1.98 | 15.13 | 261 |

*Nutrient value is with milk and sugar otherwise nutrient value is zero but they contain antioxidants.

Tea and coffee are also having caffeine in 0.02 mg and 0.06 mg respectively and tannin in 0.07 mg and 0.25 mg respectively.

## FOOD STUFFS FOR FOOD ADULTERATION

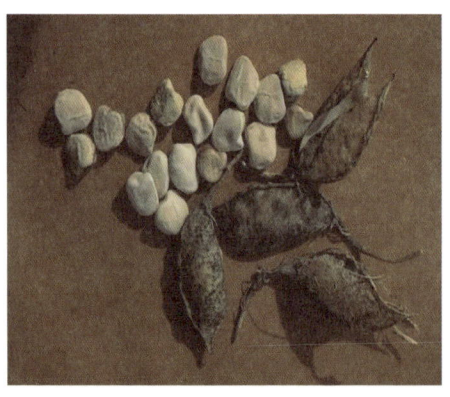
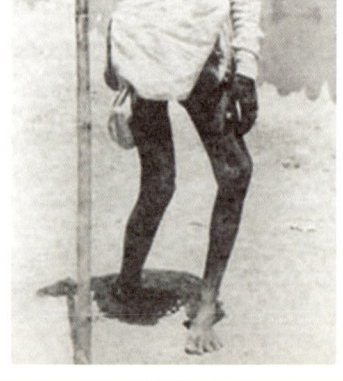

| *Lathyrus sativus* | Patient of lathyrism |

### *Lathyrus Sativus*

- It contains toxin water-soluble beta oxalyl amino alanine (BOAA), so toxin from seed is removed by soaking it in hot water and discarding that water.
- BOAA toxin cannot cross BBB, but if taken in large amount and/or for more than 2 months, it will cross the BBB.

**Disease: Lathyrism:** Age: Young men 15 to 45 years

**1. Latent stage:** No symptoms

**2. No-stick stage:** Patient walks with short jerky steps without the aid of sticks.

**3. One-stick stage:** Muscular stiffness makes it necessary to use a stick.

**4. Two-stick stage:** Due to excessive bending of knees and crossed legs, patient needs two sticks for support.

**5. Crawler stage:** There is atrophy of thigh and leg muscles. Patient is reduced to crawling by throwing his weight on his hands.

### Intervention

1. Vitamin C prophylaxis: 500 – 1000 mg daily.
2. Banning the crop
3. Removal of toxin:
   i. Steeping method: Soaking pulse in hot water for 2 hours than wash it and than dry it in the sun.
   ii. Parboiling: Improved method of detoxicating the pulse. Suitable for large scale. Soaking the pulse over night in lime water followed by boiling to destroy toxin.
4. Educating the poor community to avoid using *Lathyrus sativus* as the sole staple diet and to use it only in small quantities, if at all, in a mixture with cereals and millets.

### AFLATOXIN FUNGUS INFESTATION IN GROUNDNUT

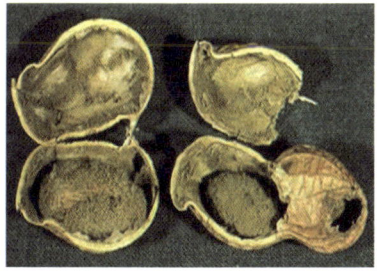 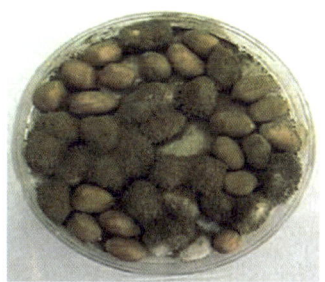

### Aflatoxin fungus infestation in maize

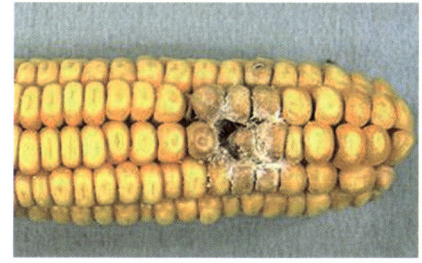 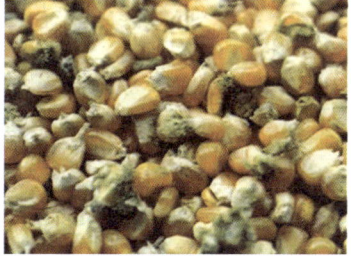

- Aflatoxins are group of mycotoxins produced by fungi, *Aspergillus flavus* and *A. parasiticus*.
- Toxin forms in proper conditions of moisture level above 16%, temperature 37°C.
- This fungus infests the food grains like groundnut, maize, parboiled rice, sorghum, wheat, cotton seed, tapioca under improper storage condition and produces aflatoxins of which $B_1$ and $G_1$ are potent hepatotoxins ($B_1$) and carcinogenic as it damages DNA.

### Prevention

- Prevention of fungal contamination of foodgrains.
- Proper storage after drying.
- Moisture content kept below 10%.
- If food gets contaminated, it must not be consumed.
- Health education
- Adoption of scientific post-harvest technology, storage and packing.

### ARGEMONE MEXICANA

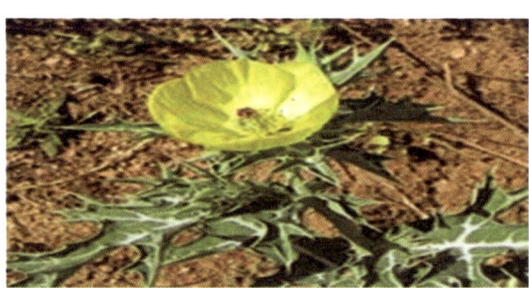

Argemone oil is orange in colour with an acid odour.

### Epidemic Dropsy

- It occurs due to contamination of mustard oil with argemone oil.
- Argemone oil contains toxic alkaloid, sanguinarine and dihydrosanguinarine, which may be responsible for DNA modifications that have carcinogenic effects.
- Other minor alkaloids present are berberine propionate, chelitrythrine and coptisine which are less toxic, which interfere with the oxidation of pyruvic acid which accumulates in blood.
- Target organs are liver, heart, kidney and lungs.

### Symptoms

- Symptoms appear within 5–20 days.
- Sudden, non-inflammatory, bilateral swelling of legs, often associated with diarrhoea, vomiting.
- Cardiovascular symptoms include dyspnoea, tachycardia, and pericardial pain.
- Skin manifestations include erythematous mottling and raised heamangioma on the skin and mucus membrane.
- Ocular manifestation include itching and burning of eyes with superficial retinal haemorrhage, disc oedema and glaucoma in some cases.
- Death occurs in 5–50 % cases due to cardiac failure.

## Detection of Argemone Oil

1. The permissible level of argemone oil in edible oil is 0.01%.
2. Nitric acid test: It is a non-specific test, detects 0.25% of argemone oil (add NA in oil →
   shake orange red color = presence of Argemone oil.)
3. Paper chromatography test: Most sensitive test. It can detect argemone oil up to 0.0001%
   concentration.
   Other tests include ferric chloride test (0.25%), cupric acid test (0.5%), and hydrochloric acid
   test which is specific test can detect up to 0.001% argemone oil in edible oil.

## Prevention

- Accidental contamination prevention by removing the argemone weeds growing among oil
  seed crops.
- We can destroy the seedlings by pulling them out of the soil during the rainy season and
  repeat the operations several times during monsoon and not allowing the plant to grow and
  shed the seeds.
- Unscrupulous dealers may be dealt with by the strict enforcement of the Prevention of Food
  Adulteration Act.
- Education of community regarding early sign of disease.

## Entomology

Question 1:    Identify the spot with reason?

Question 2:    What is the public health importance of given spot?

Question 3:    Enumerate the diseases transmitted by this arthropod?

Question 4:    What are the breeding places of this insect?

Question 5:    Describe the control measures?

Teacher's Remark ...........................................

Teacher's Sign ...........................................

## Arthropod borne diseases of health importance

| Arthropods | Disease | Vector | Causal organism | Reservoir |
|---|---|---|---|---|
| Mosquito | **Malaria** | *Anopheles* species | *Plasmodium* species | Man |
| | **Filariasis** | *Culex quinquefasciatus* | *W. bancrofti* | Man |
| | | *Mansonoides* species | *W. bancrofti* | Man |
| | | *Aedes* species | *Brugia malayi* | Man |
| | **Dengue** | *Aedes* species | Arbovirus group B | Man |
| | **Chikungunya** | *Aedes* species | Arbovirus group A | Man |
| | **Japanese encephalitis** | *Culex vishnui* group | Arbovirus group B | Mammals/birds |
| | **Yellow fever** | *Aedes* species | Arbovirus group B | Man/monkeys |
| Sandfly | **Sandfly fever** | *P. sergenti, P. papatasi* | Virus | Man |
| | **Leishmaniasis (Kala azar)** | *Phlebotomus argentipes* | *Leishmania donovani* | Man/mammals |
| | **Oriental sore** | *P. papatasi* | *L. tropica* | Man/mammals |
| Fly | **Gastroenteritis** | *M. domestica* | Specific/Non-specific organisms | Man/animal |
| | **Bacillary dysentery** | *M. domestica* | *Shigella* | Man |
| | **Amoebic dysentery** | *M. domestica* | *E. histolytica* | Man |
| | **Cholera** | *M. domestica* | *Vibrio cholerae* | Man |
| | **Typhoid** | *M. domestica* | *Salmonella typhi* | Man |
| | **Paratyphoid** | *M. domestica* | Paratyphoid A and B | Man |
| | **Viral hepatitis (A)** | *M. domestica* | HAV | Man |
| | **Poliomyelitis** | *M. domestica* | Virus | Man |
| | **Trachoma** | *M. domestica* | *C. trachomatis* | Man |
| | **Yaws** | *M. domestica* | *T. pertenue* | Man |
| Flea | **Plague (bubonic)** | *Xenopsylla* species | *Yersinia pestis* | Rodents |
| | **Endemic** | *Xenopsylla* species | *R. typhi* | Rodents |
| | **Murine typhus** | | | Domestic animal |
| | **Chiggerosis (Jigger)** | *Tunga penetrans* (chigoe) | – | – |
| | ***Dipylidium caninum*** | Ctenocephalides felis/canis | *Dipylidium caninum* | Dogs, cats, wild carnivores |
| | ***H. nana*** | X cheopis/C canis/ Pulex irritans | *H. nana* | Rats, mice |
| Louse | **Epidemic typhus** | Pediculus humanus | *R. prowazeki* | Man |
| | **Epidemic relapsing fever** | Pediculus humanus | *Borrelia recurrentis* | Man |
| | **Trench fever** | Pediculus humanus | *Bartonella quintana* | Man/animals |
| | **Dermatitis** | Pediculus humanus/ capitis | Secondary infection | Man |

*Contd.*

Arthropod borne diseases of health importance (*Contd.*)

| Arthropods | Disease | Vector | Causal organism | Reservoir |
|---|---|---|---|---|
| Tick | Kyasanur forest disease (KFD) | Hard ticks species | Arbovirus group B | Monkeys/birds |
| | Tick typhus | Hard ticks species | *R. conorii* | Dogs |
| | Tularaemia | Hard ticks species | *P. tularensis* | Rabbits/ rodents/cattle |
| | Relapsing fever | Soft tick | *B. duttoni* | Rats |
| Mite | Scabies | Sanguineus L. | *S. scabei* | Man |
| | Scrub typhus | *L. deliense* | *Orientia tsutsugamushi* | Rodents |
| | Rickettsial pox | Allodermanyssus | *R. akari* | Rodents |
| Cyclops | Dracontiasis | *Cyclops* species | *D. medinensis* | Man |
| | Fish tape worm | *Cyclops* species | *D. latum* | Fish |
| Reduviid bugs | Chagas disease | Reduviid | *T. cruzi* | Domestic animals/man |
| Tsetse flies | Trypanosomiasis | *Glossina* species | *T. gambiense* and *T. rhodesiense* | Wild animals/ cattle/man |

## BREEDING PLACES OF MOSQUITOES

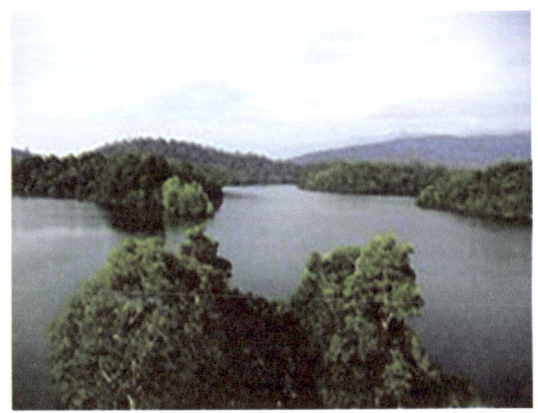

**Open field clear water river (Breeding places for *Anopheles*)**

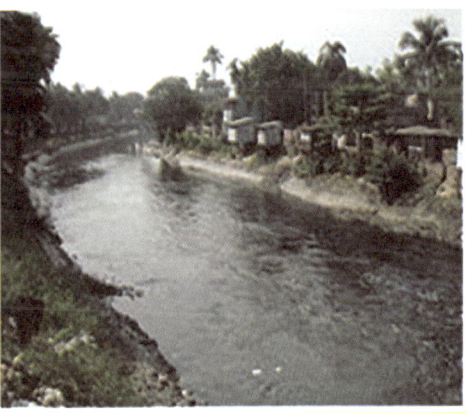

**Open field dirty water (NALA) (Breeding places for *Culex*)**

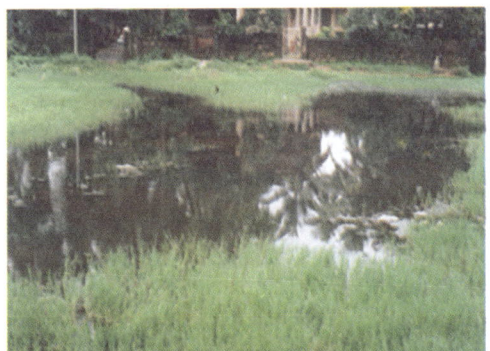

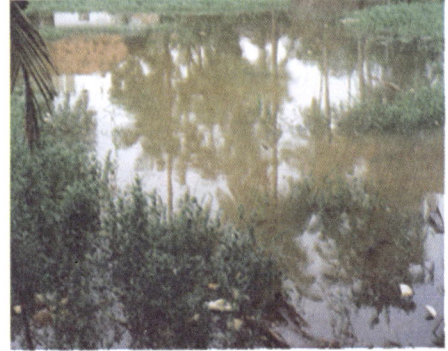

**Open field water collection with aquatic plants (Breeding places for *Mansonia*)**

## ARTIFICIAL COLLECTION OF WATER: BREEDING PLACES FOR AEDES MOSQUITOES

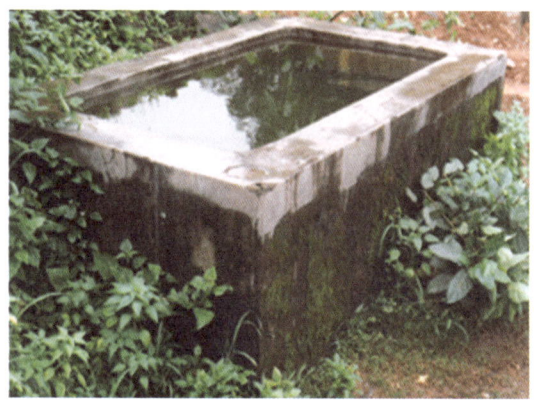

Unused well

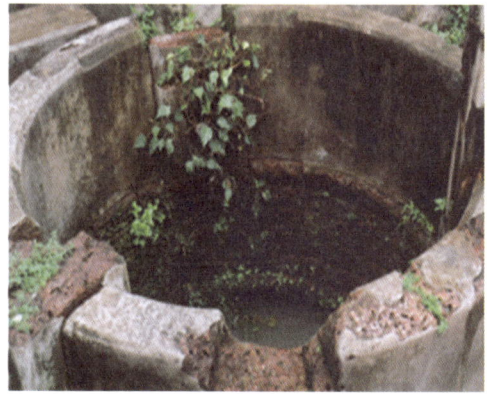

Open tank

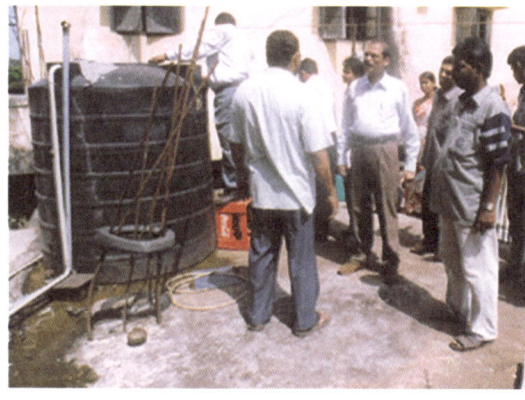

House-hold open tank

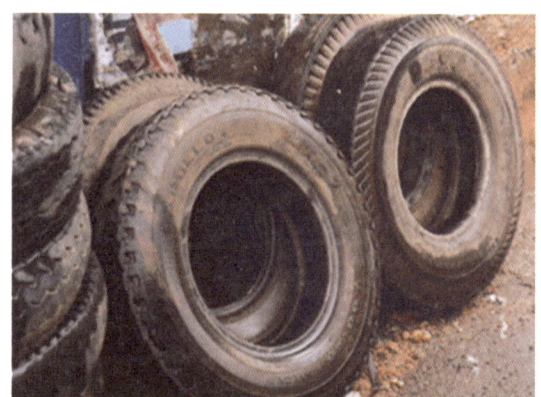

Tyres in open

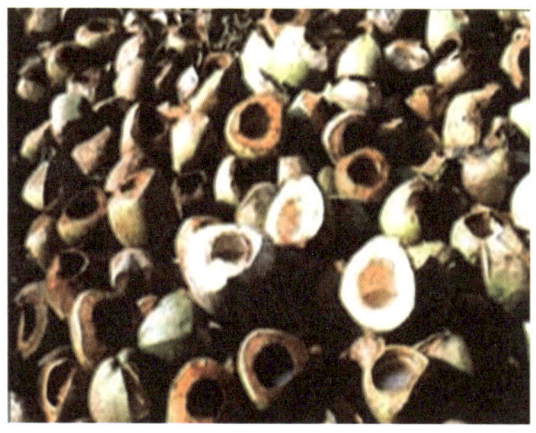

Coconut-shells in open

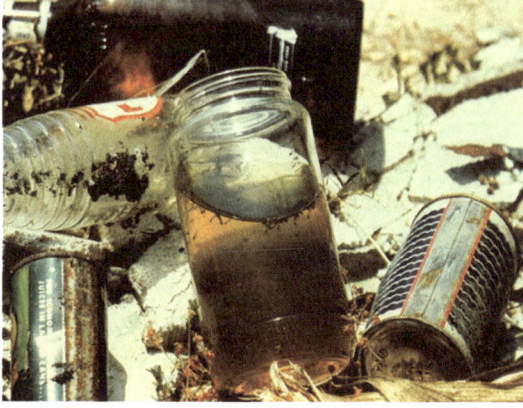

Water collection in open containers

# LIFE CYCLE OF ANOPHELES MOSQUITOES

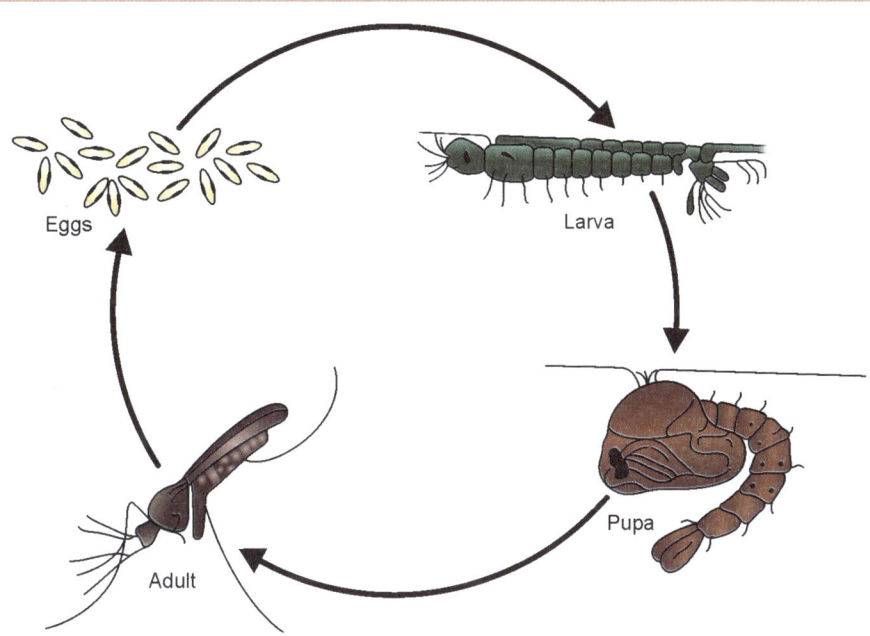

Eggs

Larva

Pupa

Adult

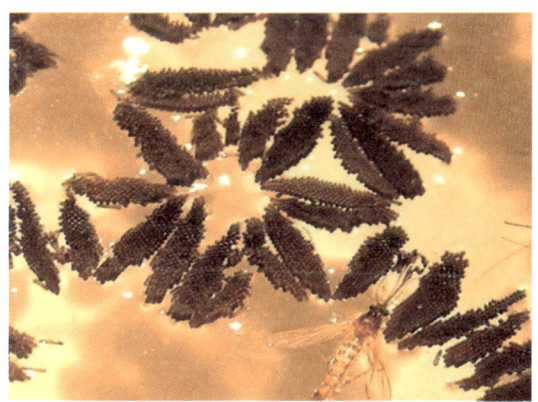

**Eggs**

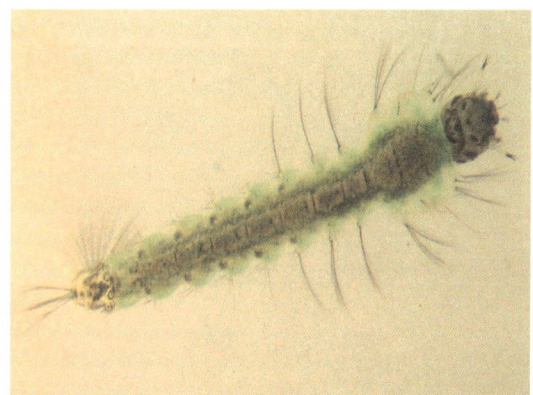

**Larva**

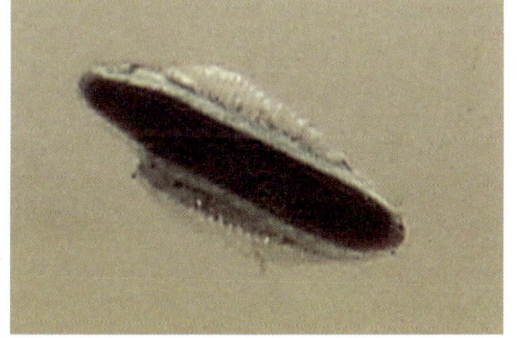

**Single egg**

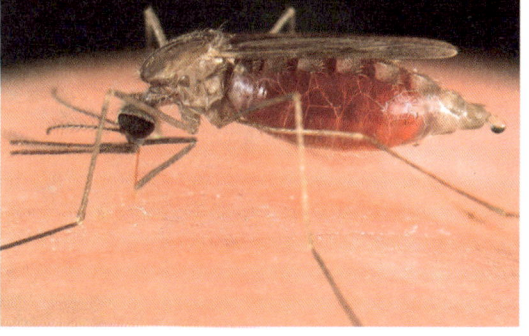

**Adult**

# CULEX

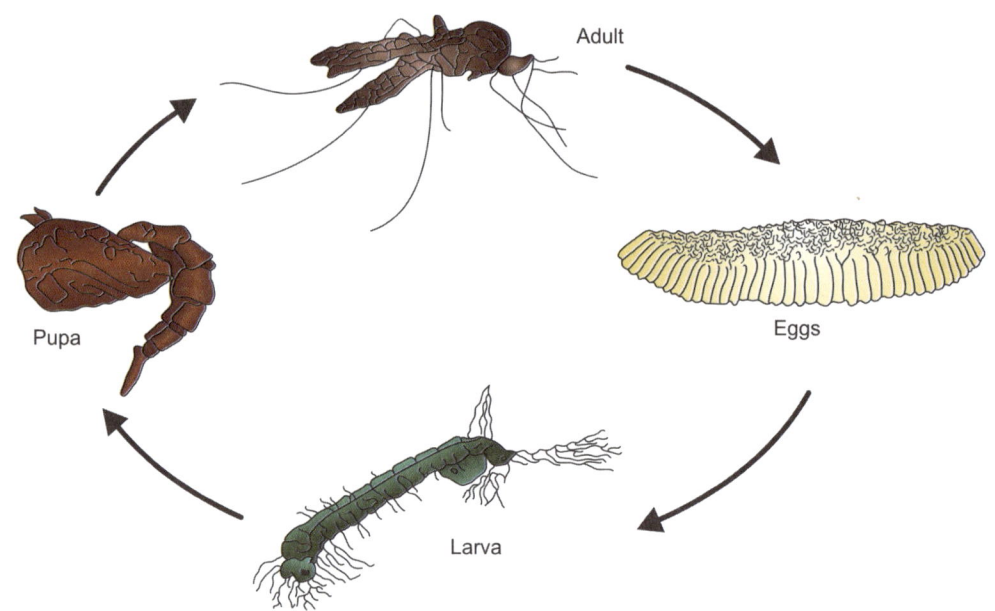

Adult

Pupa

Eggs

Larva

**Life cycle of culex**

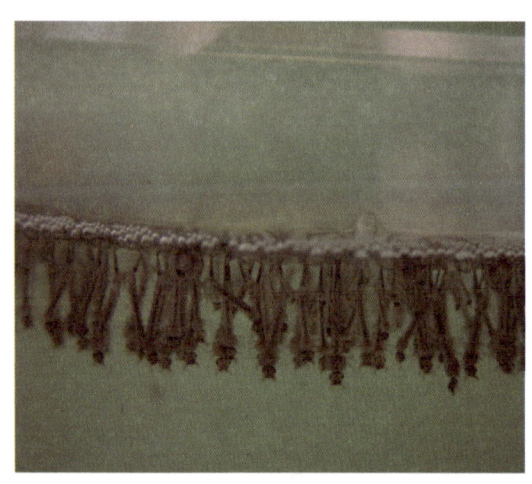

**Pupa**

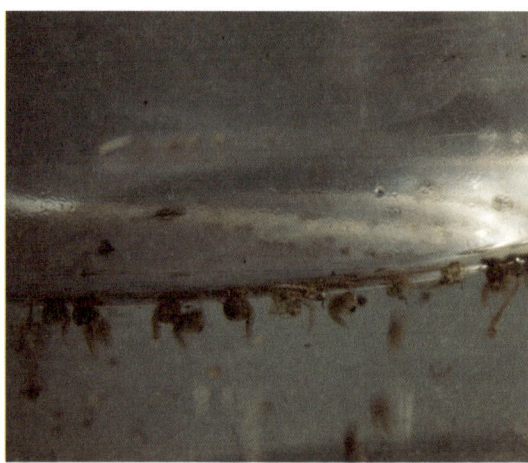

**Larvae**

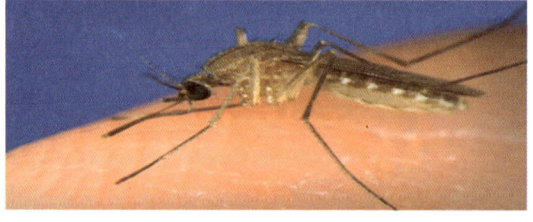

**Adult**

# LIFE CYCLE OF AEDES

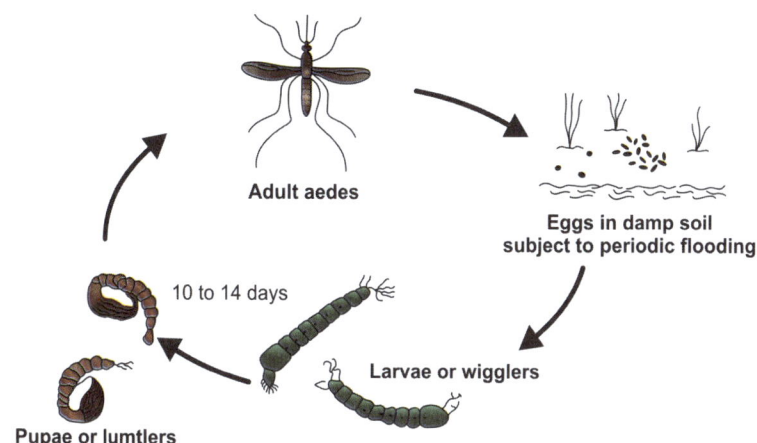

Adult aedes

Eggs in damp soil subject to periodic flooding

10 to 14 days

Larvae or wigglers

Pupae or lumtlers

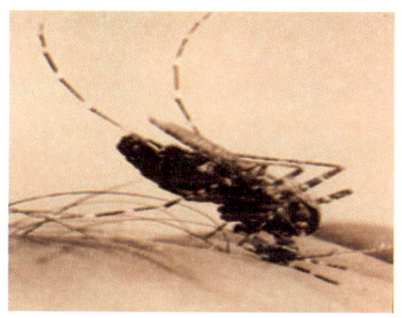

**Mansoni mosquito**

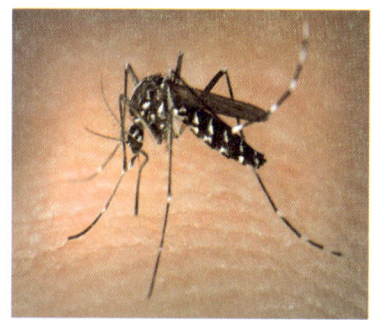

**Aedes mosquito**

| | Anopheles | Aedes | Culex |
|---|---|---|---|
| Eggs | | | |
| Larvae | | | |
| Pupae | | | |
| Adults | | | |

**Difference between Anopheles, Aedes and Culex mosquito**

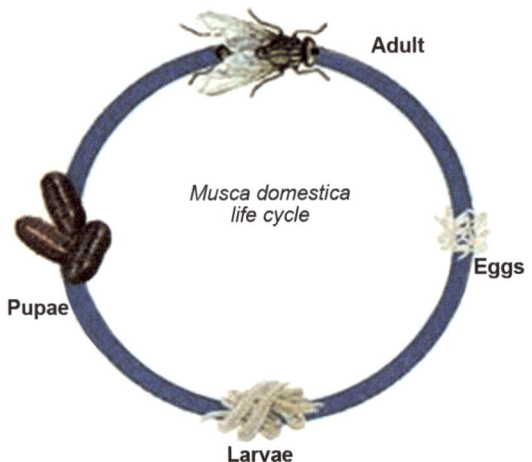

**Life cycle of house fly**

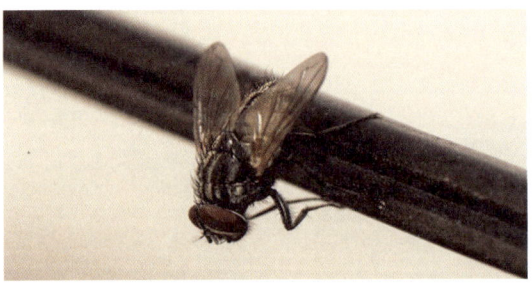

**Adult house fly**

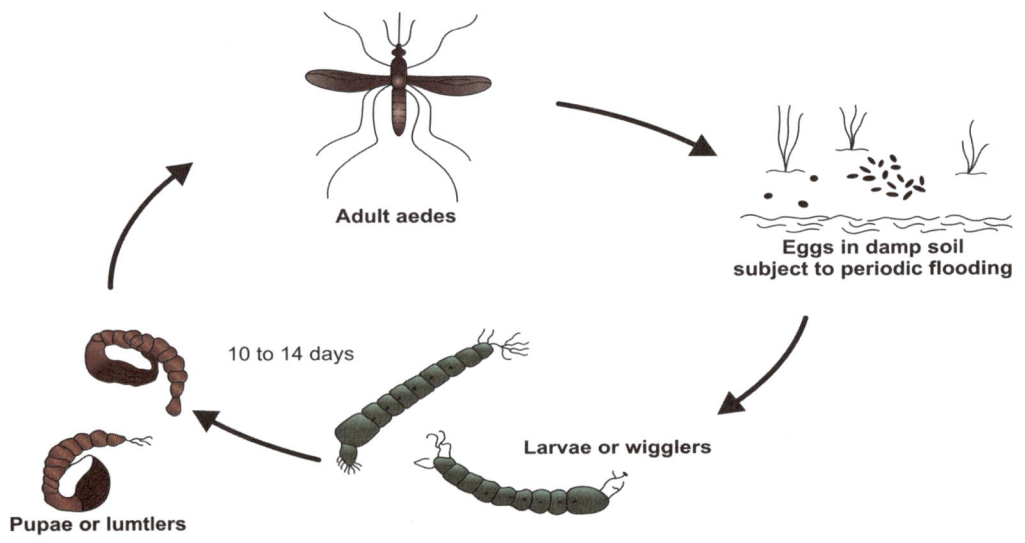

**Life cycle of sand fly**

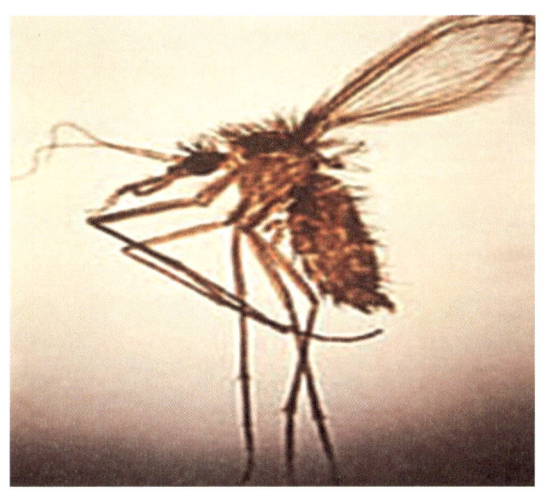

Sand fly

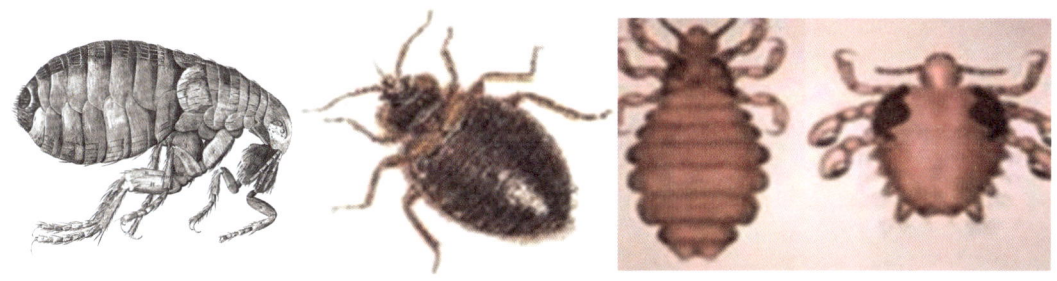

Rat flea          Bed bug          Head louse   Pubic louse

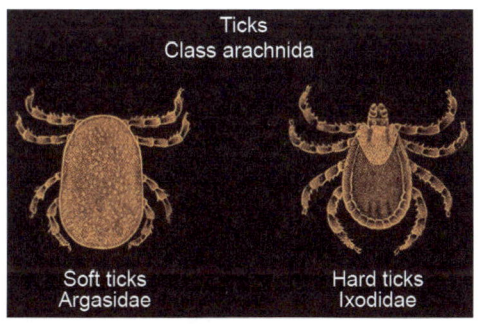

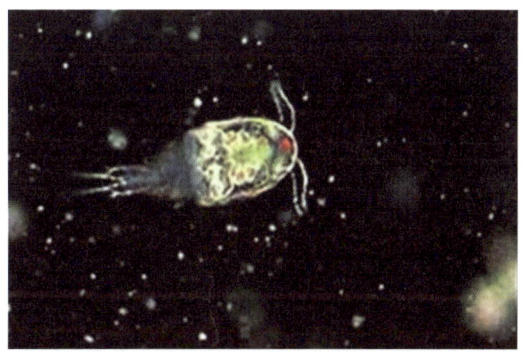

Cyclops

## Vectors

| Name of vector | Identification | Diseases transmitted | Control |
|---|---|---|---|
| **Class Insecta** | | | |
| **Anopheles** | • Proboscis and palpi are equal in length<br>• Wings are spotted<br><br>• No hairy antennae<br><br>• Busy antennae in males | **Malaria**<br>(*Plasmodium* species) | • Environmental—source reduction<br>• Chemical—insecticide spray<br>• Genetic—gene distortion<br>• Personal protection—*Mosquito net, coils, liquid, repellent creams and spray |
| **Culex** | • Palpi are smaller than proboscis<br>• Proboscis makes an acute angle with body<br>• Wings are unspotted | • Filariasis—*W. bancrofti*<br>• Japanese encephalitis<br>• Viral arthritis | • Environmental—source reduction<br>• Chemical—insecticide spray<br>• Genetic—gene distortion<br>• Personal protection—*Mosquito net, coils, liquid, repellent creams and spray |
| **Aedes** | • Palpi are smaller than proboscis<br>• Wings with white stripes on black body (Tiger mosquitoes)<br>• Broad imprecated scales | • Dengue and dengue haemorrhagic fever<br>• Chikungunya<br>• Yellow fever | • Environmental—removal of artificial water collecting receptacles<br><br>• Chemical—insecticide spray<br>• Genetic—gene distortion<br>• Personal protection—*Mosquito net, coils and repellents |
| **House fly** | • Body is covered with sticky hair (tenet hair) Large compound eyes Retractile proboscis<br>• Dark longitudinal stripes on thorax<br>• Dark and light marking on abdomen | By mechanical transmission<br>• Typhoid<br>• Cholera<br>• Gastroenteritis<br>• Amoebiasis<br>• Polio<br>• Anthrax | • Environmental sanitation and personal hygiene<br>• Hygienic disposal of refuse and human and animal excreta<br>• Screening mesh—14 holes per square inch |

*Contd.*

**Vectors** (*Contd.*)

| Name of vector | Identification | Diseases transmitted | Control |
|---|---|---|---|
| **House fly** Contd. | • Leg has a pair of pads | • Trachoma <br> • Yaws <br> • Maggots cause meioses | • Insecticides: DDT—5% <br> • Methoxychlor—5% <br> • Lindane—0.5% <br> • Larvicides: Diazinon—2% <br> • Dichlorovos—2% <br> • Dimethoate—1% <br> • 25 to 50 liter/square metre in breeding places <br> • Fly traps fly baits, ribbons and fly paper |
| **Rat flea** | • Bilaterally compressed wingless body <br> • Conical head <br> • No neck <br> • Exoskeleton with bristles <br> • Three pairs of spiny strong limbs <br> • Foot end (claws) | Bubonic plague (bite of blocked flea) <br> Endemic <br> Typhus (murine) (contamination of skin with faeces of fleas) <br> Chiggarosis | Insecticide: DDT 10% (dust where rodent moves and burrows) 5% indoor spray Dichrovos resin strip Insufflations (disinfection) of ship, aircraftsae. Rat destruction Poisonous bait, trapping, emitting hydrocyanic acid gas, rat proofing <br> Personal protection: Repellents— diethyltoluamide, benzyl benzoate |
| **Head louse** | • Having head, thorax and abdomen <br><br><br> • Body is flattened dorsoventrally <br><br> • No wings <br> • Three pairs of legs | • Epidemic typhus: *Rickettsia prowazekii* (Contact of lice faeces through abrasion or unbroken skin) <br> • Relapsing fever: *Borrelia recurrentis* (crushed fluid) <br> • Trench fever: *Rickettsia quintana* (louse faeces) | • Insecticide: DDT 1–2 gm, indane 0.25 mg <br> • Dichrovos <br> • Personal hygiene |
| **Sand fly** | • Smaller than mosquito <br><br> • Antennae long and filamented <br> • Lanceolate wings <br> • Second vein of the wing divides twice <br> • Very long 3 pairs legs | • Kala azar through bite (*L. donovani*) <br> • Sand fly fever through wound contamination with virus in saliva) <br> • Oriental sore through bite (*Leishmania tropica*) | • Source reduction: Clearing, filling of cracks and crevices <br> • Keeping cattle and poultry outside the house <br> • Not walking in bare foot |

*Contd.*

**Vectors** *(Contd.)*

| Name of vector | Identification | Diseases transmitted | Control |
|---|---|---|---|
| | • Pair of large compound eyes | | • Insecticide: DDT 1–2 gm, indane 0.25 mg (spraying is done in all breeding places)<br>• Personal protection: Sand fly net (45 mesh/inch) impregnated with pyrethrin |
| **Class Arrachnida** | | | |
| **Itch mite** | • Tortoise (oval) shaped<br>• Four short stumpy legs<br>• No wings<br>• No demarcation of body segments<br>• Body is wrinkled covered with bristles | **Scabies** (Sarcoptes scabiei) | • Using Sarcoptidae<br>• Benzyl benzoate 25%<br>• HCH (linden) 0.5%<br>• Applied to the body below the chin after scrub bath<br>• Application is repeated after 12 hours<br>• Treat all infested persons and close contacts simultaneously and similarly (blanket treatment) |
| **Soft tick** | • Oval-shaped leathery body<br>• Big head lies ventrally, not visible from above<br>• No antennae<br>• Four pairs of legs<br>• No wings<br>• No scutum | • Q fever<br>• Relapsing fever<br>• Kyasanur forest disease (KFD) —rarely<br>Both sexes transmits the disease. Transovarian transmission of infection to progeny is also present | • Source reduction: Clearing, filling of cracks and crevices<br>• Keeping cattle and poultry outside the house<br>• Not walking bare foot<br>• Wearing full clothing<br>• Chemical insecticide indane, malathion, DDT and pyrethrum dusting on infested animal<br>• Personal protection: Insecticide repellents like dibutylphthalate (DBP), diethyltoluamide (DEET), benzylbenzoate |

*Contd.*

**Vectors** (*Contd.*)

| Name of vector | Identification | Diseases transmitted | Control |
|---|---|---|---|
| Hard tick | • Body is oval<br>• Rectangular head<br>• Head, thorax, abdomen fused<br>• Four pairs of legs<br>• No antennae<br>• No wings<br>• Dorsum covered by scutum | • KFD<br>• Typhus<br>• Spotted fever<br>• Encephalitis<br>• Tularemia<br>• Tick paralysis | • Insecticides<br>  – Malathion<br>  – Lindane<br>  – DDT<br>• Personal protection<br>• Repellents: Indalone, diethyltoluamide, benzyl benzoate<br>• Periodic examination of body |
| **Class Crustacia** | | | |
| Cyclops | • Pear-shaped (cephalo-thorax and abdomen), Semitransparent body, forked tail<br>• One small pigmented eye<br>• Just visible to naked eye—1 mm size<br>• Two pairs of antennae<br>• Five pairs of legs | • Guinea worm dracunculosis (eradicated in India)<br>• Fish tapeworm | • Physical straining in muslin/nylon strainer. Boiling the drinking water to 60°C<br>• Chemical<br>  – Chlorination–5 ppm<br>  – Lime 60 grain/gallon<br>  – Abate – 1 mg liter<br>• Permanent conversion of step well providing safe drinking water Health education. |

\* +Mosquito net 25 mesh holes per sq cm

## Insecticides

Question 1: Indentify the spot with reasons.

Question 2: Write down the public health importance of given spot.

Question 3: Enumerate the component given spot.

Question 4: Write down the doses used in control measure of given insect.

Teacher's Remark .............................................

Teacher's Sign .............................................

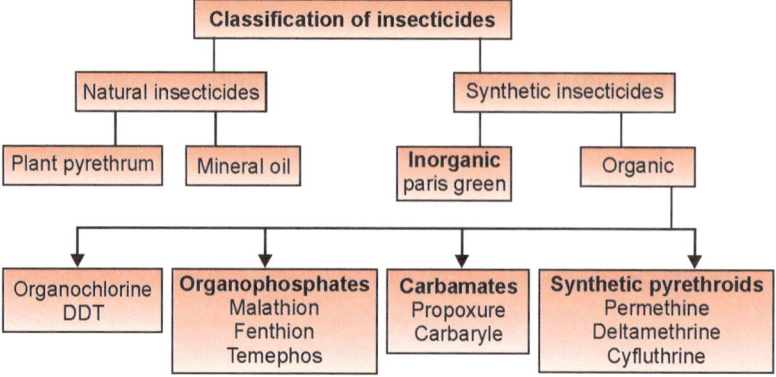

Classification of insecticides

- Natural insecticides
  - Plant pyrethrum
  - Mineral oil
- Synthetic insecticides
  - **Inorganic** paris green
  - Organic
    - Organochlorine DDT
    - **Organophosphates** Malathion Fenthion Temephos
    - **Carbamates** Propoxure Carbaryle
    - **Synthetic pyrethroids** Permethine Deltamethrine Cyfluthrine

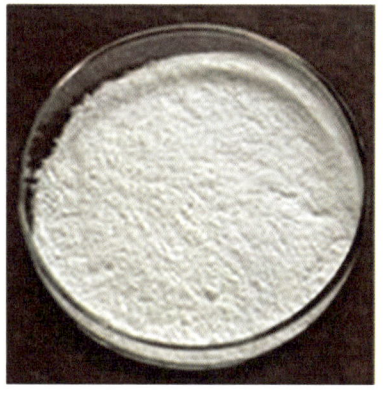
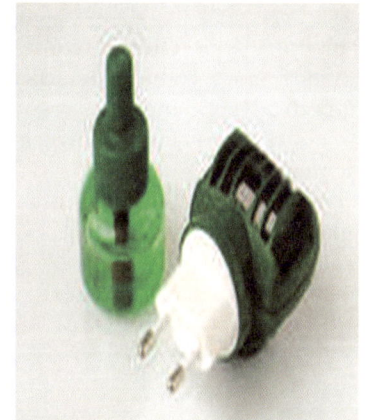
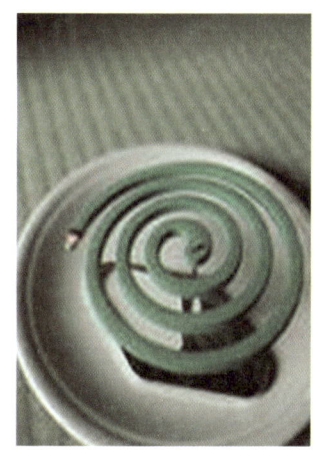

**DDT**                                    **Mosquito repellents**

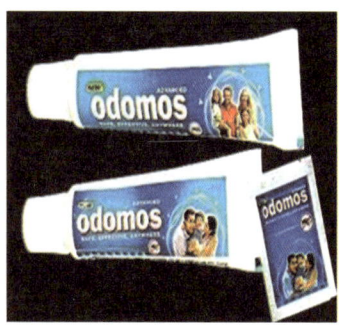
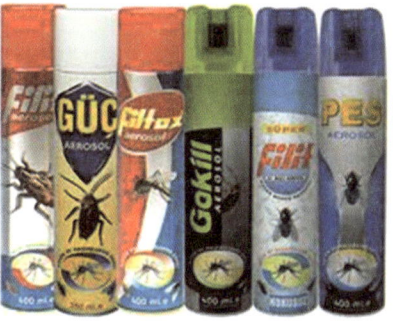
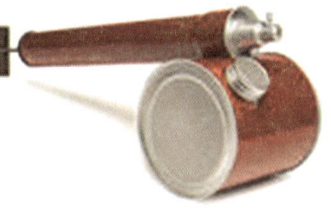

**Mosquito repellents**          **Insecticides**          **Insecticide sprayer**

## Chemicals Used for Insects Control

| Chemical for insects control | Characteristics | Dosage | Mode of action | Duration of action |
|---|---|---|---|---|
| DDT (Dichlorodiphenyl trichloroethane) | White, amorphous powder with peculiar odour | 5 % suspension 1–2 g/m² | Contact poison acting on the nervous system of the insects | 18 months but action starts decreasing after 6 months |
| Paris green Copper acetoarsenite | Emerald green Microcrystalline | 250–500 gm/acre Paris: dust in 1:5 for spray at breeding places | Stomach Poisson Larvicidal | One week |
| Mosquito coil | Smoke generated when burned | 1% Allethrin | Insecticide | Till the smoke is there |
| Allout, etc. | Vapours generated when heated | 1% Allethrin/ permethrin | Insecticide | Till the vapour is there |
| Mosquito repellent | Oil/cream with peculiar smell | N-methylphthalate or N-dimethyl-benzamide | | Till the smell is there |
| Mineral oil, e.g. kerosene | Clear liquid, peculiar odour | Film on water surface | Contact poison | Till the surface is not disturbed |
| Pyrethrum | Crystals or colourless liquid | 1% granules in water | Contact poison Pyrethrin attacks the nerves, causing paralysis followed by death | 3 months |
| Fenthion | Brown liquid; insoluble in water, slight odour of garlic | 20–40% 1g/m² | Contact poison | 3 months |
| HCH Hexachlorocy-clohexane | White powder with mustry smell, insoluble in water | Spray 20–50 mg/foot² | Insecticidal | 3 months |

# Disinfectants and Deodorants

**Question 1:** Indentify the spot with reasons.

**Question 2:** Write down the public health importance of given spot.

**Question 3:** Enumerate the composition of given spot.

**Question 4:** Enumerate the uses of given spot.

**Question 5:** Write down the doses used in various disinfection procedures.

Teacher's Remark ...........................................

Teacher's Sign ...........................................

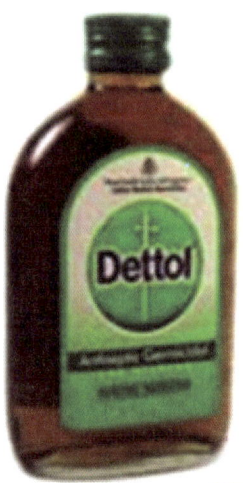
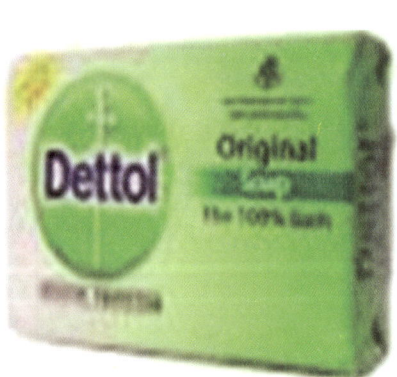
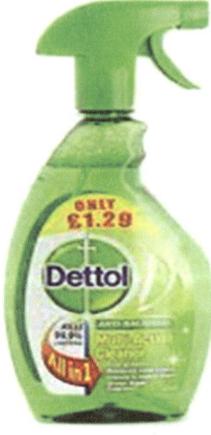
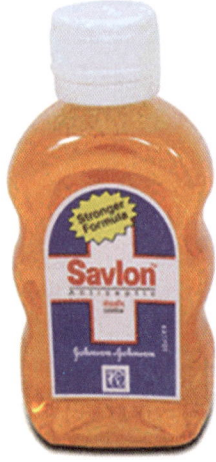
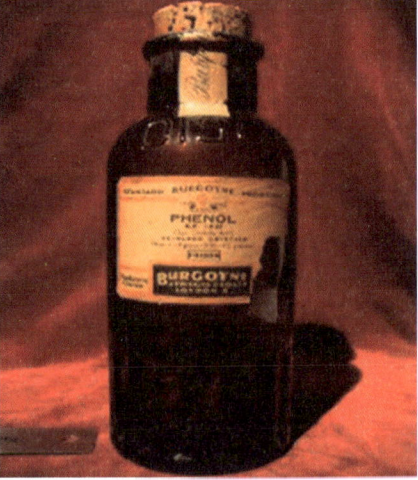
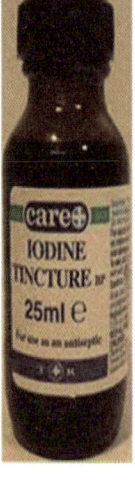
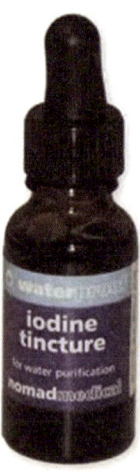

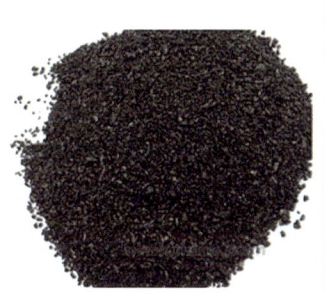 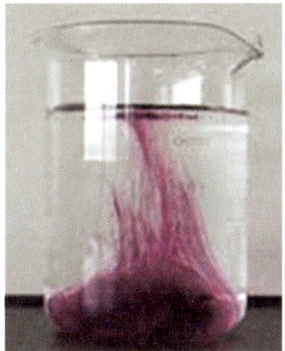 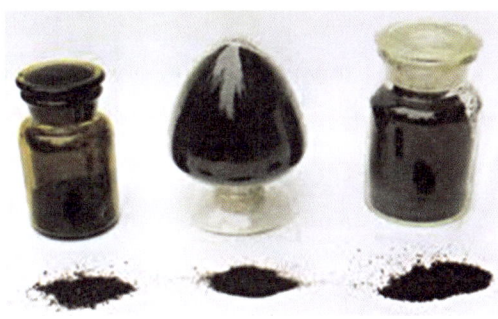

**Potassium permanganate**

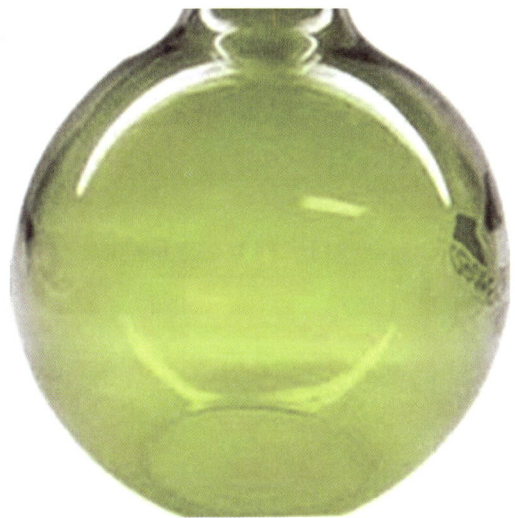 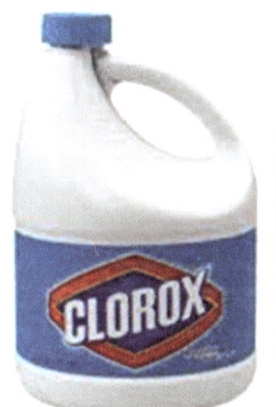 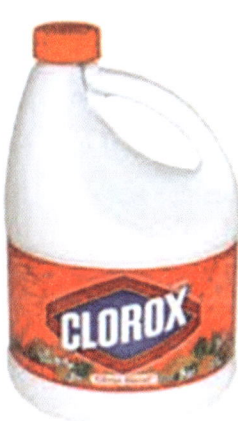

**Sodium hypochlorite**

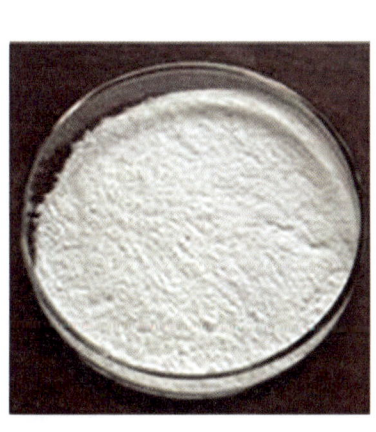 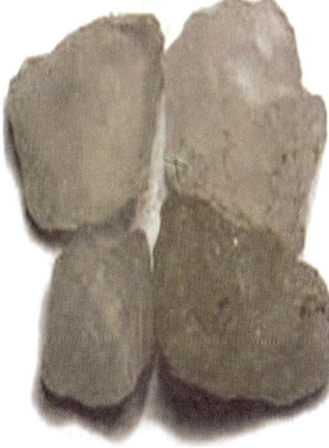 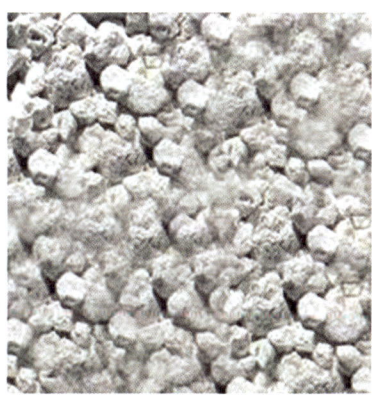

**Bleaching powder**          **Alum (Fitkary)**          **Lime (Chuna)**

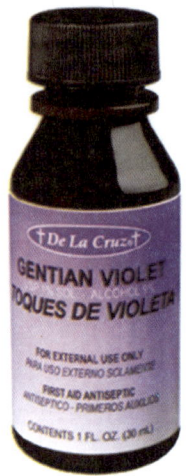
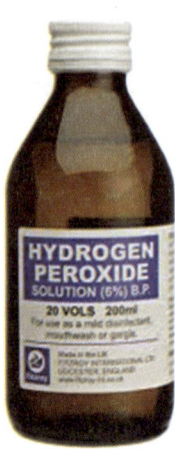

## Disinfectants/Deodorants

| Material | Features | Actions | Dosage | Uses |
|----------|----------|---------|--------|------|
| **Formaldehyde** | Tab/solution + strong Unpleasant smell | Antibacterial antiviral, antifungal | 2.5% solution 10% solution | Disinfect theaters flores |
| **Bleaching powder or chlorinated lime (CaOCl$_2$)** | White amorphous powder with pungent smell of chlorine | 25–33% available chlorine. Cl$_2$ kills all the microbes in 1–3% solution | 5% (4kg/20 lit. of water) 3–4 TSF/l | Disinfect Water |
| **Halogen tablet lime (*Chuna*)** | White tab White and stony | Germicidal, disinfectant and deodorant | 0.5 gm/20 L 10–20% solution Contact period 20 minutes | Water, water, wall and floors |
| **Dettol (cholorexylenol)** | Light yellow solution | Antiseptic | 5% contact period 15 minutes | Wounds Instruments Equipments |
| **Phenol (carbolic acid)** | Dark brown solution with aromatic smell | Disinfectant and deodorant | 5% for floors 10% for toilets | Floors and toilet |
| **Savlon (quarternary ammonium compound)** | Light yellow solution | Surface disinfectant | 5% contact period 20 minutes | Wounds Instruments Equipments |
| **Alum (*Fitkary*) Alluminium sulphate** | White and stony deodorant | Disinfectant, contact | 4–40 mg/l | Water |
| **Soap** | Cake/solution | Defoliation Cleansing action Surface acting | Period 20 minutes Lather | Floors, cloths |

## Disinfectants/Deodorants

| Material | Features | Actions | Dosage | Uses |
|---|---|---|---|---|
| Sodium hypochlorite | Colourless solution with peculiar odours | Active against all bacteria, protozoa and viruses | 0.0002% solution . | Hands Instruments Equipments |
| Tincture iodine | Brown-coloured Tab | Potent bactericidal, sporicidal, fungicidal, amoebicidal, moderate viricidal | Tincture (2 %) | Wounds |
| Providone iodine | Brown-coloured, odourless solution | Potent bactericidal, sporicidal, fungicidal, amoebicidal, moderate viricidal | 2–5 % solution iodine | Wounds Surgical procedure Praparation |
| Hydrogen peroxide | Colourless and odourless liquid | Nacent oxygen released with effervescence removes tissue debris | 6% w/v | Hands, instruments |
| Potassium permanganate | Dark purple crystals with metallic lusture | Oxidizing and astringent action | Gargle (1:4000) 1:10,000 1:100 1:50 | Potassium permanganate |
| Crystal violet (gentian-violet) | Dark blue powder or solution | Active against Gram-positive organisms | 0.5–1% solution for topical use (gentian-violet) | Crystal violet |

## Contraceptive Methods

Question 1: Identify the spot with reason

Question 2: Describe the mechanism of action

Question 3: What is the failure rate and what are its reasons?

Question 4: For how long it has its protectivity?

Question 5: What are the advantages of this method?

Question 6: What are the disadvantages of this method?

Teacher's Remark ...........................................

Teacher's Sign ...........................................

## CONTRACEPTIVE MECHANISM

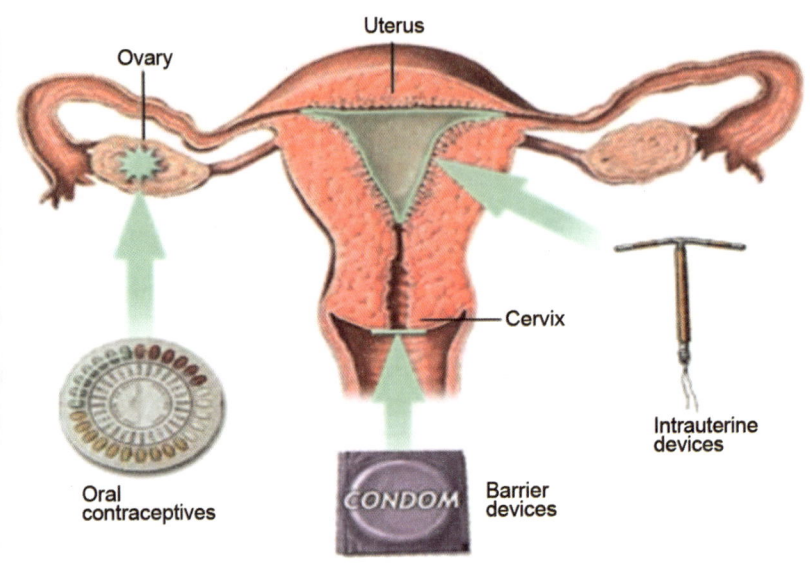

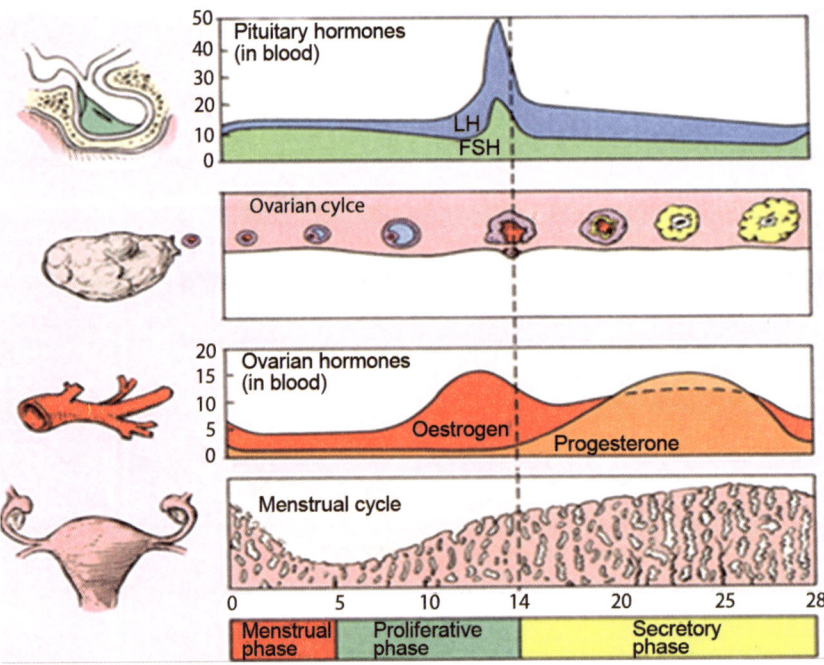

Association between pituitary hormones, ovarian cycle, ovarian hormones and menstrual cycle

## CONTRACEPTIVE DEVICES

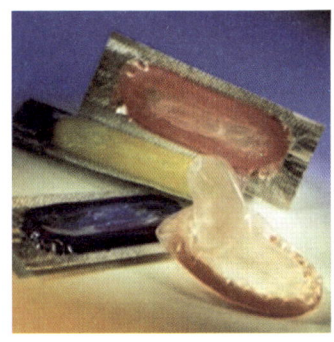 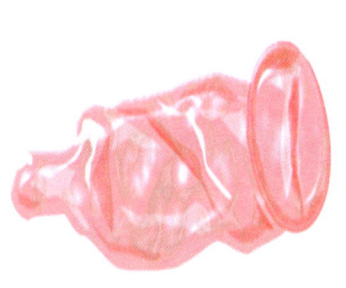 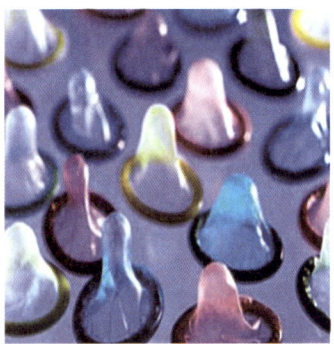

**Male condoms**

## FEMALE BARRIER DEVICES

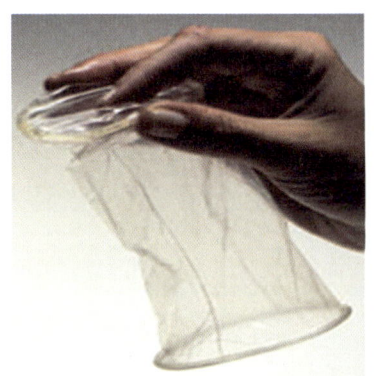 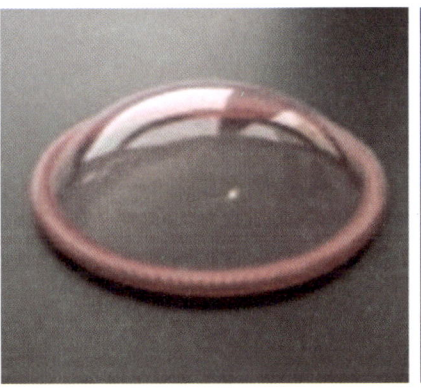 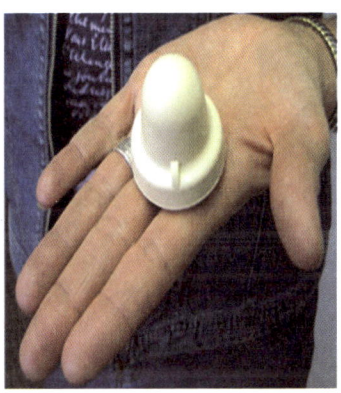

**Femidom**          **Diaphragm**          **Cervical cap**

## INTRAUTERINE DEVICES (IUDs)

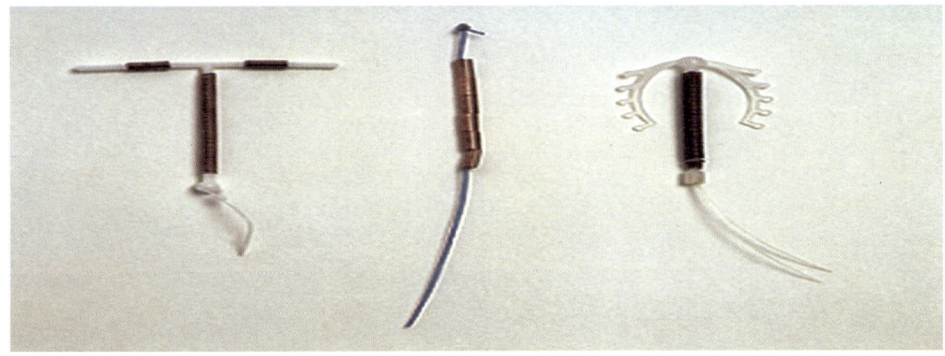

**Cu T**          **Multi-load Cu T**

## HORMONAL CONTRACEPTIVE METHODS

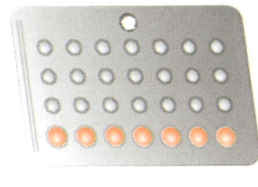 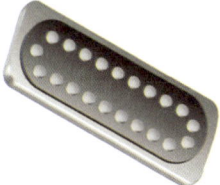

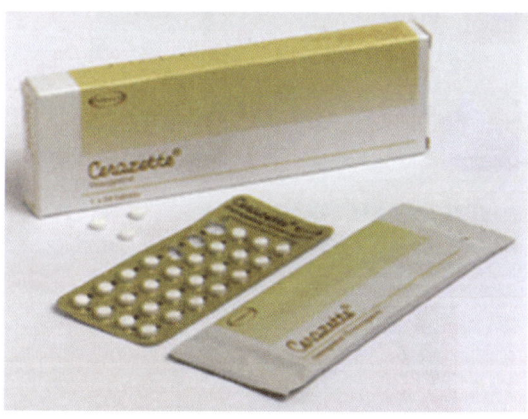

**Combined pill (Mala N)** — **Progesterone only pills**

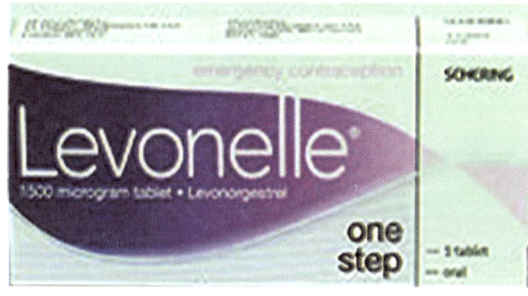

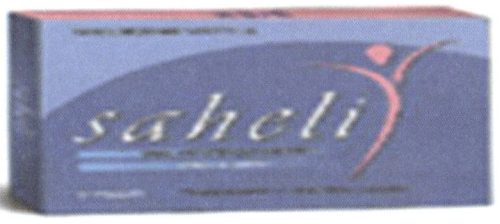

**Emergency pill** — **Once a week pill (*Saheli*)**

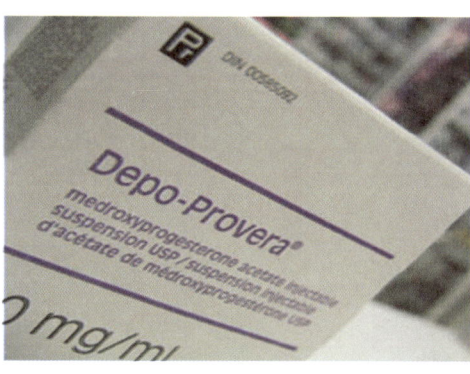

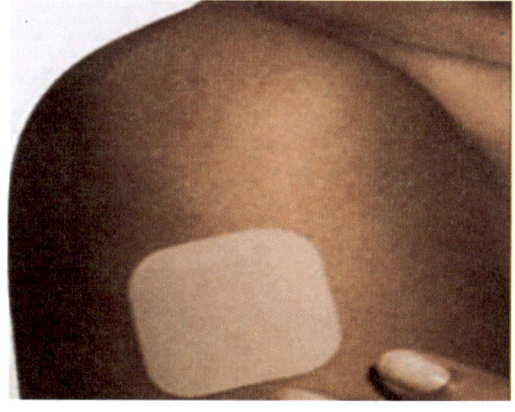

**Injectable hormonal CM** — **Intradermal hormonal patch**

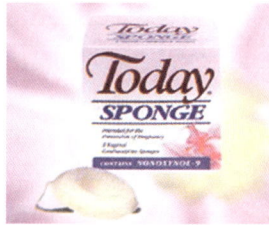 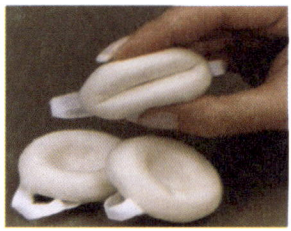

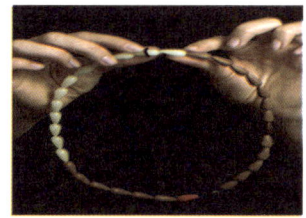

**Chemical spermicidal**          **Mala for safe period**

## HOW TO USE VARIOUS CONTRACEPTIVE DEVICES:

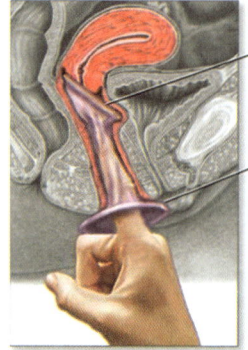

Closed end

Open end

**Female condom**

**Femidom**

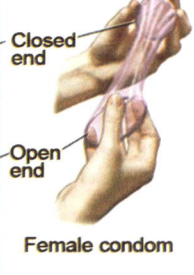

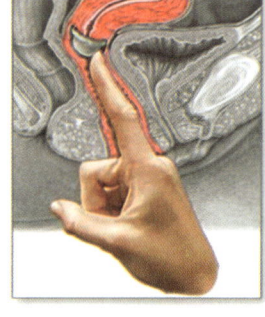

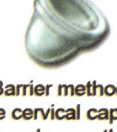

Barrier method:
The cervical cap fits
snugly over the
cervix, preventing
sperm from entering
the uterus

**Cervical cap**

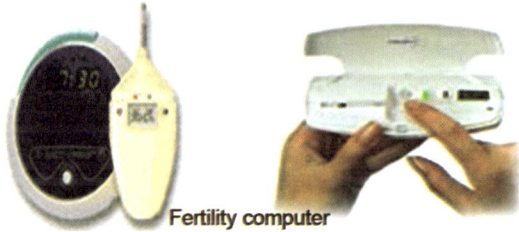

Fertility computer

Green light on the device means infertile; a red light means fertile

## MALA FOR SAFE PERIOD CALCULATION

- Red pearl indicates 1st day of menstruation
- White pearls indicate fertile periods.
- Brown pearls indicate 'safe period'.

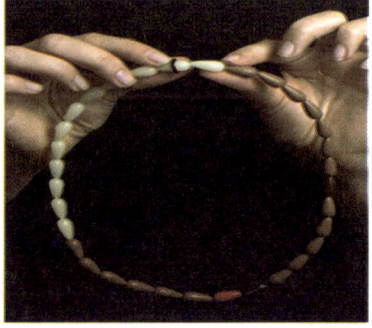

## Comparison of Contraceptive Methods

| Name of method and mechanism of action | Composition | Advantages | Disadvantages | Failure rate |
|---|---|---|---|---|
| **Barrier methods: Act as barrier in meeting of sperm to ovum** | | | | |
| Male condom | Polyurethane Plastic | Protection from STI/HIV: availability— multiple options | Reduced sensation Some users Experience allergies | 2–15% |
| Female condom | Polyurethane Plastic | Can be placed up to 8 hr in advance protection against STIs | Only 1 style currently available more costly than male condoms | 5–25% |
| Cervical cap | Silicon | Can be inserted up to 6 hr in advance Very few side effects Multiple options | Low efficacy Limited to 4 sizes Not widely available May experience allergies | 0.9–32% |
| **Chemical spermicidal: Spermicide is a chemical that kills sperms** | | | | |
| Sponges | Spermicidal Foams | Immediate and continuous protection for 24-hr period One size fits all and easy to insert | Removal tricky may experience sensitivities/ allergies to spermicide | 20–30% |
| Vaginal ring | Spermicidal with latex ring | A few side effects Can be inserted up to 6 hr in advance | Requires fitting Some users experience allergies | 6–16% |
| Diaphragm with contraceptive jelly or foam | Spermicidal latex diaphragm | A few side effects Can be inserted up to 6 hr in advance | Requires fitting Some users experience allergies | 6–16% |
| **Intrauterine devices (IUDs): Devices kept in uterus which interfere in implantation of fertilized ova and also changes the uterine wall to make it unfavourable for implantation** | | | | |
| Cu T Multiload Cu T | Copper with silicon | Longevity 5–10 years | Can be expelled or become dislodged Not recommended for women with fibroids | < 1% |
| **Hormonal: Progesterone prevents ovulation through feedback mechanism and also changes the uterine wall to make it unfavourable for implantation** | | | | |
| Combined O pills | Progesterone and oestrogen | High rate of efficacy Multiple options available | Undesirable risk and side effect profile in some women | 0.3–8% |
| Progesterone only pill (POP) | Progesterone | Regulates menstrual cycle, relatively convenient Decreased risk of POCD | | |

*Contd.*

## Comparison of Contraceptive Methods (*Contd.*)

| Name of method and mechanism of action | Composition | Advantages | Disadvantages | Failure |
|---|---|---|---|---|
| **Once a week pill** | Centcromen | Same as other pills | Less side effect than other pills | 2–8% |
| **Emergency pill** | Higher doses of progesterone | Same as other pills, only pill can protect after unprotected coitus, when taken within 72 hrs | Within 72 hrs, more effective, more side effect than other pills | 0.3–8% |
| **Vaginal ring with progesterone** | Progesterone on silicon ring | Privacy, reducing infections, protection from pregnancy, one month at a time | Contraindicated in prolapse, endometriosis susceptibility to irritation, etc. | 0.3–8% |
| **Transdermal patches** | Progesterone patch | As for pills | Higher risk profile for thromboembolic events | 0.3–8% |
| **Depo-provera injection** | Progesterone injection | Effective 24 hr following injection | Reduction in bone density, depression, and weight gain | 0.3–3% |
| **Contraceptive implants** | Progesterone implants | Longevity: 3–5 yr Fertility returns relatively quickly | Difficult to remove Scarring Spotting | 0.05% |
| **Fertility awareness methods (FAM): Time of ovulation is determined with certain signs and symptoms, so fertility period is defined to avoid intercourse** | | | | |
| **Basal body temperature (BBT)** | Temperature increases at the time of ovulation | Zero health risks or side effects | Requires significant partner education, cooperation, and daily attention | 0.6–12% |
| **Symptothermal** | Ill feeling | Enhances body awareness and partner intimacy | | |
| **Billings ovulation "Rhythm"** | Cervical mucus becomes thin Mala method avoid fertility period | Zero health risks or side effects and enhances body awareness and partner intimacy | Not ideal in perimeno-pause, lactational and women with irregular cycles | 5–25% |
| **Behavioural: Some behavioural changes required for preventing sperm to meet ova** | | | | |
| **Abstinence** | No vaginal sex | Zero health risks or side effects | Inconvenience | <1% |
| **Coitus interrupts** | Withdrawal at the time of ejaculation | Zero health risks or side effects and enhances body awareness and partner intimacy | Inconvenience | 4–27% |

*Contd.*

## Comparison of Contraceptive Methods *(Contd.)*

| Name of method and mechanism of action | Composition | Advantages | Disadvantages | Failure |
|---|---|---|---|---|
| **Sterilization: Surgical procedure is required to block meeting of sperms to ova** | | | | |
| **Female steriliza-tion, i.e. tubectomy tubal ligation** | | Permanence Cost-effective over time Effective immediately | Surgical risks | <1% |
| **Male sterlization, i.e. vasectomy** | | Permanence Cost-effective over time, less surgical risk | Not immediately effective; it may take up to 3 months to achieve sterility | <1% |

## SPECTRUM OF EFFICIENCY OF CONTRACEPTIVE METHOD WITH FOLLOWING FAILURE RATE

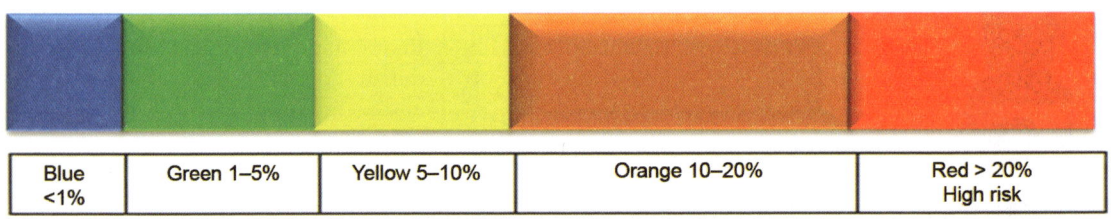

| Blue <1% | Green 1–5% | Yellow 5–10% | Orange 10–20% | Red > 20% High risk |
|---|---|---|---|---|

# Vaccines and Cold Chain Equipments

**Question 1:** What is the type of given vaccine?

**Question 2:** What are the components of the given vaccine?

**Question 3:** What are the recommendations of given vaccine?

**Question 4:** What are the contraindications of given vaccine?

**Question 5:** What are the side effects of given vaccine?

**Question 6:** Write down the rout of administration and dosage schedule of given vaccine.

**Question 7:** Write down the public health importance of this vaccine.

Teacher's Remark ...........................................

Teacher's Sign ...........................................

## BCG

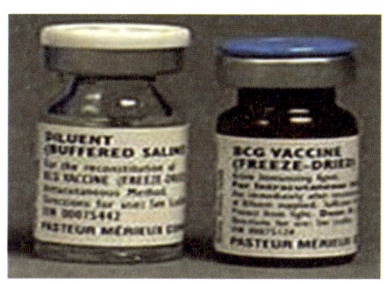

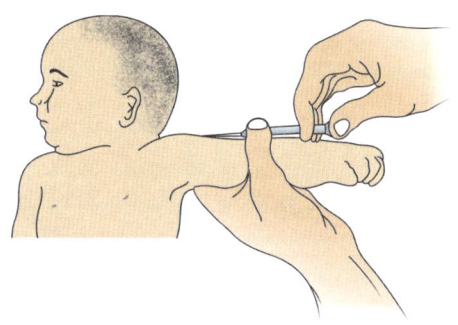

| Dose | Site |
|------|------|

## OPV

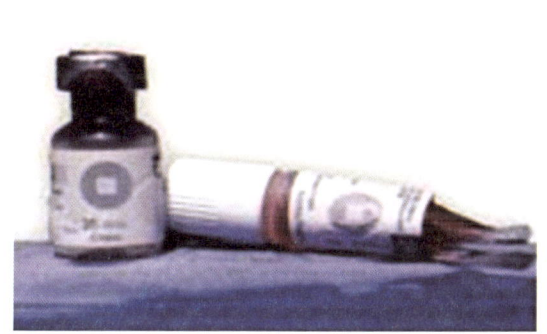

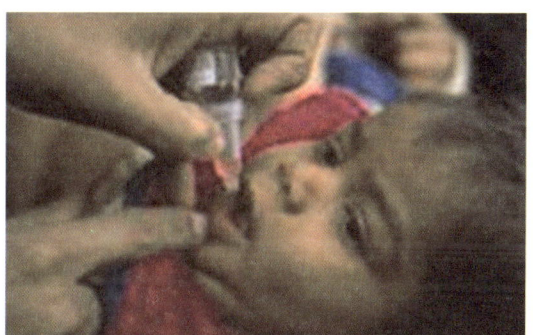

| Dose | Site |
|------|------|

## DPT

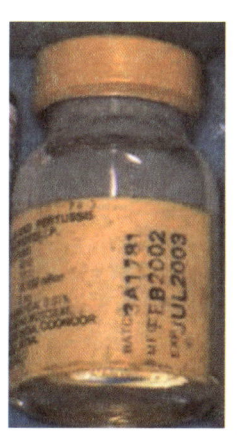

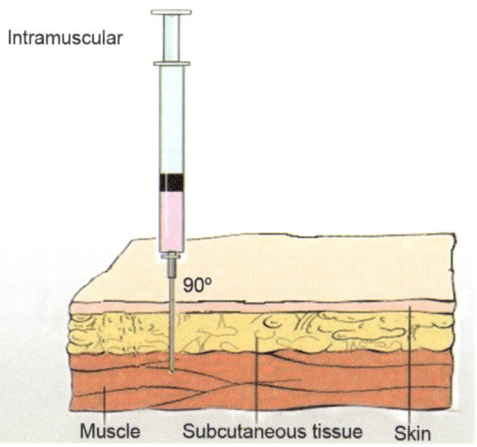

Intramuscular

90°

Muscle    Subcutaneous tissue    Skin

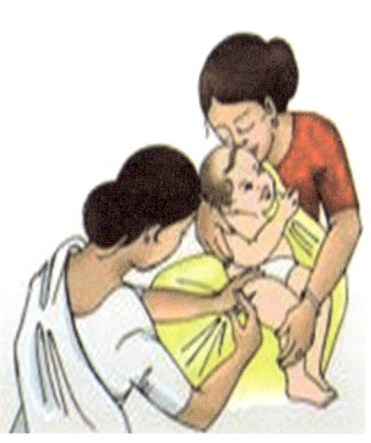

| Dose | Route | Site |
|------|-------|------|

## HEPATITIS B

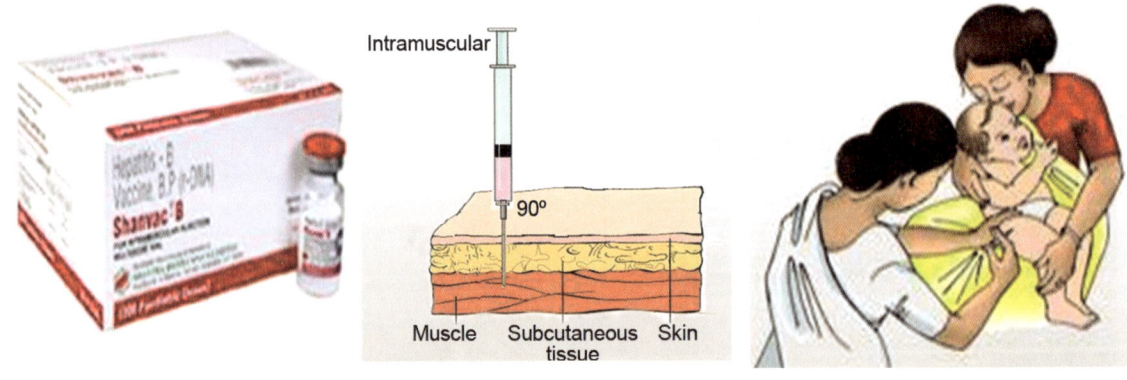

| Dose | Route | Site |

## MEASLES

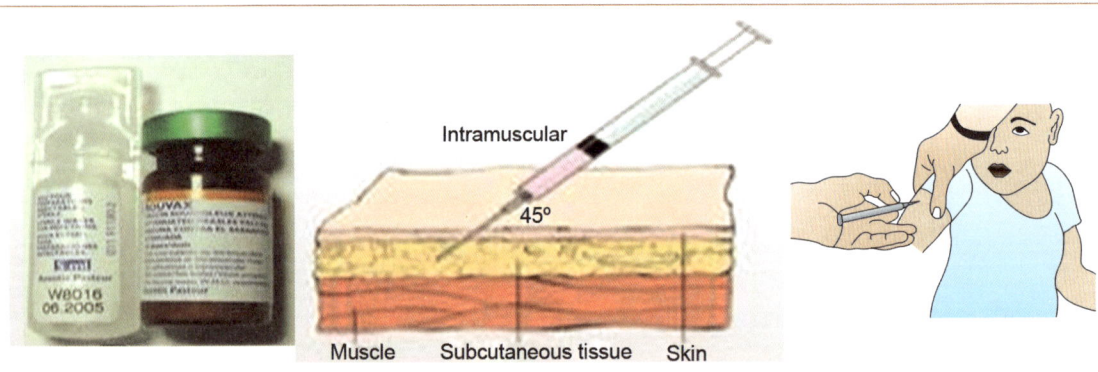

| Dose | Route | Site |

## DT

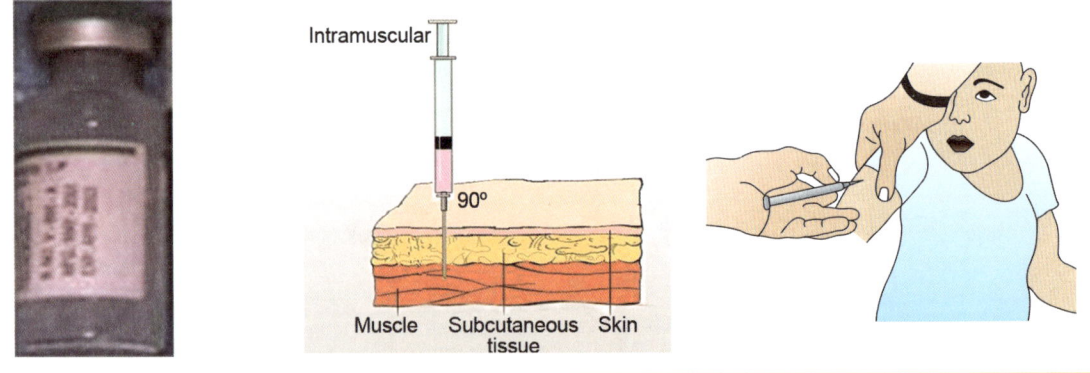

| Dose | Route | Site |

## π

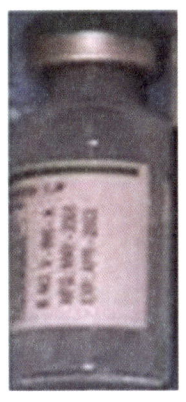 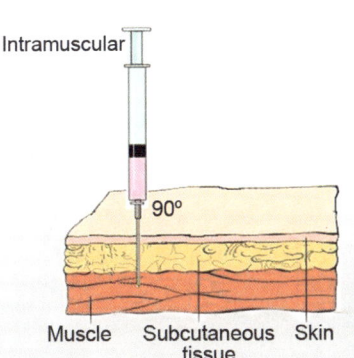 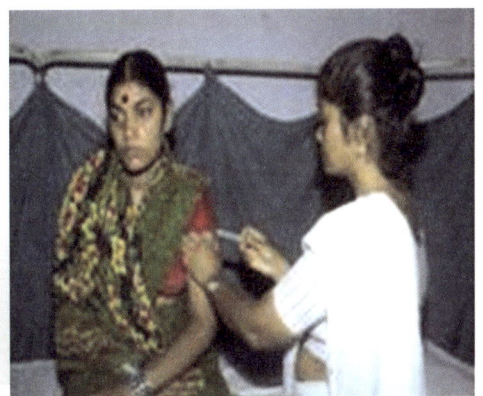

Intramuscular

90°

Muscle    Subcutaneous    Skin
         tissue

| Dose | Route | Technique |

## VITAMIN A

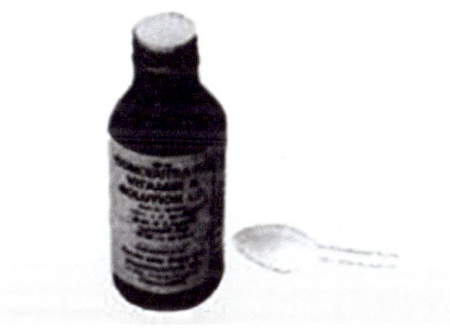 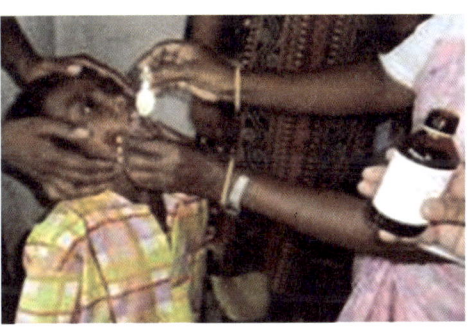

| Dose | Route |

## Vaccination Under UIP

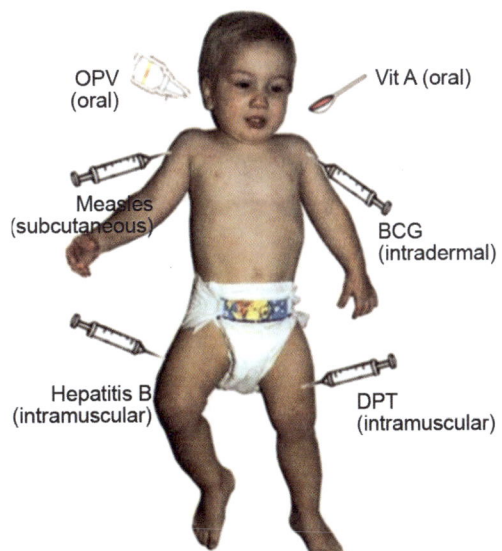

OPV
(oral)

Vit A (oral)

Measles
(subcutaneous)

BCG
(intradermal)

Hepatitis B
(intramuscular)

DPT
(intramuscular)

## Vaccines

| Name of vaccine (for disease) | Type of vaccine | Composition | Route of adm. and dose schedule | Efficacy | Remark |
|---|---|---|---|---|---|
| BCG (tuberculosis) | Live bacterial Freezed dried | *Mycobacterium bovis* Danish 1331 0.1 million bacilli/ dose 10 Doses = 1 mg/ml Diluent-NS | 0.1 ml ID at left deltoid region at birth or as early as possible | 70 – 80% Almost life-long | PSR, ulceration, lymph-adenitis<br><br>Abscess |
| OPV (Polio) | Live trivalent | $10^6$ type I TCID 50 $10^5$ type II TCID 50 $10^{5.5}$ type III TCID 50 20 doses (2 ml) | 2 drops orally = 0 + 1st dose–6 wks 2nd dose–10 wks 3rd dose–14 wks booster doses at 11/2 yr and 5 yrs | 100% life time | Very rarely Vaccine associated poliomyelitis Warm food is avoided for half an hr |
| DPT (diphtheria, pertussis, tetanus) | Triple vaccine | 0.5 ml have diphtheria toxoid 20 Lf tetanus toxoid, 0.5 Lf pertussis killed–20,000 million Alluminium phosphate–2.5 mg Thiomesol–0.01% | 0.5 ml Deep IM 1st dose – 6 wks 2nd dose–10 wks 3rd dose–14 wks booster doses at 11/2 yrs and 5 yrs (DT only at 5 yrs) | For diphtheria and tetanus 95–99% But for pertussis 70–90% for 6 years | PSR fever rarely convulsions |
| Measles (measles) | Live attenuated freezed dried | 5000 TCID 50 Edmonsten zagreb strain of measles virus | 0.5 ml SC at 9 months of age | 95% almost lifelong | PSR fever Rashes ± |
| TT (tetanus) | Toxoid monovalent | 25 Lf of toxoid | 0.5 ml IM 1st–stat 2nd dose 1 month 3rd dose 6 month | 99% 5 years | PSR fever ± Urticaria ± |
| MMR (measles mumps rubella) | Live attenuated viral Trivalent | 1000 TCID 50 EZ measles V. 5000 TCID 50 MumpsV. (Urbe Am9) 1000 TCID 50 Rubella V. (w1RA27/3) | 0.5 ml deep SC Single dose at 15–18 months | Measles–95% Mumps –98% Rubella 100% | PSR fever, convulsions, Rhino-pharyngitis |
| Hepatitis B | Plasma derived vaccine | 20 micrograms of HBsAg/ml | Child .5 ml/Adult 1 ml 1st–stat 2nd dose 1 month 3rd dose 6 month | 95% for 5 years | PSR jaundice ± |
| Hepatitis A | Formaldehyde inactivated HDCV | MM 175 Hep. A Strain **Adult**–1440 ELISA U/ml **Junior**–720 ELISA units in 0.5 ml (1–18 yrs) | 1–18 years 0.5 ml IM >18 year 1 ml IM single dose Single booster after 6–12 months | 98% for about 20 yrs | PSR fever |

*Contd.*

## Vaccines *(Contd.)*

| Name of vaccine (for disease) | Type of vaccine | Composition | Route of adm. and dose schedule | Efficacy | Remark |
|---|---|---|---|---|---|
| Typhoid | Typhoral live Typhim Vi – killed | Typhoral Ty 21 Typhim Vi | Day 1, 3, 5 orally capsule 0.5 ml IM (single dose) booster after every 3 years | 67–95% 75–100% For 3 years | GIT upset Rashes PSR rashes |
| Meningitis | Purified bacterial polysaccharide antigen | Meningococcal Capsular poly-saccharide (A and C) 50 ug | 0.5 ml deep SC every 3 years | 90% for 3 years | PSR fever |
| HIB (*H.influenzae*) | Hib titer— Haemophilus polysaccharide 25 microgram | *Haemophilus influenzae* type B Capsular polysaccharide 25 ug | 0.5 ml IM (deep SC) 1st dose–6 wks 2nd dose–10 wks 3rd dose–14 wks Booster 11/2 years | 95–99% | PSR rarely GB syndrome (1:1 lakh) |
| Rubella | Live attenuated | Wistar RA 27/3 Strain 1000 CCID | 0.5 ml deep SC/IM Single time | 100% | PSR, fever |
| Chickenpox | Live attenuated Freezed dried | Oka strain of varicella zoster $3.3^{10}$ PFU/0.5 ml | 0.5 ml SC up to 1 yr – 1 Dose > 1 yr– 2 dose 4 wks apart | 70% | Fever, rash |
| DTP+ HEP+ HIB | Pentavalent Freezed dried | Same as DPT, Hep B and influenza | 0.5 ml IM 1st dose–6 wks 2nd dose–10 wks 3rd dose—14 wks | 90% | PSR Fever |
| Influenza | Trivalent Killed V | Type $A_1 – H_3N_2$ 15 ug Type $A_2 – H_1 N_1$ 15 ug Type B 15 ug/dose | 0.5 ml SC | 90% for 3–6 months | |
| Rotateq (Rotavirus) | Tetravalent Rheosus Rotavirus | G1, G2, G3 and G4 serotypes | 0.5 ml SC 1st–2 months 2nd – 4 months 3rd 6 months | 80–95% | Mild diarrhoea |
| Pneumococcal | Polyvalent (23 Valent) | Purified Capsular polysaccharide antigens of 23 valents | 0.5 ml SC/IM > 2 yrs – 3 dose 4 wks apart | 60–90% | |
| Cholera | Killed bacterial | $6^{10}$ classical Ogava + $6^{10}$ classical Inaba + 0.5% phenol/ml | 1–10 yrs–0.25 ml >10 yr – 0.5 ml SC 2 dose 4–6 wks apart, booster every 6 month | 50% for 3–6 months | Mild diarrhoea, fever |
| Japanese encephalitis | Inactivated | Nakayama strain | 0.5 ml SC Doses-0, 7th, 30th day + B 365th day | 97% for 3 yrs | PSR |

*Contd.*

## Vaccines (*Contd.*)

| Name of vaccine (for disease) | Type of vaccine | Composition | Route of adm. and dose schedule | Efficacy | Remark |
|---|---|---|---|---|---|
| HDCV (rabies) | Human diploid Cell strain | 2.5 IU/ml | 1 ml IM at deltoid region on 0,3,7,14,28 and 90*days | 99.99% for 3–5 years | – |
| PVRV (rabies) | Vero cell culture vaccine | 5 IU/ml | 0.5 ml IM at deltoid region on 0,3, 7, 14, 28 and 90*days | 99.99% For 3–5 years | – |
| PCEV (rabies) | Purified chick embryo vaccine | 2.5 IU/ml | 1 ml IM at deltoid region on 0, 3, 7, 14, 28 and 90*days | 99.99% For 3–5 years | Sensitivity |
| PDEV (rabies) | Duck embryo cell culture vaccine | 2.5 IU/ml | 1 ml IM at deltoid region on 0, 3, 7, 14, 28 and 90*days | 99.99% for 3–5 years | Sensitivity |

*in case if given with passive immunity

# Cold Chain Equipments

Question 1: Identify the spot with reason.

Question 2: Describe the different components of given spot.

Question 3: What are uses of given spot?

Question 4: What temperature it maintains usually?

Question 5: For how long it maintains temperature in case of electricity failure?

Teacher's Remark ...........................................

Teacher's Sign ...........................................

Cold chain is needed to keep the required temperature maintain from manufacturer to beneficiaries.

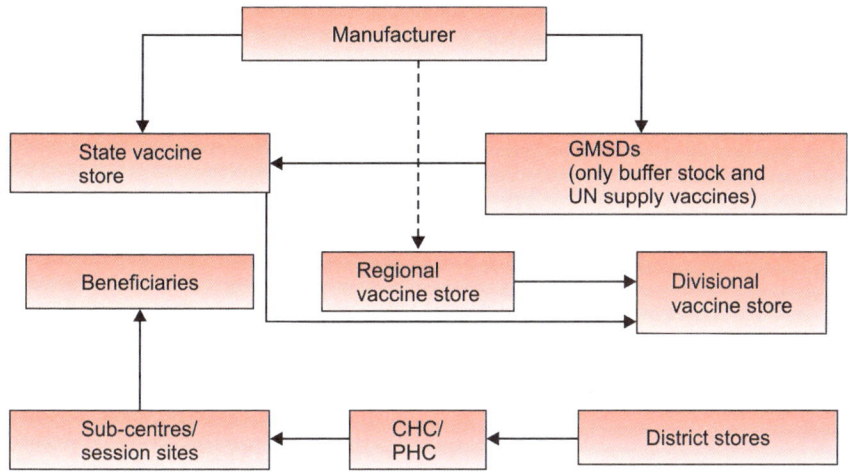

Vaccine production and distribution in India

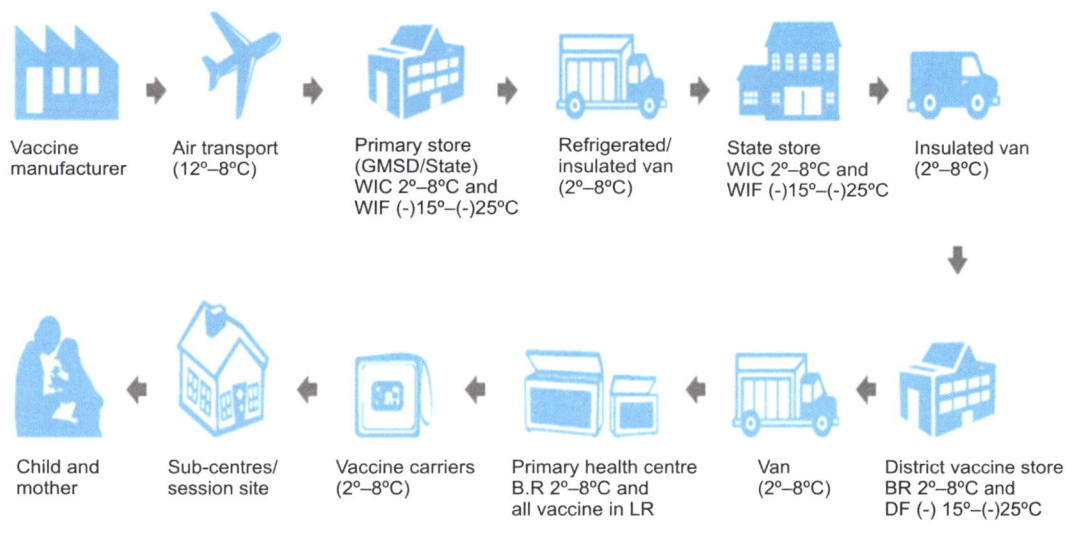

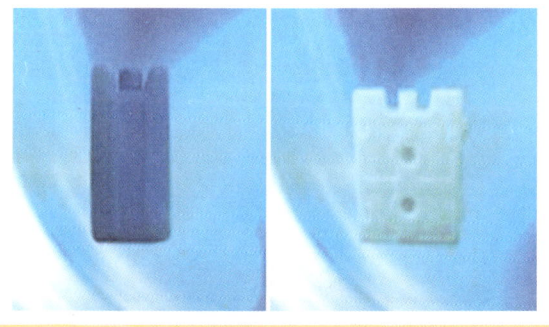

**Plastic ice pack**

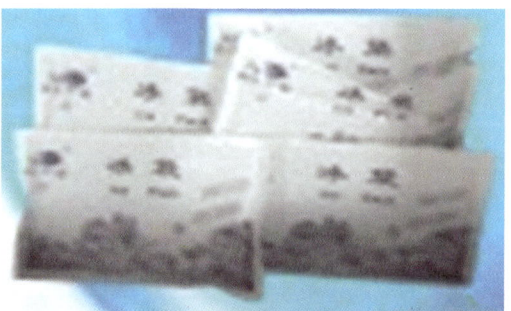

**Gel ice pack**

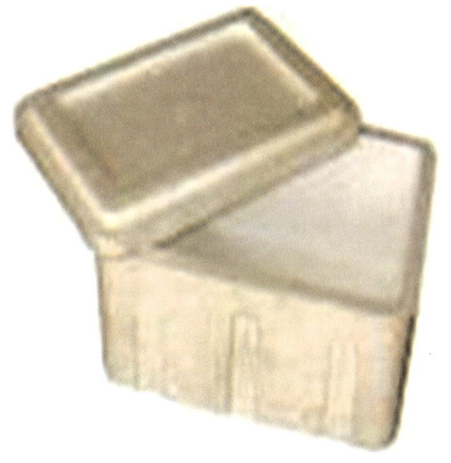

Thermocole box

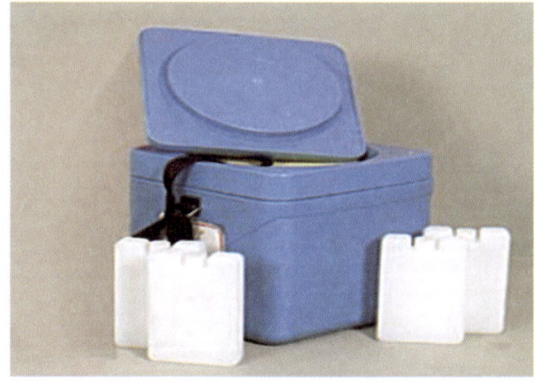

Vaccine carrier

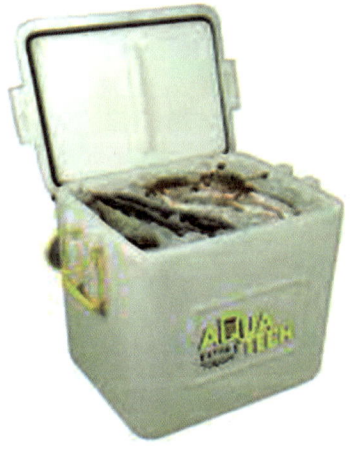

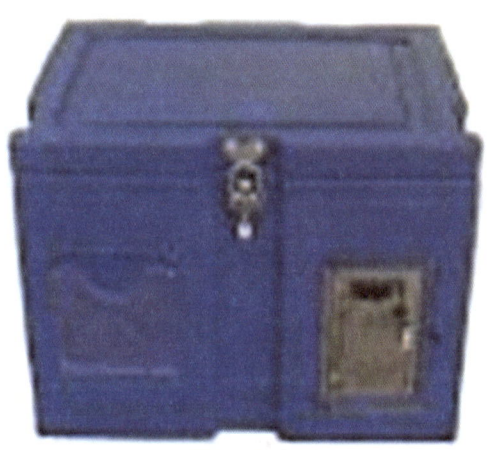

Cold boxes

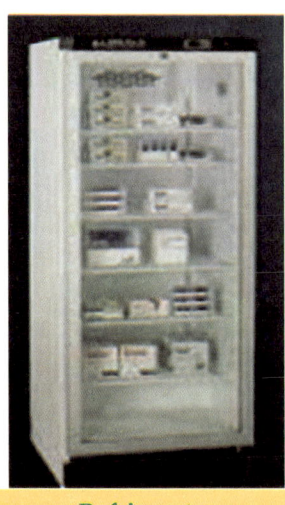

Refrigerator

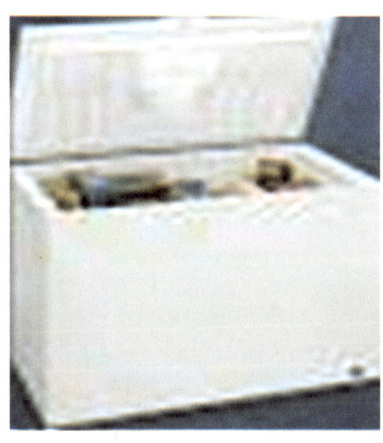

Deep freezer

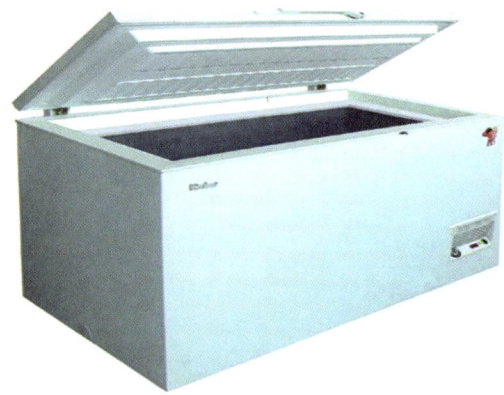

Ice lined refrigerator (ILR)

## Cold Chain Equipments

| Name of equipment | Parts | Use | Efficiency | *Remark |
|---|---|---|---|---|
| Ice packs | Flat plastic bottles or packed gel ice prepared by freezing water in it | For lining walls of vaccine carriers and cold boxes at vaccination camp | 2 hrs if in open | Do not add salt to water, should be fully frozen |
| Thermocole boxes | Thermocole box No ice packs | Transportation of vaccines for short duration | 3 hrs | Ice cubes at the bottom, shorten cold life |
| Day carrier | Insulated plastic box with 2 ice packs | Transportation of vaccines at SC for camp | 6–8 hrs | 1 ice pack at the bottom and 1 at the top |
| Vaccine carrier | Insulated plastic box with 4 ice packs | Transportation of vaccines at SC for camp | 2 days | Fully frozen ice pack lining |
| Cold boxes | Insulated plastic box lined with about 24 ice packs | Transportation of vaccines from regional stores to state/district | 5 days | Lined with ice packs, ice pack at bottom and at top also |
| Refrigerator | Freezer—Icepacks Cabinet—Vaccines Door—Water Bottles | Storage of vaccine at PHC | One month | Fix plug to socket Socket filled water bottles Dedicated use Twice a day temp. Check |
| Deep freezer | Top opening equip. No freezer | Storage of polio and measles vaccine at PHC, CHC and district hospitals | 3 months | Fix plug to socket Filled water bottles Daily temp. check |

*Contd.*

## Cold Chain Equipments *Contd.*

| Name of Equipment | Parts | Use | Efficiency | *Remark |
|---|---|---|---|---|
| ILR | Top opening equip. No freezer lined with frozen ice packs or ice tubes | Storage of vaccine at PHC, CHC and district hospitals | 3 months | Fix plug to socket Filled water bottles Daily temp. check |

*Ice packs should be fully frozen

Put vaccine vials and ampoules in a plastic bag and close it with rubber band

'T' series of vaccine (DPT, DT and TT) should not be in touch of ice packs, so place some packing material in between.

'T' series of vaccine (DPT, DT and TT) should not be kept at bottom in ILR.

Tightly close lid.

Keep away from direct sunlight.

Handle with care.

At SC, no vaccine should be stored.

At PHC, not more than one month vaccine should be stored.

At district hospital, not more than three months vaccine should be stored.

## Photographs and other Miscellaneous Spots

Question 1: Indentify the spot with reasons.

Question 2: Write down the public health importance.

Question 3: Write down preventive measure of this disease.

Teacher's Remark .............................................

Teacher's Sign .............................................

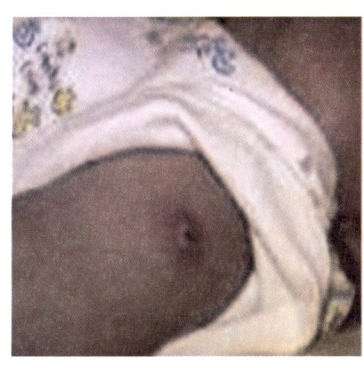
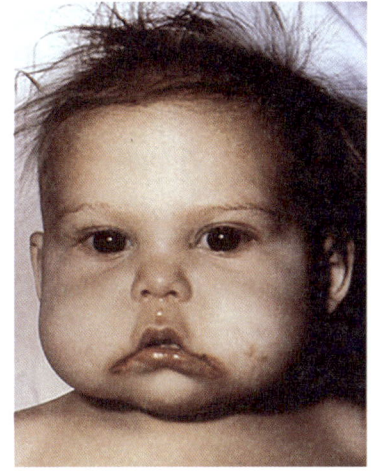
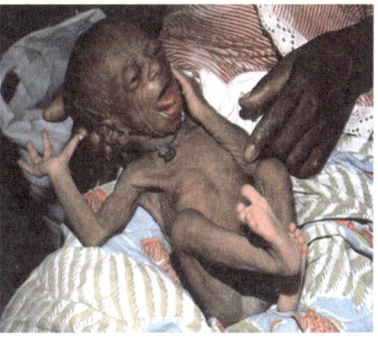

1. BCG boil      2. PEM—Kwashiorkor (moon face)    3. PEM—marasmus child

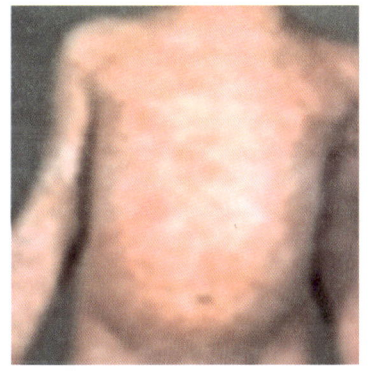
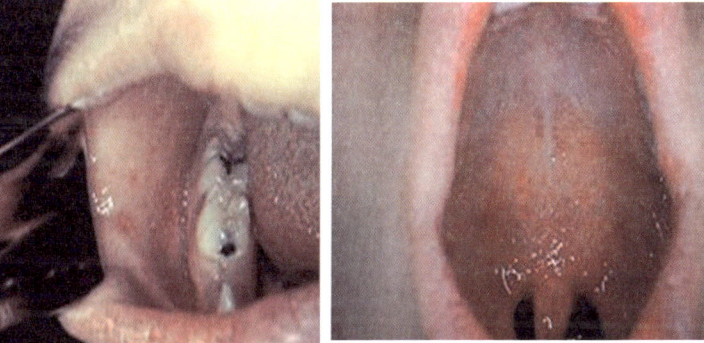

4. Measles               5. Measles—Koplic spot

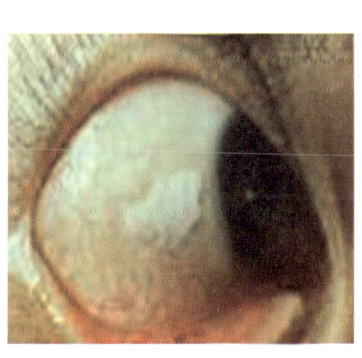
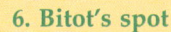
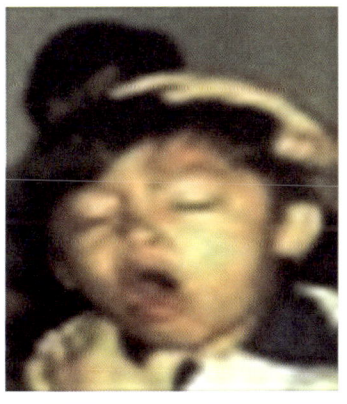
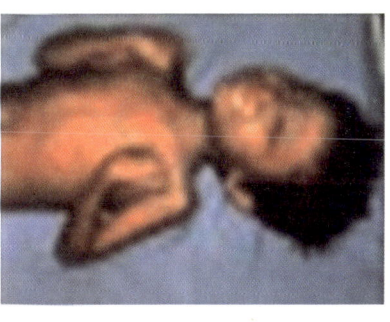

6. Bitot's spot        7. Whooping cough        8. Neonatal tetanus

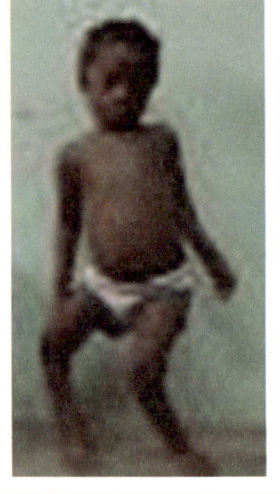

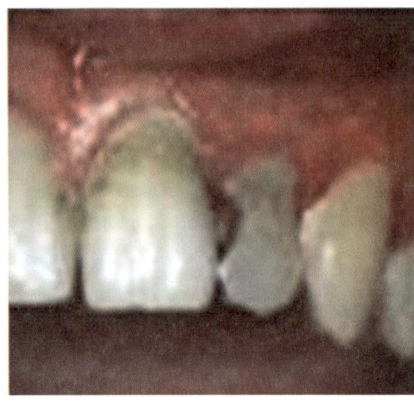

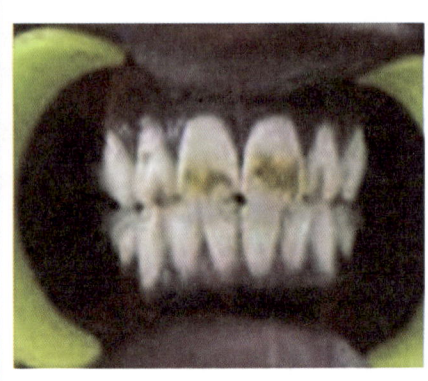

| 9. Rickets | 10. Caries | 11. Fluorosis |

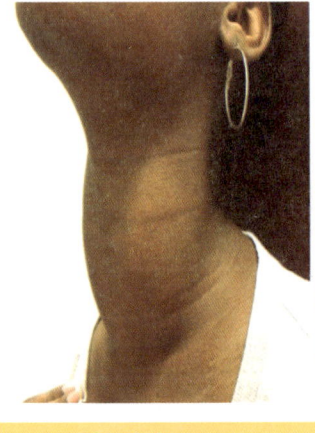

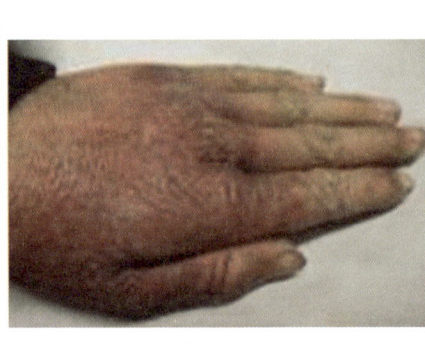

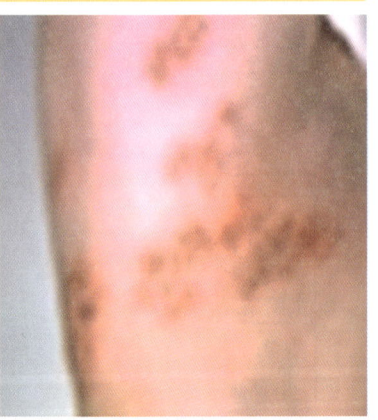

| 12. Goitre | 13. Pellagra | 14. Herpes |

## (1) Mamta Card
## ANC Part

### गर्भावस्था के दौरान नियमित जांच अनिवार्य है

| | |
|---|---|
| **पंजीकरण** | पहली तिमाही में स्वास्थ्य केन्द्र में पंजीकरण कराएं। |
| **प्रसवपूर्व जांच** | पंजीकरण के बाद कम से कम तीन बार प्रसव पूर्व जांच अवश्य कराएं। |
| **रक्तदाब, रक्त, पेशाब** | प्रत्येक जांच के समय रक्तदाब और रक्त व पेशाब की जांच करवाएं। |
| **वजन** | प्रत्येक जांच के समय अपना वजन अवश्य करवाएं। गर्भावस्था में कम से कम 10-12 कि.ग्रा. वजन बढ़ना चाहिये। गर्भावस्था के अन्तिम 6 महीनों में हर महीने कम से कम एक कि.ग्रा. वजन अवश्य बढ़ना चाहिए। |
| **टेटनस टॉक्साॅयड के टीके** | टेटनस टॉक्साॅयड के दो टीके लगवाएं। पहला टीका गर्भावस्था की पुष्टि होने पर और दूसरा टीका एक माह के बाद। (तिथि भरें) |
| **आयरन गोलियां** | कम से कम 3 महीने तक प्रतिदिन आयरन व फोलिक एसिड की एक गोली अवश्य खाएं। कुल मिलाकर कम से कम 100 गोलियां खाना आवश्यक है। (दी गई गोलियों की मात्रा एवं तिथि भरें) |

### गर्भावस्था के दौरान देखभाल

- विभिन्न प्रकार के खाद्य पदार्थों का सेवन करें।
- अधिक मात्रा में भोजन करें- लगभग सामान्य आहार से एक चौथाई ज्यादा।
- आंगनवाड़ी केन्द्र से मिले पूरक पोषाहार को नियमित रूप से खाएं।
- दिन में कम से कम 2 घण्टे विश्राम करें।
- इसके अलावा रात में 8 घंटे सोएं।
- केवल आयोडीन युक्त नमक का उपयोग करें।

**हर प्रसवपूर्व जांच पर पोषण परामर्श सुनिश्चित करें**

---

### प्रसव पूर्व देखभाल
#### पूर्व गर्भावस्था में प्रसूति संबंधी जटिलता
**कृपया सही जवाब पर निशान (✓) लगाएं**

| | | |
|---|---|---|
| क. एपीएच ☐ | ख. एक्लेम्पसिया ☐ | ग. पीआईएच ☐ *(Preg. Induced Hypertension)* |
| घ. रक्त की कमी ☐ | ड. बाधित प्रसव ☐ | च. पीपीएच ☐ |
| छ. एलएससीएस ☐ | ज. शिशु में जन्मजात दोष ☐ | झ. अन्य ☐ |

#### पिछला विवरण
**कृपया सही जवाब पर निशान (✓) लगाएं**

| | | |
|---|---|---|
| क. तपेदिक ☐ | ख. उच्च रक्तदाब ☐ | ग. हृदय रोग ☐ |
| घ. मधुमेह ☐ | ड. दमा ☐ | च. अन्य ☐ |

#### जांच

| सामान्य अवस्था | दिल | फेफड़े | स्तन |
|---|---|---|---|
| | | | |

#### प्रसव पूर्व जांच

| | 1 | 2 | 3 | 4 |
|---|---|---|---|---|
| तिथि | | | | |
| कोई समस्या | | | | |
| पीओजी (सप्ताह) *(Period of Gestation)* | | | | |
| वजन (कि.ग्रा.) | | | | |
| नब्ज की गति | | | | |
| रक्तदाब | | | | |
| पीलापन | | | | |
| सूजन | | | | |
| गोलियां | | | | |

#### उदर जांच

| | | | | |
|---|---|---|---|---|
| भ्रूण की लंबाई सप्ताह/से.मी. | | | | |
| बनावट/गर्भस्थिति | | | | |
| गर्भस्थ शिशु का हिलना-डुलना | सामान्य/ कम/ नहीं | सामान्य/ कम/ नहीं | सामान्य/ कम/ नहीं | सामान्य/ कम/ नहीं |
| गर्भस्थ शिशु की प्रति मिनट हृदय गति | | | | |
| पी/वी यदि किया गया हो | | | | |

#### आवश्यक जांच

| | | | | |
|---|---|---|---|---|
| हीमोग्लोबिन | | | | |
| मूत्र एल्ब्युमिन | | | | |
| मूत्र शर्करा | | | | |
| एन.एन.एम. के हस्ताक्षर | | | | |

रक्त ग्रुप एवं आरएच प्रकार ☐    तिथि ☐ / /

#### वैकल्पिक जांच

गर्भावस्था में मूत्र की जांच ☐    तिथि ☐ / /
एचबीएस एजी ☐    तिथि ☐ / /
*(Hepatitis B Surface Antigen)*
रक्त शर्करा ☐    तिथि ☐ / /

**गांव के निर्धारित मासिक में बच्चा स्वास्थ्य और पोषण दिवस में शामिल हों**

**Mamta Card......**

## High-risk Pregnancy and Intranatal Care

## Postnatal Care

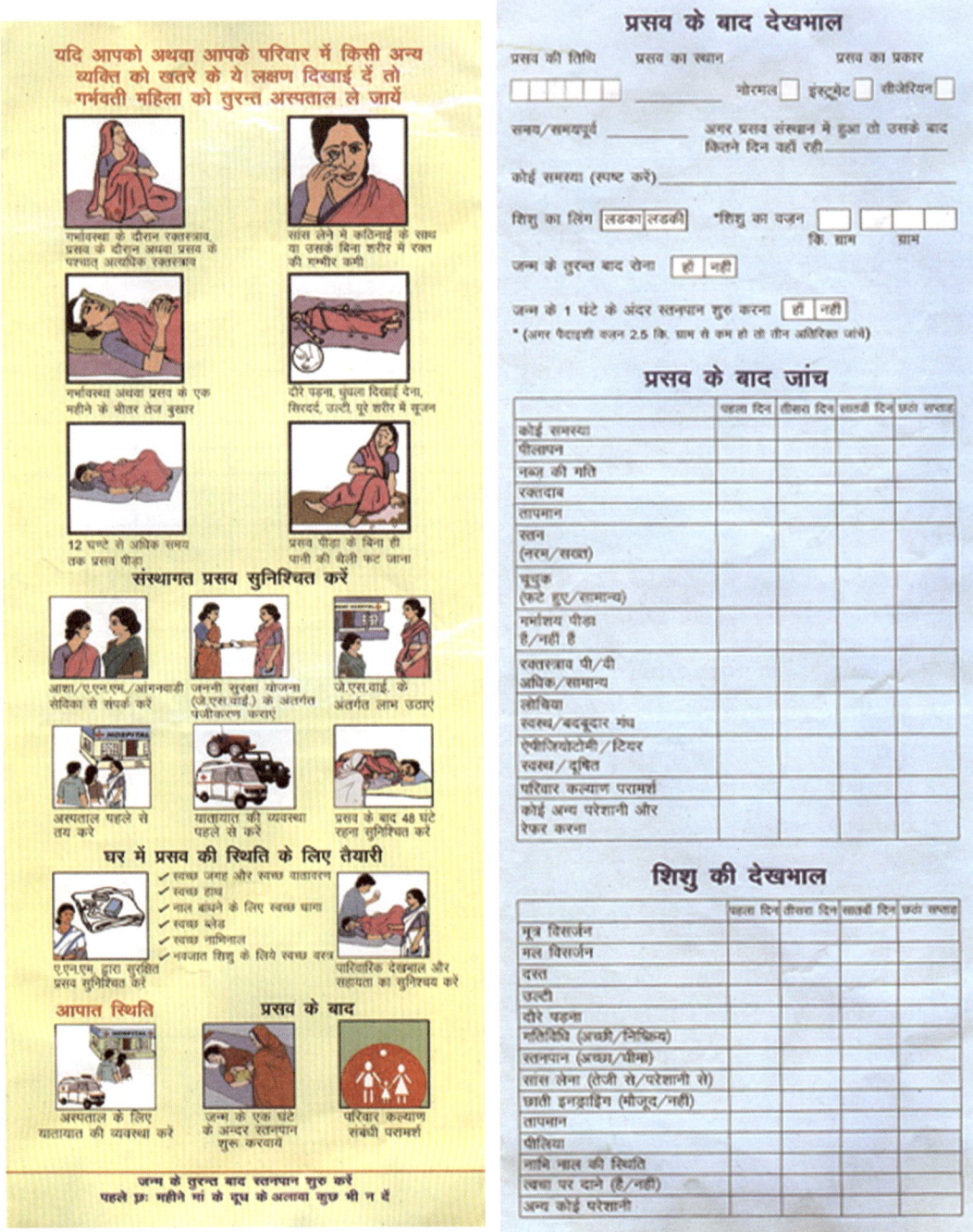

## Mamta Card......

## Newborn Care

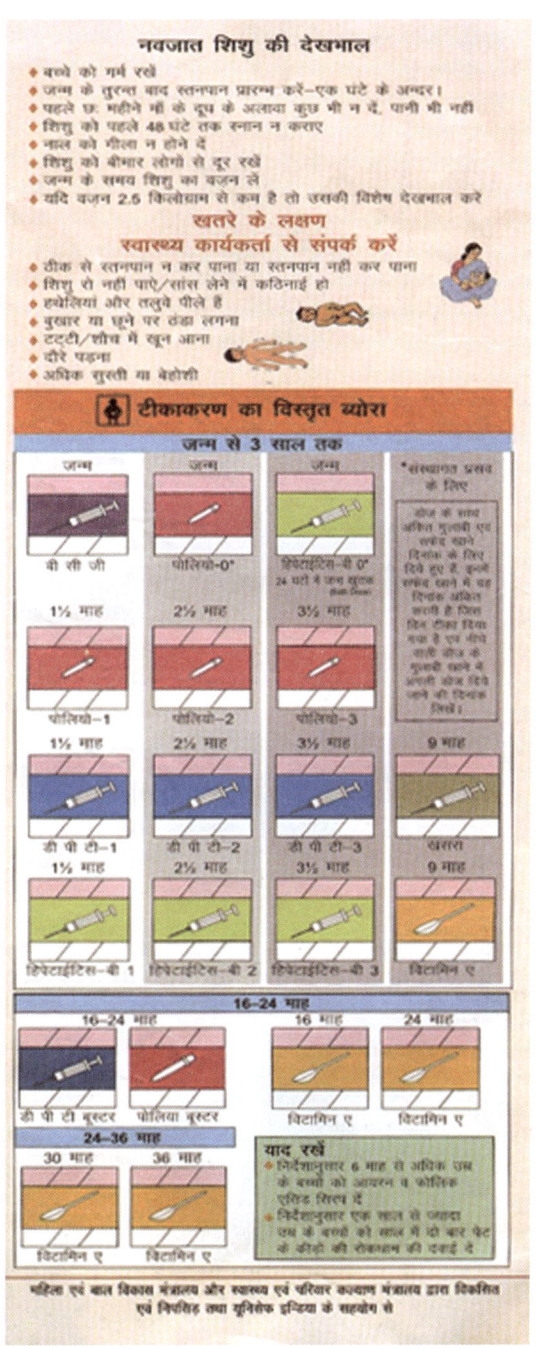

### Mamta Card......
### Infant Care

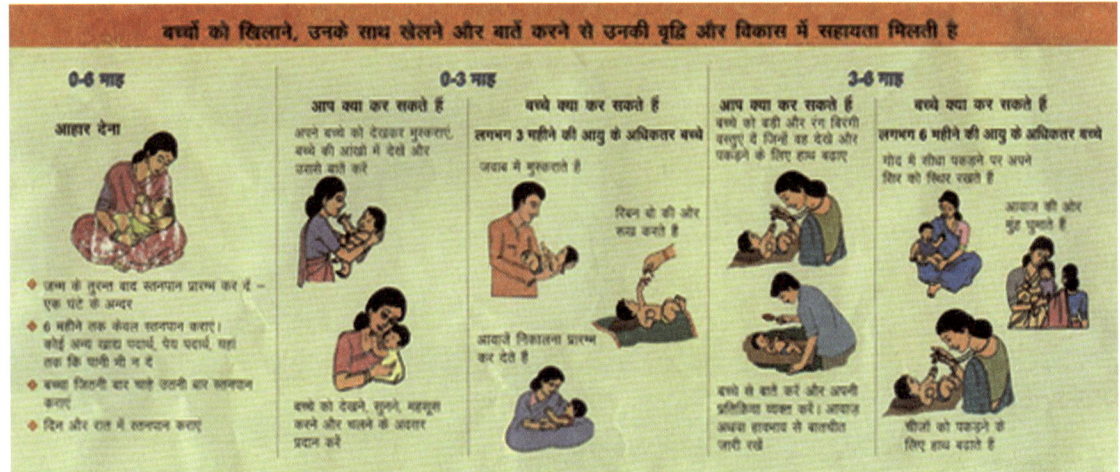

**1st 6 Months**

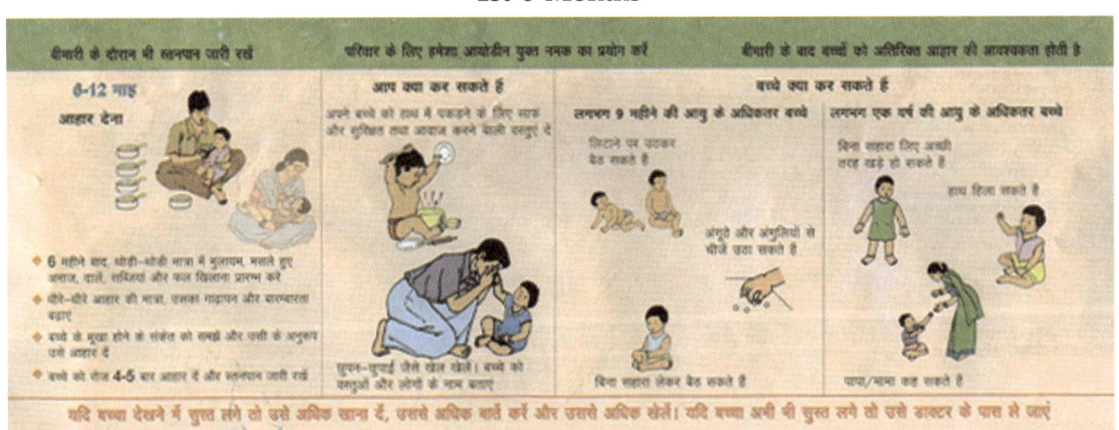

**6 Months to 12 Months**

### Mamta Card......
### Under-five Care

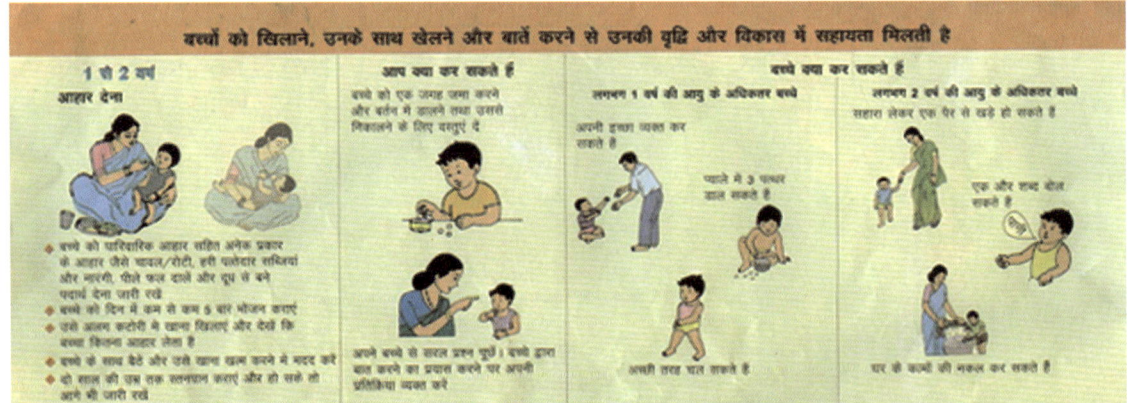

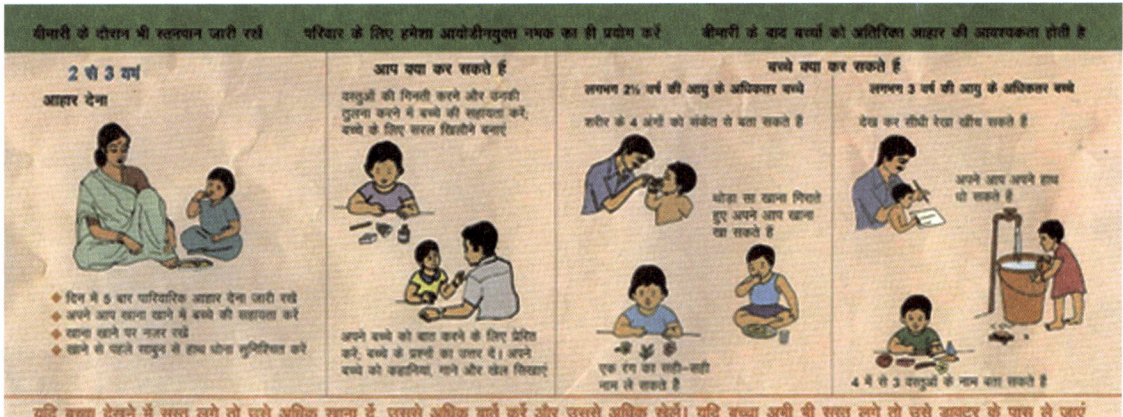

## ORS Packets

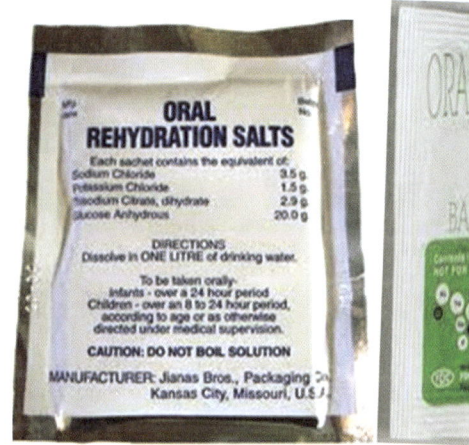

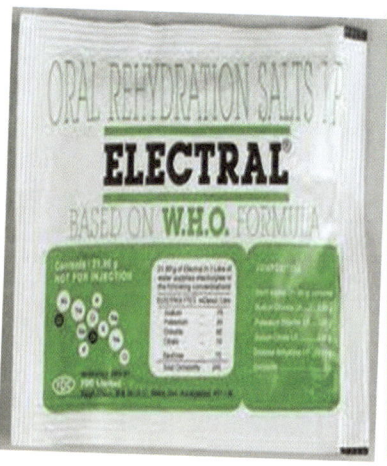

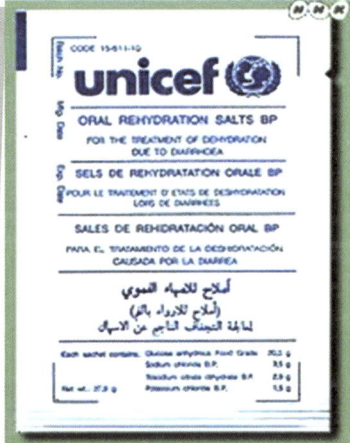

## Road to Health Card

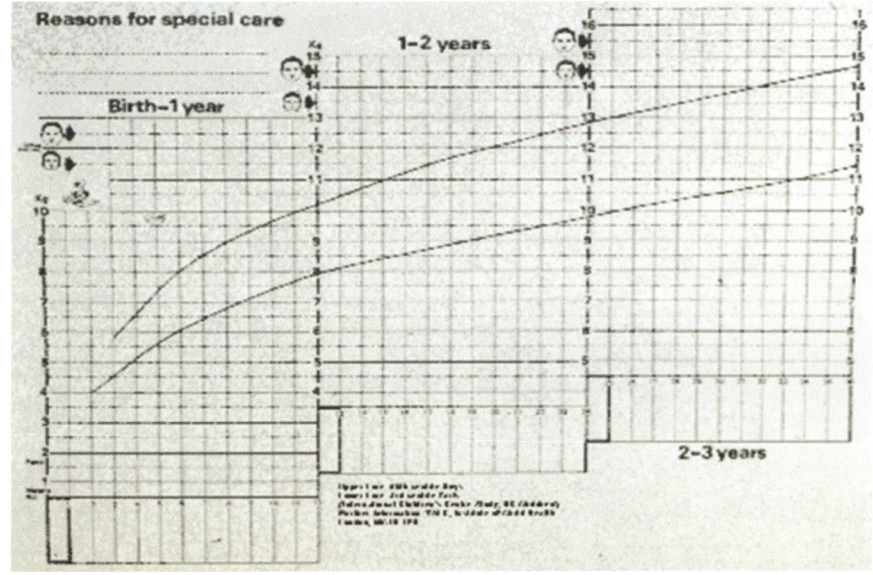

## Partograph

1
2
3
4
5
6
7
8
9
10
11
12

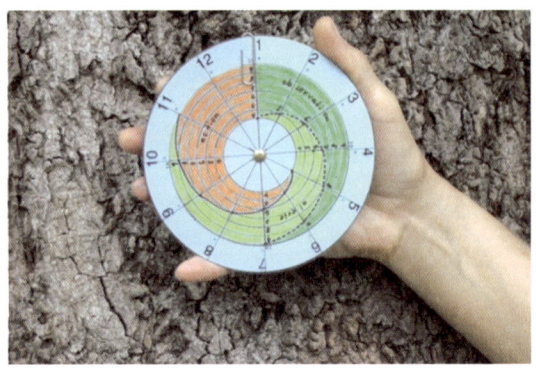

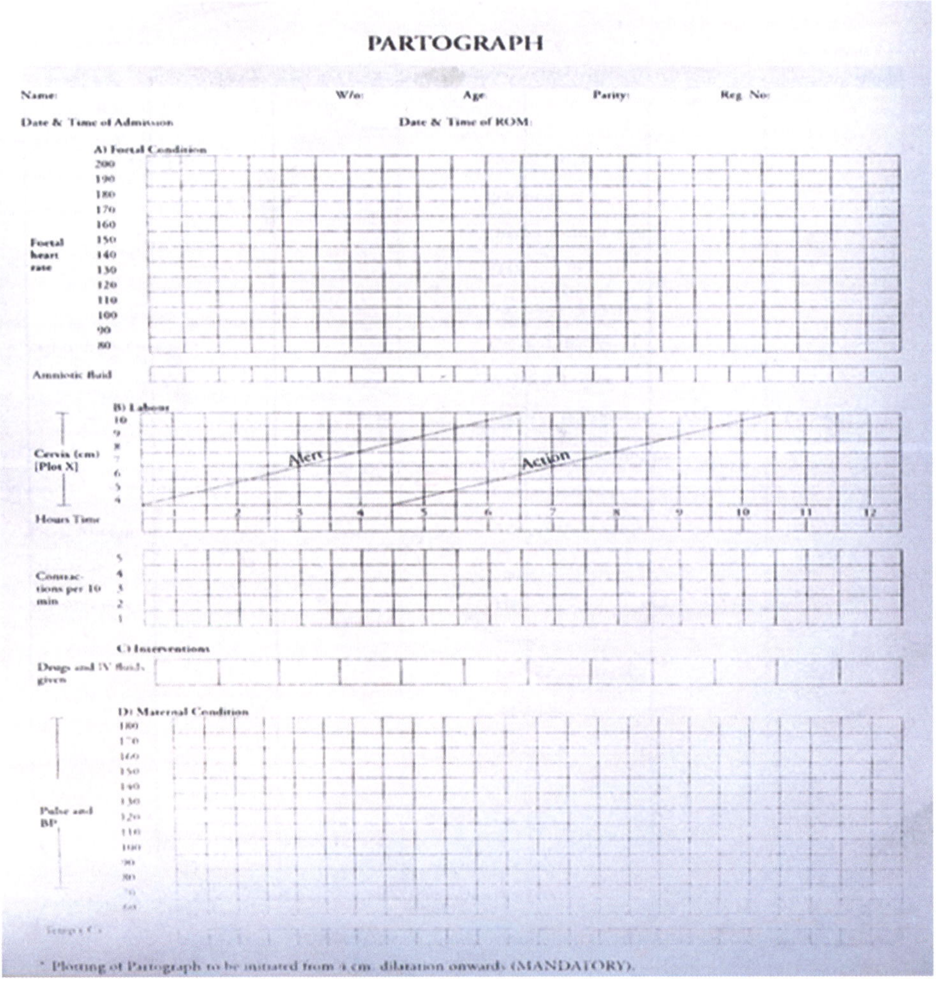
PARTOGRAPH
Name:
W/o:
Age:
Parity:
Reg. No:
Date & Time of Admission
Date & Time of ROM:
A) Foetal Condition
200
190
180
170
160
150
140
130
120
110
100
90
80
Foetal heart rate
Amniotic fluid
B) Labour
10
9
8
7
6
5
4
Cervix (cm) [Plot X]
Alert
Action
Hours Time
1
2
3
4
5
6
7
8
9
10
11
12
5
4
3
2
1
Contractions per 10 min
C) Interventions
Drugs and IV fluids given
D) Maternal Condition
180
170
160
150
140
130
120
110
100
90
80
70
60
Pulse and BP
Temp (°C)
* Plotting of Partograph to be initiated from 4 cm. dilatation onwards (MANDATORY).

# Kishori Card

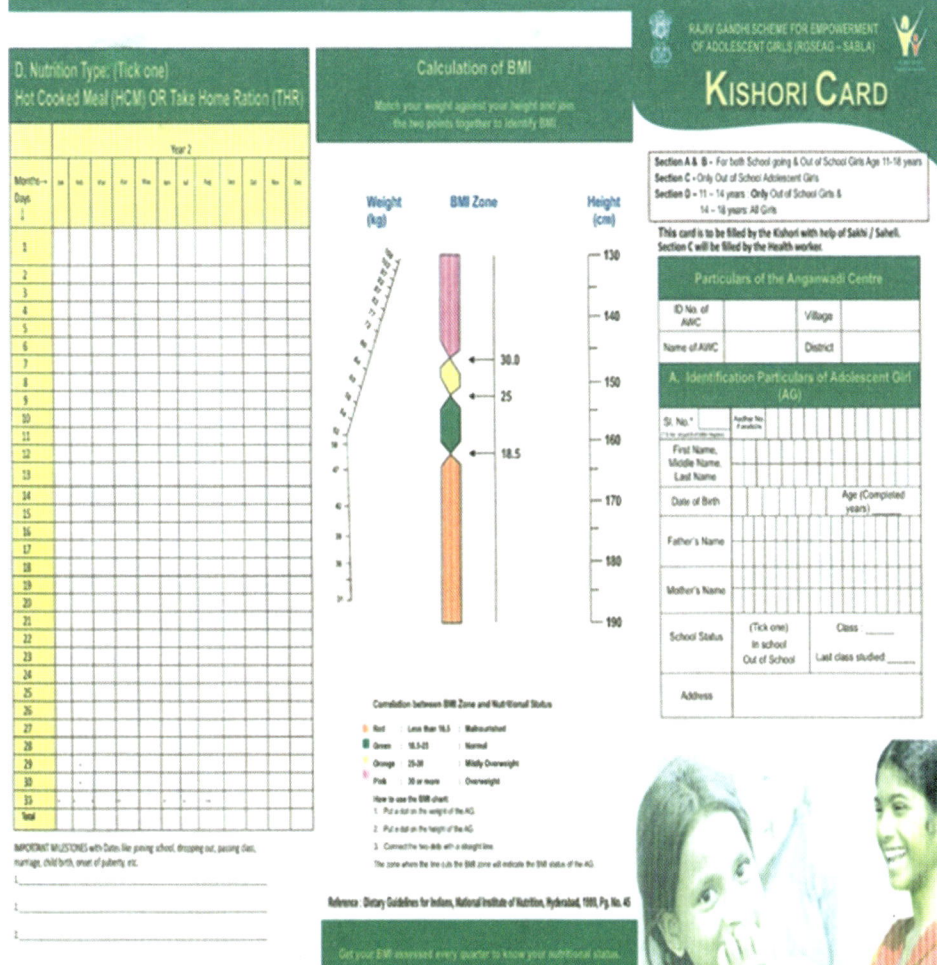

## Immunization Card

| B. Guidance / Counselling Sessions (No. of Sessions attended)** | | | | | |
|---|---|---|---|---|---|
| Quarters | | | Year 1 | | |
| Topic | | | | | |
| Nutrition & Health Education sessions (minimum 2 in a quarter) | | | | | |
| Family Welfare, ARSH & child care practices sessions (minimum 3 in a quarter) | | | | | |
| Life Skill Education sessions (minimum 2 in a quarter) | | | | | |
| Exposure visit (attach details) -post offices, bank,/ police station, etc (minimum 2 to each of them in one year) | | | | | |

| Quarters | Year 2 | | | |
|---|---|---|---|---|
| | 1st (Apr-June) | 2nd (Jul-Sept) | 3rd (Oct-Dec.) | 4th (Jan-Mar.) |
| Topic | | Write date | | |
| Nutrition & Health Education sessions (minimum 2 in a quarter) | | | | |
| Family Welfare, ARSH & child care practices sessions (minimum 3 in a quarter) | | | | |
| Life Skill Education sessions (minimum 2 in a quarter) | | | | |
| Exposure visit (attach details) -post offices, bank/police station, etc (minimum 2 to each of them in one year ) | | | | |

** For each Guidance/ Counselling session attended, put date in the relevant column against the relevant topic.

MESSAGES

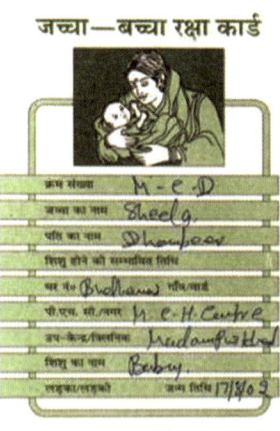

| C. Health Services | | | | | |
|---|---|---|---|---|---|
| Quarters | | | Year 1 | | |
| Date of Health Check-up | | | | | |
| Height (in cms.) | | | | | |
| Weight (in Kgs ) | | | | | |
| BMI *** | | | | | |
| Status: N - Normal M - Malnourished | | | | | |
| No. of IFA Tablets | Provided | | | | |
| | Consumed | | | | |
| Referral Services received | (Write whichever is correct) Yes | | | | |
| | No | | | | |

| Quarters | Year 2 | | | |
|---|---|---|---|---|
| | 1st (Apr-June) | 2nd (Jul-Sept) | 3rd (Oct-Dec.) | 4th (Jan-Mar.) |
| Date of Health Check-up | | | | |
| Height (in cms.) | | | | |
| Weight (in Kgs.) | | | | |
| BMI *** | | | | |
| Status N - Normal M - Malnourished | | | | |
| No. of IFA Tablets | Provided | | | | |
| | Consumed | | | | |
| Referral Services received | (Write whichever is correct) Yes | | | | |
| | No | | | | |

*** Formula : BMI (in kg/m²) = Weight (in kg) ÷ (Height in m)²
(BMI below 18.5 is underweight and BMI between 18.5 & 23.5 is normal – see chart on leaf 6)

D. Nutrition Type: (Tick one)
Hot Cooked Meal (HCM) OR Take Home Ration (THR)

IMPORTANT MILESTONES with Dates like joining school, dropping out, passing class, marriage, child birth, onset of puberty, etc.

1. _____
2. _____
3. _____

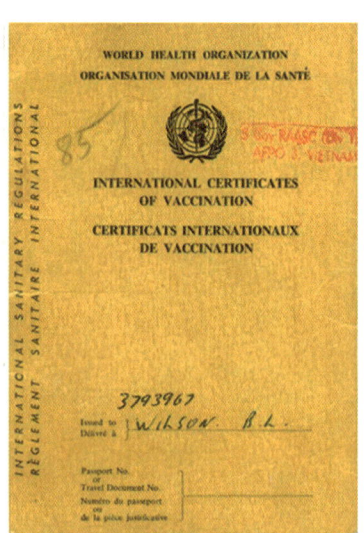

जच्चा—बच्चा रक्षा कार्ड

क्रम संख्या  M-e-D
जच्चा का नाम  Sheela
पति का नाम  Dhorbeer
शिशु होने की सम्भावित तिथि
वार्ड नं (Budhana) गाँव/वार्ड
पी.एम. सी./नगर  H-e-H-Centre
उप-केन्द्र/चिकित्सक  Mudampur Hosp.
शिशु का नाम  Baby
लड़का/लड़की  जन्म तिथि 17/8/02

राष्ट्रीय टीकाकरण मिशन
भारत सरकार

WORLD HEALTH ORGANIZATION
ORGANISATION MONDIALE DE LA SANTÉ

INTERNATIONAL SANITARY REGULATIONS
RÈGLEMENT SANITAIRE INTERNATIONAL

85

INTERNATIONAL CERTIFICATES OF VACCINATION

CERTIFICATS INTERNATIONAUX DE VACCINATION

3793967
Issued to
Délivré à  WILSON. B.L.

Passport No.
or
Travel Document No.
Numéro du passeport
ou
de la pièce justificative

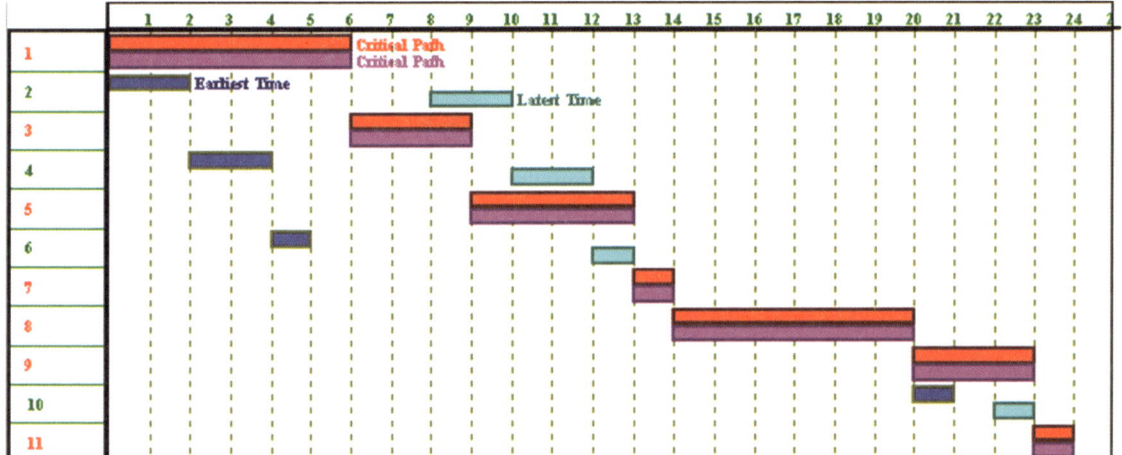

**Gantt Chart**

## Measuring Tools

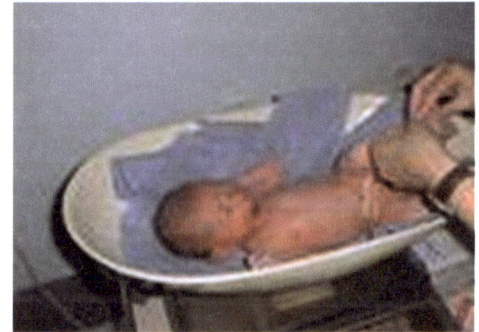

Infant weighing machine

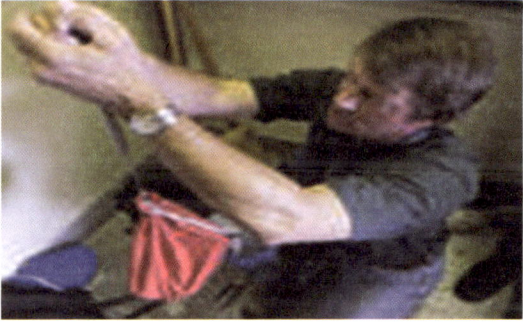

Under-five weighing machine

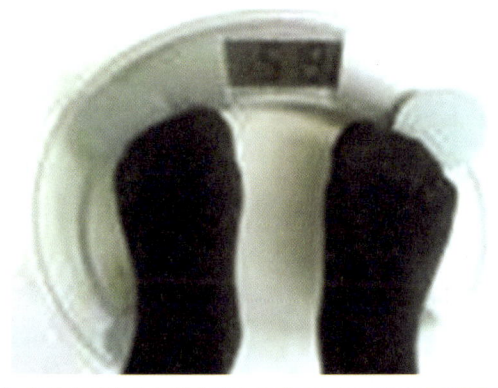

Adult weighing machine

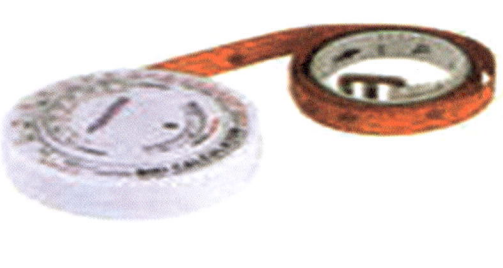

Measuring tape

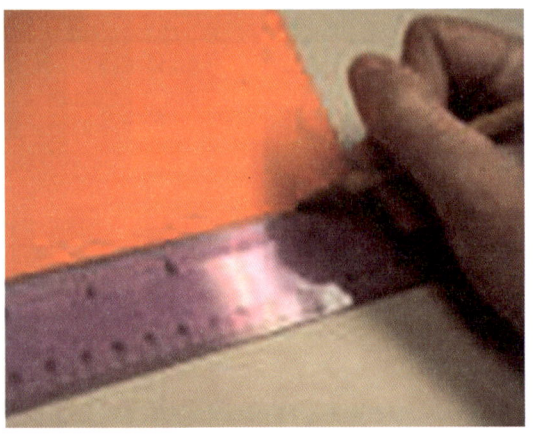

Litre–measuring

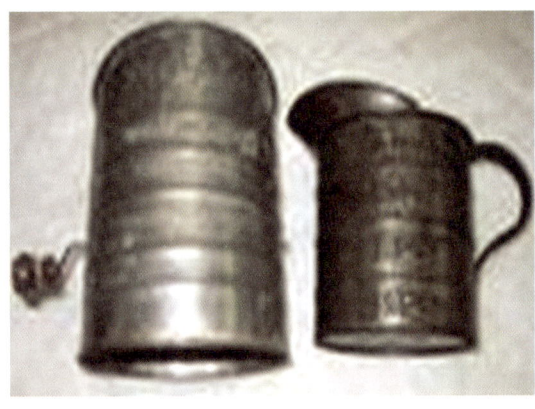

Liquid

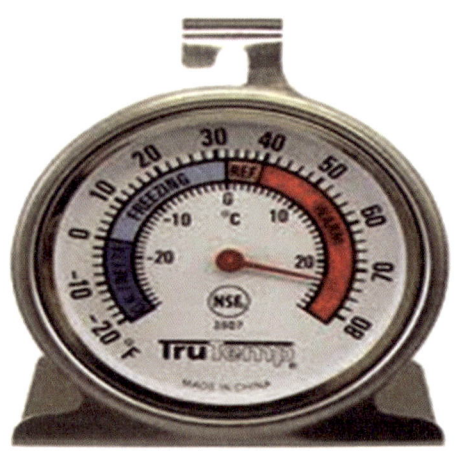

Dial thermometer

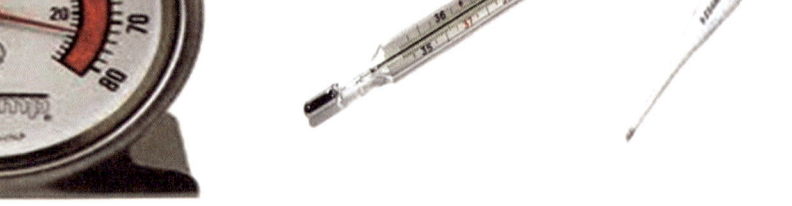

Thermometers

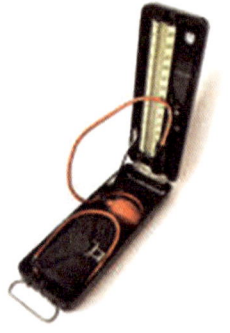

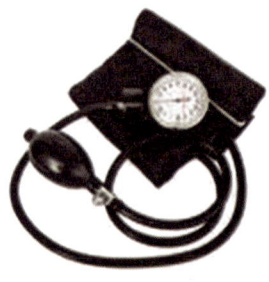

Blood pressure instruments

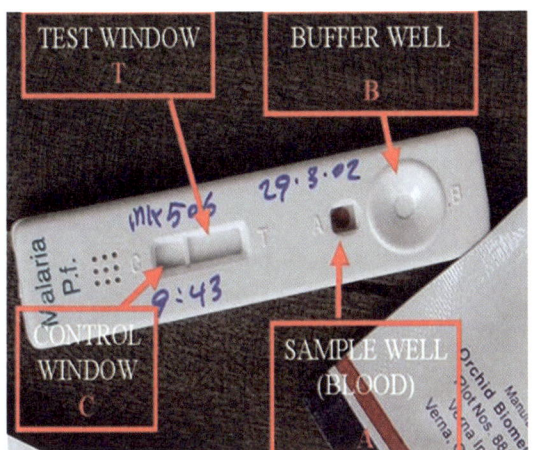

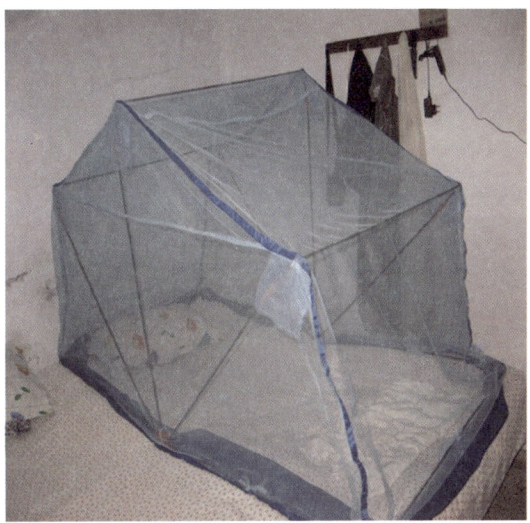

**Malaria rapid test kit**

**Mosquito net**

### Malaria Rapid Test Kit

To test malaria through rapid test.

### Mosquito Net

- Offers protection against mosquito bites during sleep.
- The size of single hole in the net should not be more than 0.0475 inch.
- The numbers of holes in one square inch of net should be 150.
- Use of insecticide treated mosquito net is also available nowadays.

## MOSQUITO REPELLENTS

### Mosquito Coil

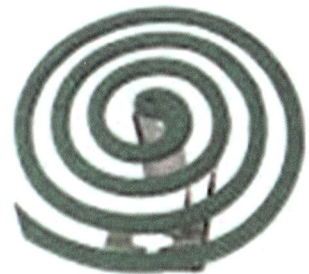

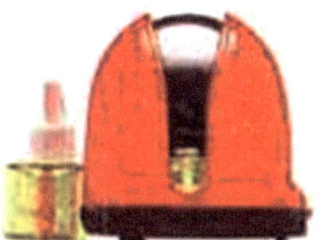

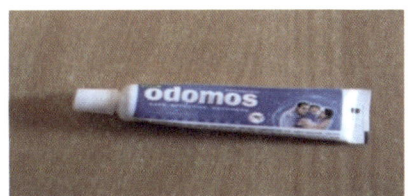

**Mosquito coil**      **Mosquito repellent liquid**      **Mosquito repellent cream**

- Mosquito repellents have insect repellent diethyl benzamide.
- Odomos have insect repellent diethyl benzamide 12%.
- Mosquito coil and mosquito repellent liquid repellent insect through fumes.
- Cream applied on exposed skin.
- It remains active against mosquitoes for 18–20 hours.

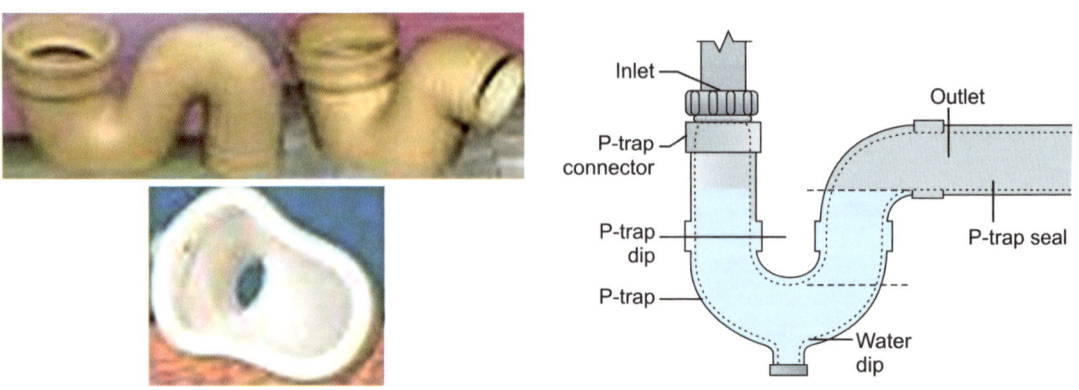

**P-Trap for water closet toilet**

## Miscellaneous Spots

| Name of spot | Public health importance |
|---|---|
| Mamta Card—ANC part | *To monitor ANC |
| Mamta Card—Intranatal part | *To monitor intranatal during delivery |
| Mamta Card—PNC part | *To monitor PNC |
| Mamta Card—Newborn care | *To monitor newborn care |
| Mamta Card—Under five care | *To monitor under-five children |
| Partograph | To monitor labour during intranatal care |
| Kishori card | To monitor health of adolescent girl |
| Road to health | Find out the growth of a child. Early detection of malnutrition, health education about child growth and malnutrition |
| Immunization card | *To monitor vaccination |
| International vaccination certificate | Certificate for vaccination required |
| Gantt chart | Chart showing activities involve with their time schedule in a project |
| Infant weighing machine | To weigh infant to know weight of infant |
| Under-five weighing machine | To weigh under-five children to know weight |
| Adult weighing machine | To weigh adult to know weight |
| Measuring tape | To measure length like mid arm circumference, chest circumference, etc. |
| Measuring liquid | To measure liquid like water, milk, medicine syrup, etc. |
| Thermometer | To measure temperature. Dial thermometer is used to measure temperature in ice-line refrigerator, vaccine carrier, etc. |
| Blood pressure instruments | To measure blood pressure |
| Malaria rapid test kit | To diagnose malaria |
| Mosquito net | It is for personnel protection measure from mosquitoes |

*Contd.*

*Contd.*

| Name of spot | Public health importance |
|---|---|
| Mosquito coil | Mosquito repellents |
| All-out | Mosquito repellents |
| Odomos | Mosquito repellents |
| Horrock's apparatus | Used for finding required amount of bleaching powder for given sample of water |
| P-Trap | Bent pipe used in water seal type of sanitary latrines. It holds water so acts as water seal, so prevent smell and access of flies to faeces |

*Details is given in chapter 'case study and family study'

# 5     Field Visits

## Field Visits

1. Urban health training centre (UHTC)
2. Rural health training centre (RHTC)
3. Anganwari centre
4. Subcentre
5. Primary health centre
6. Community health centre
7. District hospital
8. District tuberculosis centre
9. Integrated counselling and testing centre (ICTC)
10. Hospital waste facility
11. Water filtration plant
12. Sewage treatment plant

Teacher's Remark .........................................
Teacher's Sign .........................................

## Visit to UHTC

Name of UHTC _____            Date _____

Address _____

MOIC name with mobile no _____

Concerned medical college _____

Building: Own/rented

IEC material displayed: Yes/No         Area map displayed: Yes/No

Tour programme of HWs displayed: Yes/No     Suggestion box: Yes/No

| Staff IPHS standard (16) | At present UHTC | Reason of *Problem, if any |
|---|---|---|
| 1 Assisstant Professor Comm. Medicine | | |
| 1 Senior Demonstrator Comm. Medicine | | |
| 1 Medical Officer | | |
| 1 Public Health, Nurse | | |
| 1 Health Assistant, Female | | |
| 1 Health Assistant, Male | | |
| 1 Health Worker, Female | | |
| 1 Health Assistant, Male | | |
| 1 Medical Social Worker | | |
| 1 Laboratory Technician | | |
| 1 IV Class | | |
| 1 Sweeper | | |
| **Physical structure (IPHS standard)** | **At present UHTC** | **Reason of *problem, if any** |
| Centrally located | | |
| Area 73.50 to 100.20 sq. mts | | |
| Waiting area with displays | | |
| Clinic room | | |
| Examination room (1950 × 3000 mm) | | |
| Minor OT | | |
| Laboratory (3800 × 2700 mm) | | |
| General store: Office room | | |
| Immunization/FP/counselling area | | |
| Toilet (1950 × 1200 mm) | | |
| **Support services (IPHS standard)** | **At present UHTC** | **Reason of *problem, if any** |
| Electricity | | |
| Water | | |
| Telephone | | |
| **Record maintenance (IPHS standard)** | **At present UHTC** | **Reason of *problem, if any** |
| ANC register | | |

*Contd.*

*Contd.*

| Record maintenance (IPHS standard) | At present UHTC | Reason of *problem, if any |
|---|---|---|
| PNC register | | |
| Eligible couple register | | |
| Target couple register | | |
| Infant register | | |
| Under-five register | | |
| Family planning register | | |
| Family survey register | | |
| Outdoor register | | |
| Stock and issue register | | |
| Training register | | |
| Laboratory register | | |
| Field visit register | | |
| Supervisory visit register | | |

*Problem is the difference between what is required and what is present.

## Last Year's Performance

| Variable | Estimated | Achieved | Reason of *problem, if any |
|---|---|---|---|
| Pregnancy registration | | | |
| ANC visit | | | |
| PNC visit | | | |
| Eligible couple | | | |
| BCG vaccination | | | |
| OPV vaccination | | | |
| DPT vaccination | | | |
| Measles vaccination | | | |
| TT Pregnant vaccination | | | |
| Patients seen | | | |
| Referred patient | | | |
| Trainings conducted of MBBS students | | | |
| Trainings conducted of interns | | | |
| Trainings conducted of MD (Comm. Med.) | | | |

*Problem is the difference between what is required and what is present.

Brief conclusive descriptive notes: _____

**Teacher's Remark** .........................................
**Teacher's Signature** .........................................

## Visit to RHTC

Name of RHTC _____         Date _____

Address _____

MOIC name with mobile no _____

Concerned medical college _____

Building: Own/rented

IEC material displayed: Yes/No         Area map displayed: Yes/No

Tour programme of HWs displayed: Yes/No         Suggestion box: Yes/No

| Staff IPHS Standard (16) | At present RHTC | Reason of *Problem if any |
|---|---|---|
| 1 Assisstant Professor Comm. Medicine | | |
| 1 Senior Demonstrator Comm. Medicine | | |
| 1 Medical Officer | | |
| 1 Public Health, Nurse | | |
| 1 Health Assistant, Female | | |
| 1 Health Assistant, Male | | |
| 1 Health Worker, Female | | |
| 1 Health Assistant, Male | | |
| 1 Medical Social Worker | | |
| 1 Laboratory Technician | | |
| 1 Driver | | |
| 2 IV Class | | |
| 2 Sweepers | | |
| **Physical structure (IPHS standard)** | **At present RHTC** | **Reason of *problem, if any** |
| Centrally located | | |
| Area 73.50 to 100.20 sq.mts | | |
| Waiting area with displays | | |
| Labour room (3800 × 4200 mm) | | |
| Clinic room (3300 × 3300 mm) | | |
| Examination room (1950 × 3000 mm) | | |
| Wards 5.5 × 3.5 m each (4–6 beds) | | |
| Minor OT | | |
| Laboratory (3800 × 2700 mm) | | |
| General store | | |

*Contd.*

*Contd.*

| Physical structure (IPHS standard) | At present RHTC | Reason of *problem, if any |
|---|---|---|
| Immunization/FP/counselling areas | | |
| Office room 3500 × 3000 mm | | |
| Dirty utility room | | |
| Boundary wall with gate | | |
| Toilet (1950 × 1200 mm) | | |
| Residential accommodation for staff | | |
| 2 Residential accommodations for interns, separate for girls and boys | | |
| **Support services (IPHS standard)** | **At present RHTC** | **Reason of *problem, if any** |
| Electricity with generator backup | | |
| Water | | |
| Telephone | | |
| Garden (optional) | | |
| **Record maintenance (IPHS standard)** | **At present RHTC** | **Reason of *problem, if any** |
| ANC register | | |
| Deliveries conducted at centre register | | |
| Deliveries assisted by HWF register | | |
| PNC register | | |
| Family survey register | | |
| Eligible couple register | | |
| Target couple register | | |
| Infant register | | |
| Under-five register | | |
| Family planning register | | |
| Outdoor register | | |
| Notifiable disease register | | |
| Malaria blood smear register | | |
| Stock and issue register | | |
| Training register | | |
| Field visit register | | |
| Supervisory visit register | | |

*Problem is the difference between what is required and what is present.

## Last Year's Performance

| Variable | Estimated | Achieved | Reason of *problem, if any |
|---|---|---|---|
| Pregnancy registration | | | |
| ANC visits | | | |
| Deliveries conducted/assisted | | | |
| Referred pregnancy PNC visit | | | |
| Eligible couple | | | |
| BCG vaccination | | | |
| OPV vaccination | | | |
| DPT vaccination | | | |
| Measles vaccination | | | |
| TT pregnant vaccination | | | |
| Patient seen | | | |
| Referred patient | | | |

Brief conclusive descriptive notes: _____

**Teacher's Remark** ........................................

**Teacher's Signature** ........................................

## Visit to Aganwadi Centre

Name of Anganwadi Centre _____          Date _____

Address _____

Name of AWW with mobile no _____

Name of *Mahila Supervisior* with mobile no _____

Concerned ICDS Block _____

Building: Own/Rented

No. of rooms: 1 | 2 | 3 | > 3

IEC material displayed: Yes/No          Suggestion box: Yes/No _____

| Staff IPHS standard | At present AWC | Reason of *problem, if any |
|---|---|---|
| AWW | | |
| Helper | | |
| @Optional worker ASHA | | |

*Contd.*

Contd.

| Physical structure | At present AWC | Reason of *problem, if any |
|---|---|---|
| Centrally located | | |
| Pre-school education room | | |
| Examination room | | |
| Cooking supplementary nutrition room | | |
| Toilet | | |
| Support services | | |
| Laboratory—Diastix | | |
| Laboratory—Uristix | | |
| Supplementry food | | |
| Cooking utensils | | |
| Utensil for SN distribution | | |
| Electricity | | |
| Water | | |

*Problem is the difference between what is required and what is present

@optional worker is for coordination from NRHM

| Record maintain IPHS standard | At present SC | Reason of *problem, if any |
|---|---|---|
| ANC register | | |
| Eligible couple register | | |
| Lactating women register | | |
| Infant register | | |
| 1 to 3 years child register | | |
| 3 to 6 years child register | | |
| Supplementary nutrition stock register | | |
| *Poshahar Vitran* register | | |
| Pre-school enrolment register | | |
| Malnutrition child register | | |
| ANM visit register | | |
| Health check-up register | | |
| Referred cases register | | |
| Supervisory visit register | | |

## Last year's performance

| Variable | Estimated | Achieved | Reason of *problem, if any |
|---|---|---|---|
| ANC registration | | | |
| Eligible couple | | | |
| Infant registered | | | |
| 1 to 3 years child registered | | | |
| 3 to 6 years child registered | | | |
| Supplementary nutrition stock (months) | 3 Months | | |
| Immunization complete for age | | | |
| Under weight | | | |
| Malnutrition (> 2 SD but < 3 SD) | | | |
| Malnutrition (> 3 SD) | | | |
| *Poshahar vitran* | | | |
| Pre-school enrolled | | | |
| ANM visits | | | |
| TT pregnant vaccination | | | |
| Supervisory visits | | | |
| Referred cases | | | |

Brief conclusive descriptive notes: _____

**Teacher's Remark** .........................................

**Teacher's Signature** .........................................

## Visit to Subcentre

Name of SC _____          Date _____
Address _____
Name of in charge with mobile no _____
Concerned PHC _____          Concerned CMHO Office at _____
Building: Own/rented          No. of rooms:
IEC material displayed: Yes/No          Area map displayed: Yes/No
Tour programme of HWs displayed: Yes/No          Suggestion box: Yes/No

| Staff IPHS standard | At present SC | Reason of *problem, if any |
|---|---|---|
| 2 Health worker, female | | |
| Health worker, male | | |
| @Optional worker | | |
| **Physical structure IPHS standard** | **At present SC** | **Reason of *problem, if any** |
| Centrally located | | |

*Contd.*

Contd.

| | | |
|---|---|---|
| Area 73.50 to 100.20 sq. mts | | |
| Waiting area 3300 × 2700 mm) with displayes | | |
| Labour Room (4050 × 3000 mm) | | |
| Clinic Room (3300 × 3300 mm) | | |
| Examination room (1950 × 3000 mm) | | |
| Toilet (1950 × 1200mm) | | |
| Residential accommodation | | |
| Support services IPHS standard | | |
| Laboratory—Diastix | | |
| Laboratory—Uristix | | |
| Electricity | | |
| Water | | |
| Telephone | | |
| Transport | | |
| Monitoring TBA, VHG and ASHA | | |

*problem is the difference between what is required and what is present.
@Optional worker is for cleanliness of centre and is paid ₹ 100/month by ANM from contingency fund.

| Record maintain IPHS standard | At present SC | Reason of *problem, if any |
|---|---|---|
| ANC Register | | |
| Deliveries conducted at centre register | | |
| Deliveries assisted by HWF register | | |
| PNC register | | |
| Eligible couple register | | |
| Target couple register | | |
| Infant register | | |
| Under-five register | | |
| Family planning register | | |
| Outdoor register | | |
| Notifiable disease register | | |
| Malaria blood smear register | | |
| Stock and issue register | | |
| Training register | | |
| Dai's register | | |
| Field visit register | | |
| Supervisory visit register | | |

## Last Year's Performance

| Variable | Estimated | Achieved | Reason of *problem, if any |
|---|---|---|---|
| Pregnancy registration | | | |
| ANC visit | | | |
| Deliveries conducted/assisted | | | |
| Referred pregnancy | | | |
| PNC visit | | | |
| Eligible couple | | | |
| BCG vaccination | | | |
| OPV vaccination | | | |
| DPT vaccination | | | |
| Measles vaccination | | | |
| TT pregnant vaccination | | | |
| Patient seen | | | |
| Referred patient | | | |

Brief conclusive descriptive notes: _____

**Teacher's Remark** .......................................

**Teacher's Signature** .......................................

### Visit to PHC

Name of PHC                                                        Date _____

Address _____

MOIC name with mobile no _____

Concerned CMHO Office at _____

Building: own/rented

IEC material Displayed: Yes/No                    Area map displayed: Yes/No

Tour programme of HWs displayed: Yes/No                    Suggestion box: Yes/No

| Staff IPHS standard (16) | At present PHC | Reason of *problem, if any |
|---|---|---|
| 2 Medical Officer | | |
| 1 Nurse – Midwife | | |
| 1 Block Extension Educator | | |
| 1 Health Assistant, Female | | |
| 1 Health Assistant, Male | | |
| 1 Health Worker, Female | | |

*Contd.*

*Contd.*

| 1 Health Assistant, Male | | |
|---|---|---|
| 1 Upper Division Clerk | | |
| 1 Lower Division Clerk | | |
| 1 Laboratory Technician | | |
| 1 Driver | | |
| 4 IV Class | | |
| **Physical structure IPHS standard** | **At present PHC** | **Reason of \*problem, if any** |
| Centrally located | | |
| Area 73.50 to 100.20 sq. mts | | |
| Waiting area (3300 × 2700 mm) with displayes | | |
| Labour room (3800 × 4200 mm) | | |
| Clinic room (3300 × 3300 mm) | | |
| Examination room (1950 × 3000 mm) | | |
| Wards 5.5 × 3.5 m each (4–6 beds) | | |
| Minor OT | | |
| OT (optional) | | |
| Laboratory (3800 × 2700 mm) | | |
| General store: | | |
| Immunization/FP/counselling area: | | |
| 3000 × 4000 mm | | |
| Office room 3500 × 3000 mm | | |
| Dirty utility room | | |
| Boundary wall with gate | | |
| Toilet (1950 × 1200 mm) | | |
| Residential accommodation | | |
| **Support services IPHS standard** | **At present PHC** | **Reason of \*problem, if any** |
| Electricity with generator backup | | |
| Water | | |
| Telephone | | |
| Transport | | |
| Garden (optional) | | |
| **Record maintain IPHS standard** | **At present PHC** | **Reason of \*problem, if any** |
| ANC register | | |
| Deliveries conducted at centre register | | |
| Deliveries assisted by HWF register | | |

*Contd.*

*Contd.*

| | | |
|---|---|---|
| PNC register | | |
| Eligible couple register | | |
| Target couple register | | |
| Infant register | | |
| Under-five register | | |
| Family planning register | | |
| Outdoor register | | |
| Notifiable disease register | | |
| Malaria blood smear register | | |
| Stock and issue register | | |
| Training register | | |
| Dais' register | | |
| Field visit register | | |
| Supervisory visit register | | |

*Problem is the difference between what is required and what is present.

## Last Year's Performance

| Variable | Estimated | Achieved | Reason of *problem, if any |
|---|---|---|---|
| Pregnancy registration | | | |
| ANC visit | | | |
| Deliveries conducted/assisted | | | |
| Referred pregnancy | | | |
| PNC visit | | | |
| Eligible couple | | | |
| BCG vaccination | | | |
| OPV vaccination | | | |
| DPT vaccination | | | |
| Measles vaccination | | | |
| TT pregnant vaccination | | | |
| Patient seen | | | |
| Referred patient | | | |

Brief conclusive descriptive notes: _____

**Teacher's Remark** ...........................................

**Teacher's Signature** ...........................................

## Visit to CHC

Name of CHC _____          Date _____

Address _____

MOIC name with mobile no _____

Concerned CMHO office at _____

Building: Own/Rented

IEC material displayed: Yes/No          Area map displayed: Yes/No

Pharmacy for drug dispensing and storage: Yes/No          Registration counters: Yes/No

Facilities displayed: Yes/No          Suggestion box: Yes/No

| Staff IPHS standard (31) | At present CHC | Reason of *problem, if any |
|---|---|---|
| 1 General surgeon(MS/DNB Gen Surg.) | | |
| 1 General physician (MD/DNB Gen Med.) | | |
| 1 Gynaecologist (MS/DNB Gynae.) | | |
| 1 Paediatrician (MD/DNB/DCh Paed.) | | |
| 1 Anaesthetic (MD/DNB/DA Anaesthesia) | | |
| 1 Block surveillance officer (MD/DPH ) | | |
| 1 Eye surgeon (MS/DNB Ophth) | | |
| 1 Ophthalmic assistant | | |
| 7 Staff nurse | | |
| 1 PHN | | |
| 1 ANM | | |
| 1 Laboratory technician | | |
| 1 Radiographer | | |
| 1 Pharmacist/computer | | |
| 1 Clerk | | |
| 4 (as per need) Data entry operater /stastistical assistant/OT attendent/OPD attendent/ chaukidar/mali/dresser | | |
| 1 Dhobi | | |
| 2 Ward boys | | |
| 3 Sweepers | | |

*Problem is the difference between what is required and what is present

| Physical structure IPHS standard | At present CHC | Reason of *problem, if any |
|---|---|---|
| Centrally located | | |
| Waiting area with displayes | | |
| 6 OPDs | | |
| 1 Emergency/casualty room | | |
| 2 Wards (separate for males and females) | | |
| Minor OT | | |
| OT with associated facilities | | |
| Laboratory (3800 × 2700 mm) | | |
| CSSD (sterilization and sterile store) | | |
| General store | | |
| Immunization/counselling area | | |
| Office room (3500 × 3000 mm) | | |
| Dirty utility room | | |
| Boundary wall with gate | | |
| 2 Toilets (1950 mm × 1200 mm) | | |
| Residential accommodation | | |
| **Support services IPHS standard** | **At present CHC** | **Reason of *problem, if any** |
| Electricity with generator backup | | |
| Laundry | | |
| Water | | |
| Telephone | | |
| Transport | | |
| Garden | | |
| **Record maintain IPHS standard** | **At present CHC** | **Reason of *problem, if any** |
| ANC register | | |
| Deliveries conducted at centre register | | |
| Deliveries Assisted by HWF register | | |
| PNC register | | |
| Eligible couple register | | |
| Target couple register | | |
| Infant register | | |
| Under-five register | | |

*Contd.*

*Contd.*

| | | |
|---|---|---|
| Family planning register | | |
| Outdoor register | | |
| Notifiable disease register | | |
| Malaria blood smear register | | |
| Stock and issue register | | |
| Training register | | |
| Dais' register | | |
| Field visit register | | |
| Supervisory visit register | | |

*Problem is the difference between what is required and what is present

## Last year's Performance

| Variable | Estimated | Achieved | Reason of *problem, if any |
|---|---|---|---|
| Pregnancy registration | | | |
| ANC visit | | | |
| Deliveries conducted/assisted | | | |
| Referred pregnancy | | | |
| PNC visit | | | |
| Eligible couple | | | |
| BCG vaccination | | | |
| OPV vaccination | | | |
| DPT vaccination | | | |
| Measles vaccination | | | |
| TT Pregnant vaccination | | | |
| Patient seen | | | |
| Referred patient | | | |

Brief descriptive notes: _____

Teacher's Remark .........................................

Teacher's Signature .........................................

## Visit to District Hospital

Name of district hospital _____          Date _____

Address _____

PMO name with mobile no _____

Concerned CMHO office at _____

Building: Own/Rented

IEC material displayed: Yes/No          Area map displayed: Yes/No

Pharmacy for drug dispensing and storage: Yes/No   Registration counters: Yes/No

Facilities displayed: Yes/No          HMC: Yes/No

Hospital waste facility: Yes/No          If Yes, What...............

Citizen charter: Yes/No Suggestion box: Yes/No

| Staff IPHS standard (60) | At Present DH (300 Beded) | Reason of *problem, if any |
|---|---|---|
| 1 Hospital superintendent (PMO) | | |
| 3 Medical specialist | | |
| 3 Surgery specialists | | |
| 6 O and G specialists | | |
| 3 Paediatricians | | |
| 2 ENT Surgeons | | |
| 2 Orthopaedician | | |
| 2 Opthalmologists | | |
| 6 Anaesthetists | | |
| 1 Psychiatrist | | |
| 1 Dermatologist | | |
| 1 Radiologist | | |
| 2 Pathologists | | |
| 1 Microbiologist | | |
| 20 Casualty doctors | | |
| 1 Dental surgeon | | |
| 1 Forensic expert | | |
| 1 Public health manager | | |
| 4 AYUSH physician[2] | | |
| **Paramedical staff (total 207)** | **At present** | **Reason of *problem, if any** |
| 100 Staff nurses | | |
| 30 Hospital workers (OP/ward + OT + blood bank) | | |

*Contd.*

*Contd.*

| Paramedical Staff (Total 207) | At present | Reason of *problem, if any |
|---|---|---|
| 20 Sanitary workers | | |
| 2 Ophthalmic assistants | | |
| 2 Social workers/counsellors | | |
| 1 Cytotechnician | | |
| 1 ECG technician | | |
| 1 ECHO technician | | |
| 1 PFT technician | | |
| 1 Audiometrician | | |
| 12 Laboratory technicians ( lab + blood bank) | | |
| 4 Laboratory attendants (hospital worker) | | |
| 1 Dietician | | |
| 4 Maternity assistants (ANM) | | |
| 3 Radiographers | | |
| 2 Dark room assistants | | |
| 8 Pharmacists | | |
| 2 Physiotherapists | | |
| 8 Matrons | | |
| 1 Statistical assistant | | |
| 2 Medical records officers | | |
| 1 Electrician | | |
| 1 Plumber | | |
| Administrative staff (28) | At present | Reason of *problem, if any |
| 1 Manager | | |
| 1 Junior administrative officer | | |
| 2 Office superintendents | | |
| 2 Office assistants | | |
| 5 Assistants | | |
| 3 Junior assistants/typists | | |
| 1 Accountant | | |
| 3 Record clerks | | |
| 2 Computer operators | | |
| 2 Drivers | | |
| 2 Peons | | |
| 2 Security staff | | |

*Contd.*

*Contd.*

| Operation theatre staff (26) | At present | Reason of *problem, if any |
|---|---|---|
| 11 Staff nurses | | |
| 10 OT assistants | | |
| 5 Sweepers | | |
| **Blood bank/storage staff** | **At present** | **Reason of *problem, if any** |
| 5 Staff nurses | | |
| 2 Male nursing assistants (MNA)/FNA | | |
| 1 Lab technician | | |
| 2 Sweepers | | |
| **Physical structure IPHS standard** | **At present DH** | **Reason of *problem, if any** |
| Area of 65–85 m$^2$ per bed | | |
| Circulation areas (3.5 m height) | | |
| OPD block | | |
| Waiting area with displays | | |
| 6 OPDs | | |
| 1 Emergency/casualty room | | |
| 1 Nursing station | | |
| Blood bank | | |
| Pharmacy | | |
| Physiotherapy | | |
| Diagnostic block | | |
| Clinical laboratory | | |
| Imaging/radiodiagnosis | | |
| ICU ward | | |
| Nurses station | | |
| Indoor block | | |
| 2 Wards (separate for male and female) | | |
| OT block | | |
| Minor OT | | |
| 3 OT with associated facilities | | |
| Delivery suite unit | | |
| Labour room | | |
| Neonatal room | | |
| Others | | |

*Contd.*

*Contd.*

| | | |
|---|---|---|
| Hospital kitchen | | |
| CSSD (sterilization and sterile store) | | |
| General store | | |
| Immunization/counselling area | | |
| Trauma centre | | |
| Medical gas room | | |
| Seminar room | | |
| Administrative block | | |
| Office rooms | | |
| **Support services IPHS standard** | **At present DH** | **Reason of *problem, if any** |
| Electricity with generator backup | | |
| Equipment room | | |
| Laundry | | |
| Water | | |
| Dirty utility room | | |
| Boundary wall with gate | | |
| 2 Toilet (1950 × 1200 mm) | | |
| Residential accommodation | | |
| Telephone with intercom | | |
| Garden | | |
| Parking | | |

*Problem is the difference between what is required and what is present.

Brief descriptive notes: _____

**Teacher's Remark** ........................................

**Teacher's Signature** ........................................

**Visit to Integrated Counselling and Test Centre (ICTC)**

Name of centre _____          Date of visit: _____

Address of the centre: _____

Name of MOIC with mobile no _____

Building: Own/rented

No. of rooms:

IEC material displayed: Yes/No          Suggestion box: Yes/No

| Staff | At present ICTC | Reason of *problem, if any |
|---|---|---|
| MOIC | | |
| MO | | |
| Technician | | |
| Counsellor male | | |
| Counsellor female | | |

| Services | At present ICTC | Reason of *problem, if any |
|---|---|---|
| Detection of STI/HIV | | |
| Counselling | | |
| Pretest counselling | | |
| Post-test counselling | | |
| Reactive counselling | | |
| Non-reactive counselling | | |
| Beneficiaries | | |
| Person for STI/HIV testing | | |

| Physical structure | At present ICTC | Reason of *problem, if any |
|---|---|---|
| Waiting area with displays | | |
| Sitting arrangements | | |
| Counselling room | | |
| Health education room with TV and video room, health education material | | |
| Toilet (1950 × 1200 mm) | | |

| Support services | At present ICTC | Reason of *problem, if any |
|---|---|---|
| Electricity | | |
| Water | | |
| Toilet | | |

| Records | At present ICTC | Reason of *problem, if any |
|---|---|---|
| HIV test register with codes | | |
| HIV test result register with codes | | |
| Pretest counselling register | | |
| Post-test counselling register | | |
| Reactive counselling register | | |
| Non-reactive counselling register | | |

*Problem is the difference between what is required and what is present.

## Last Year's Performance

| Variable | Estimated | Achieved | Reason of *problem, if any |
|---|---|---|---|
| Voluntary reported | | | |
| Referred by parent/spouse HIV Pt | | | |
| Patients of other departments | | | |
| Victims of sex abuse | | | |

*Contd.*

*Contd.*

| | | | | |
|---|---|---|---|---|
| Homosexuals | | | | |
| Commercial sex workers | | | | |
| Risk behaviour group | | | | |
| Number of clients counselled by one counsellor | | | | |
| Number of counselling | | | | |
| Sessions per day per counsellor | | | | |

Brief conclusive descriptive notes: _____

Teacher's Remark ...........................................

Teacher's Signature ...........................................

## VISIT TO HOSPITAL WASTE FACILITIES

### Autoclaves

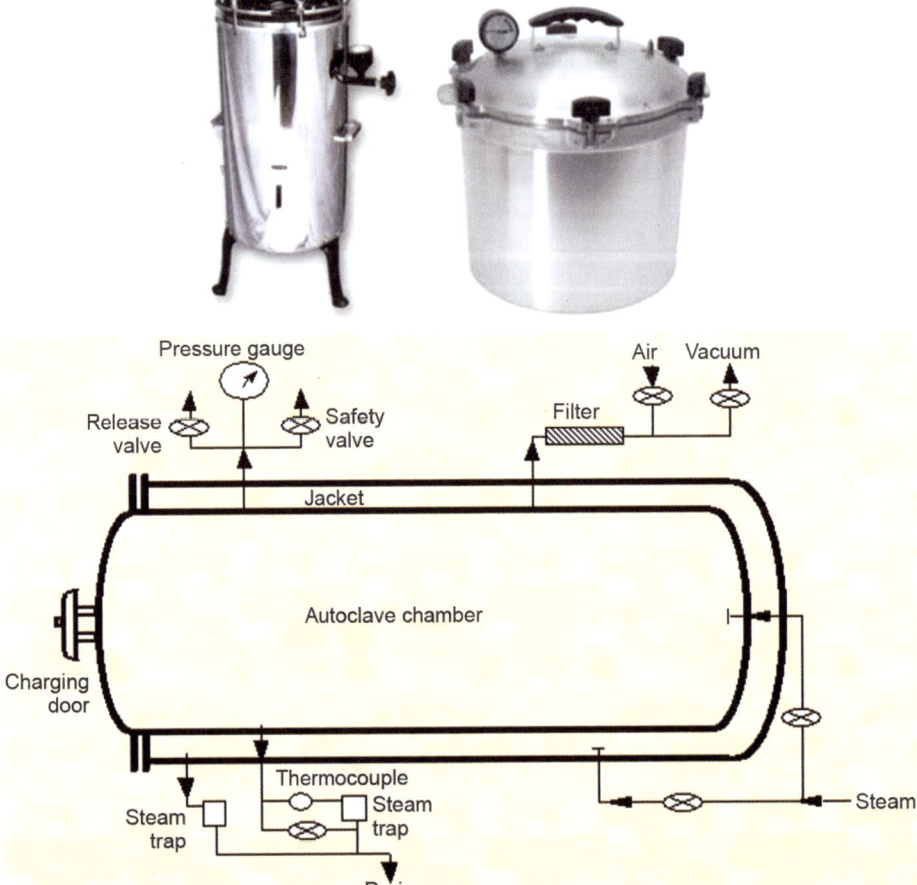

## Standard for Autoclaving

- Gravity flow autoclaving:
  - Temp > than 121°C and 15 pound per sq inch (psi) pressure for 60 min.
  - Temp > than 135°C and 31 pound per sq inch (psi) pressure for 45 min.
  - Temp > than 149°C and 52 pound per sq inch (psi) pressure for 30 min.

- Vacuum autoclaving:
  - Temp > than 121°C and 15 pound per sq inch (psi ) pressure for 45 min.
  - Temp > than 135°C and 31 pound per sq inch (psi) pressure for 30 min.

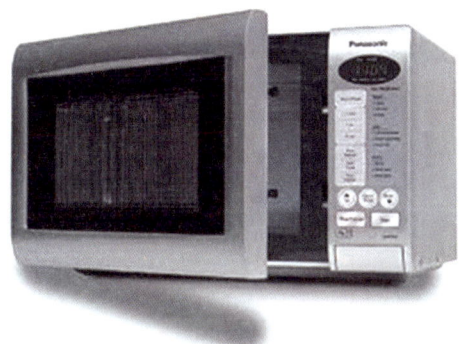 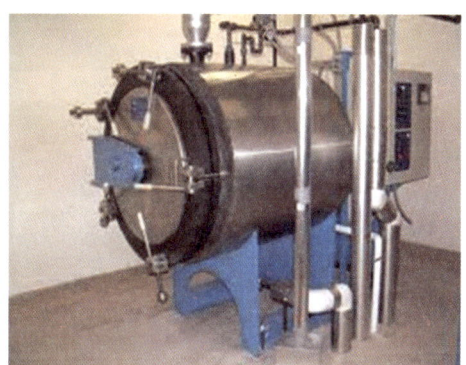

| Microwave | Hydroclave |

**Microwave** is an appliance that heats by dielectric heating accomplished with microwave type electromagnetic radiation that is used to rotate and heat polarized molecules in food. Microwave radiation is between common radio and infrared frequencies, being usually at 2.45 gigahertz (GHz)—a wavelength of 122 millimetres (4.80 in)—or, in large industrial/commercial ovens, at 915 megahertz (MHz)—328 millimetres (12.9 in).

A microwave converts only part of its electrical input into microwave energy. A typical consumer microwave oven consumes 1100 W of electricity in producing 700 W of microwave power, an efficiency of 64%.

Microwave heating is more efficient on liquid water than on frozen or dense sustances, where the movement of molecules is more restricted.

**Hydroclave:** It is an appliance that used to treat waste by dry as well as wet heat after shredding into small particles.

## INCINERATOR

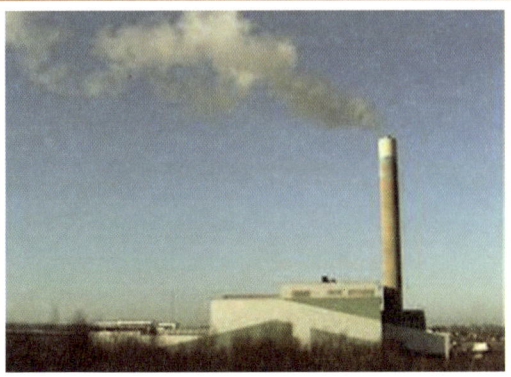

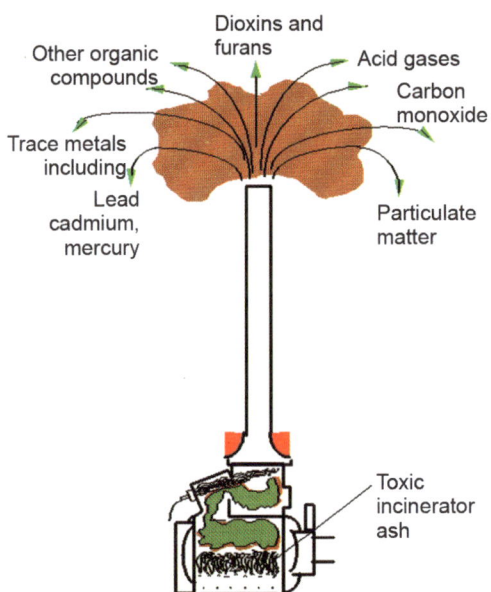

**Incinerator** is a cemented constructed plant for hospital waste disposals.

A controlled combustion process, waste is completely oxidized and harmful microorganisms present in it are destroyed/denatured under high temperature. Volume of waste is reduced markedly and converted to ash.

### Standard for Incineration

- Minimum height of the stack should be 30 metres above the ground.
- Above emission limits should be achieved.
- Waste to be incinerated not to be disinfected with chlorine substance.
- Chlorinated plastics should not be incinerated.
- Toxic metals in incineration ash should be limited to within regulatory quantities.
- Only low sulphur fuels like LDO/LSHS to be used as fuel.
- The common treatment facility (CTF) should be located away from human habitation.

Brief conclusive descriptive note about hospital waste facilities: _____

**Teacher's Remark** .........................................
**Teacher's Signature** .........................................

## WATER FILTRATION PLANT

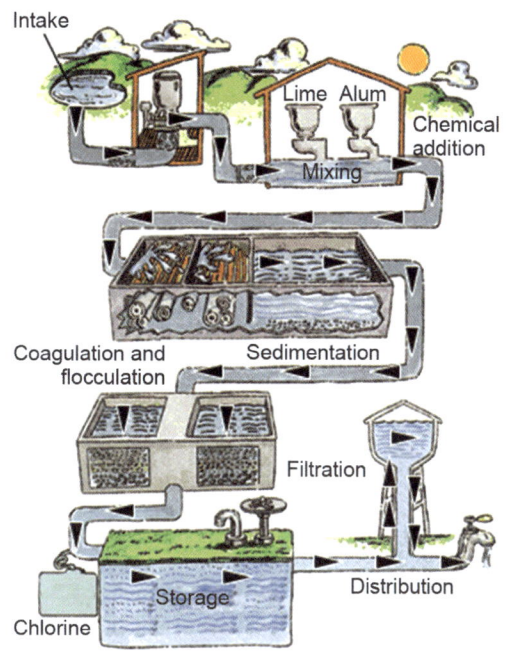

Name of plant _____          Date of visit: _____
Address of the plant: _____
Name of O/IC with mobile no _____
Building: Own/rented
No. of rooms:
IEC material displayed: Yes/No          Suggestion box: Yes/No

| Staff | At present plant | Reason of **problem, if any |
|---|---|---|
| Water work's Manager | | |
| Water work's Engineer | | |
| Water work's technician | | |
| Peon | | |
| Any other specify | | |
| **Physical structure** | At present *W/NW | Reason of **problem, if any |
| Waiting area with displays | | |
| Water testing lab | | |
| Source of raw water | | |
| Pumping method | | |
| Toilet (1950 × 1200 mm) | | |
| **Components of main plant** | | |
| Pre-filtration storage chamber | | |

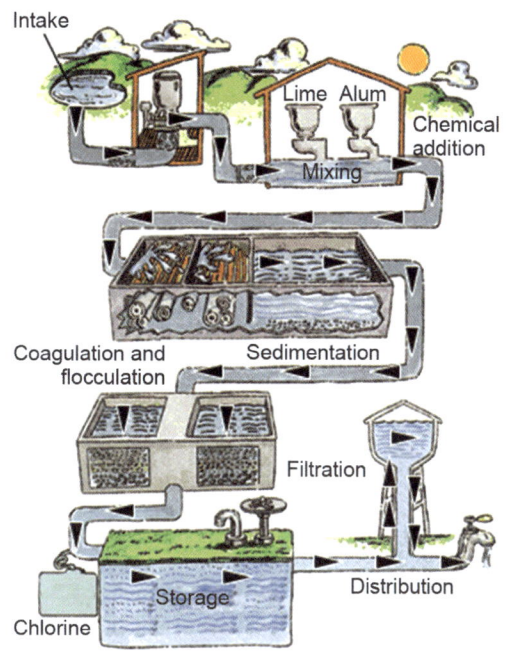 *Contd.*

*Contd.*

| | | |
|---|---|---|
| Mixing chamber (allum and lime) | | |
| Coagulation and flocculation chamber | | |
| Sedimentation chamber | | |
| Filtration chamber | | |
| Chlorination | | |
| Post-filtration storage chamber | | |
| Tank for distribution | | |
| **Support services** | **At present ICTC** | **Reason of **problem, if any** |
| Electricity | | |
| Water | | |
| Toilet | | |
| **Record maintain** | **At present ICTC** | **Reason of **problem, if any** |
| Water testing register | | |
| Log book | | |

*Working/Not working

**Problem is the difference between what is required and what is present.

## Last Year's Performance
## Water Testing at Source

| S. no. | Date of tests | Procedure used | Test result |
|---|---|---|---|
| | | | |
| | | | |

## Water Testing at Distribution

| S. no. | Date of tests | Procedure used | Test result | Reason of *problem, if yes | Action taken |
|---|---|---|---|---|---|
| | | | | | |
| | | | | | |
| | | | | | |

*Problem is the difference between what is required and what is present.

## Back Washing

| S. no. | Date of backwash | Procedure used | Duration |
|---|---|---|---|
| | | | |
| | | | |

Brief conclusive descriptive notes: _____

**Teacher's Remark** .......................................

**Teacher's Signature** .......................................

**Water purification** is the process of removing undesirable chemicals, biological contaminants, suspended solids and gases from contaminated water.

The goal is to produce water fit for a specific purpose. Most water is purified for human consumption (drinking water), but water purification may also be designed for a variety of other purposes, including meeting the requirements of medical, pharmacological, chemical and industrial applications.

In general, the methods used include physical processes such as filtration, sedimentation, and distillation, biological processes such as slow sand filters or biologically active carbon, chemical processes such as flocculation and chlorination and the use of electromagnetic radiation such as ultraviolet light.

The purification process of water may reduce the concentration of particulate matter including suspended particles, parasites, bacteria, algae, viruses, fungi and a range of dissolved and particulate materials derived from the surfaces that water may have made contact with after falling as rain.

The standards for drinking water quality are typically set by governments or by international standards. These standards will typically set minimum and maximum concentrations of contaminants for the use that is to be made of the water.

### SEWAGE TREATMENT PLANT

**Sewage treatment** is the process of removing contaminants from wastewater and household sewage, both runoff (effluents) and domestic.

Its objective is to produce an environmentally safe fluid waste stream (or treated effluent) and a solid waste (or treated sludge) suitable for disposal or reuse (usually as farm fertilizer).

## Sewage Treatment Generally Involves Three Stages

1. **Primary treatment** consists of temporarily holding the sewage in a quiescent basin where heavy solids can settle to the bottom while oil, grease, etc. solids float to the surface. The settled and floating materials are removed and the remaining liquid may be discharged or sent to secondary treatment.

2. **Secondary treatment** removes dissolved and suspended biological matter.

3. **Tertiary treatment** is sometimes defined as anything more than primary and secondary treatment in order to allow rejection into a highly sensitive or fragile ecosystem. Treated water is sometimes disinfected chemically or physically prior to discharge into a stream, river, bay, etc. or it can be used for agricultural purposes.

Brief descriptive note: _____

**Teacher's Remark** .........................................

**Teacher's Signature** .........................................

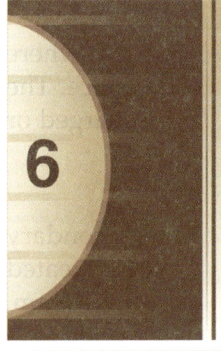

# 6 Water Sampling, Examination and Treatment

## COLLECTION OF WATER FOR INDIVIDUAL USES
- Collect from a safe source
- Store in a container with contamination safeguards
- Find out quality of water through sampling and examination
- Treat to reduce microbial contamination
  - Physical treatments
  - Chemical treatments
  - Combined physical-chemical treatments

### Safe Water

Water is termed safe when it does not harm the consumer even when ingested over prolonged periods. It must be:
  a. Free of pathogenic organisms
  b. Free from harmful chemical substances
  c. Acceptable to taste and appearance
  d. Usable for domestic purposes
If not safe, it can lead to following diseases.

### Water-related Diseases

| Type | Cause | Diseases |
|------|-------|----------|
| Water, born diseases | Ingestion of contaminated water | Amoebic and bacillary dysentery, cholera, typhoid, viral hepatitis A/E/C, leptospirosis, giardisis, schistosomiasis, dracunculosis, ascariasis, etc. |
| Water-based diseases | Contact of contaminated water | Scabies, dermatitis, trachoma, conjunctivitis infestation and diseases transmitted by louse, flea, ticks, etc. |
| | Helping in breeding of diseases transmitting agents | Mosquito, born diseases, fly-born diseases, cyclops-born diseases, etc. |

*Contd.*

*Contd.*

| Type | Cause | Diseases |
|---|---|---|
| Lack of water | Deficiency of water | Dehydration |
| | Poor personnel hygiene | Scabies, dermatitis, trachoma, conjunctivitis infestation and diseases transmitted by louse, flea, ticks, etc. |
| Excess of water | Flood | Accidents due to flood disaster |
| | Contamination of water | Diseases due to ingestion of contaminated water |
| | | Diseases due to contact of contaminated water |

## Source of Water

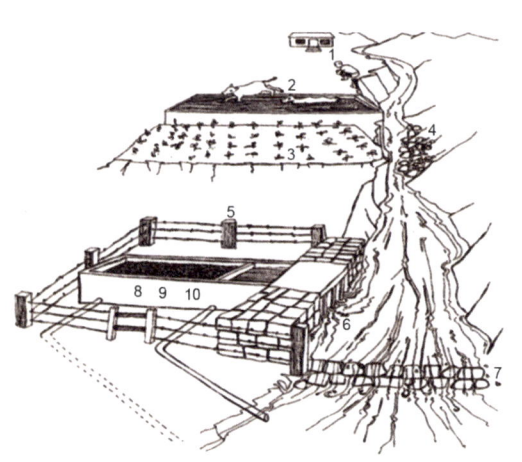 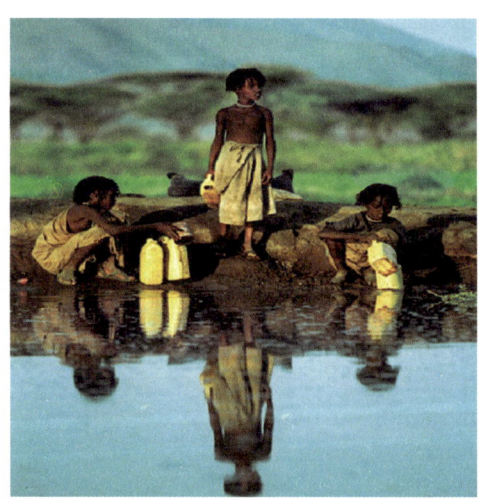

**Surface water**

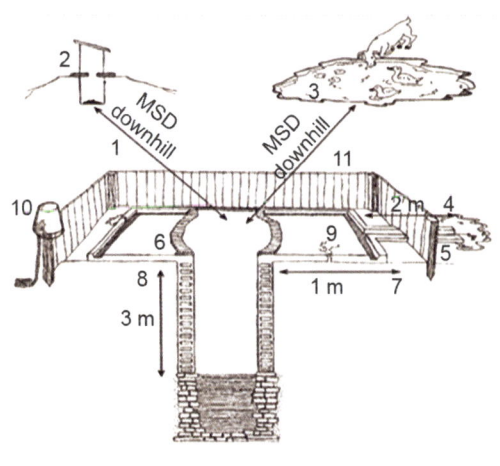 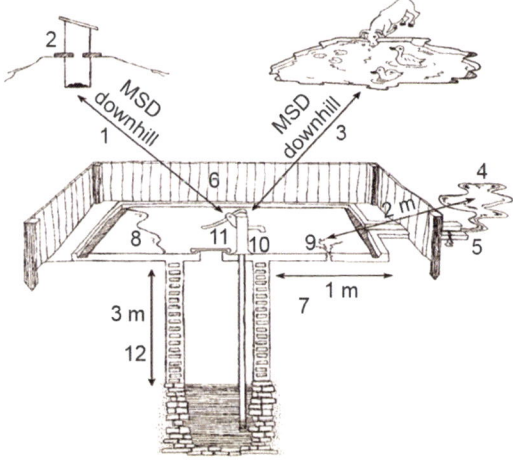

**Open dug well**          **Covered dug well with hand pump**

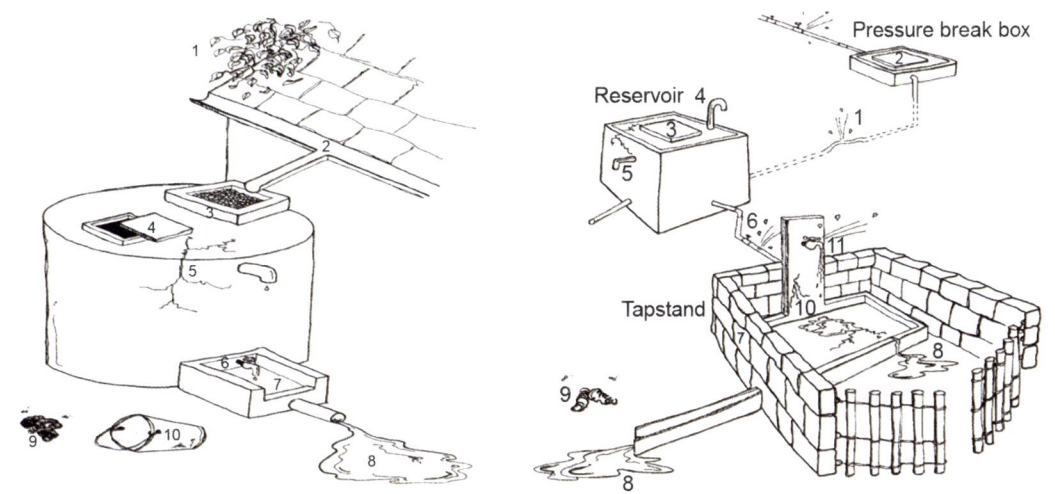

| Tanka-rain water collection | Piped water supply |

Surface water, open dug well water is **not at all safe** for drinking.

Covered dug well with hand pump and *tanka* water **may be used** for drinking.

Treated piped water is **safe for drinking until unless it is not leaked**.

### Collection of Water Sample

### Collection of Water for Physical and Chemical Examination

- Take transparent beverage bottles.
- Clean the bottle with distilled water.
- Clean the bottle with chromic acid cleaning mixture (chromic acid mix = 1 lit. conc.$H_2SO_4$ + 35 ml. sod. chromate).
- About 2.5 litres water should be collected.
- Sample should be examined within 72 hrs.

### Collection of Water for Microbial Examination

- Sampling points and sampling frequency should be preplanned.
- Sample should be collected, stored and dispatched in suitable sterilized glass bottles.
- Enough volume (at least 200 ml) of water should be taken.
- Sodium thiosulphate added to dechlorinated.
- Prevent contamination.
- Properly labelled.

### Method of Collection of Sample

| Steps | Tap water | Dug well | Surface water |
|---|---|---|---|
| 1. | Clean the tap | Take a 250 ml capacity bottle | Take a 250 ml capacity bottle |
| 2. | Open tap for 1–2 mts for highest flow then sterilize tap with sprit lamp | Put some sodium thiosulphate in a sterilized bottle | Put some sodium thiosulphate in a sterilized bottle |

*Contd.*

*Contd.*

| Steps | Tap water | Dug well | Surface water |
|---|---|---|---|
| 3. | Open tap for 1–2 mts for medium flow | Tie bottle mouth with string and stone as shown in figure | Open the mouth of bottle |
| 4. | Open sterilized bottle with aseptic technique | Dip the bottle into the well | Dip the bottle into the well water 20 cm deep from surface |
| 5. | Fill bottle with water leaving air space | Fill bottle with water leaving air space | Fill bottle with water leaving air space |
| 6. | Close the bottle | Close the bottle | Close the bottle |
| 7. | Label it properly | Label it properly | Label it properly |

## Collection of Water Sample

### Sampling from Tap Water

**a. Clean the up**
Remove from the tap any attachments that may cause splashing. Using a clean cloth, wipe the outlet to remove any dirt.

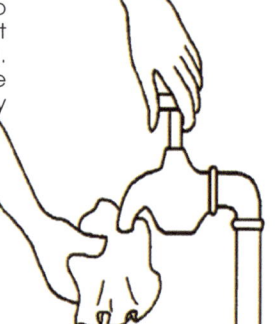

**b. Open the tap**
Turn on the tap at maximum flow and let the water run for 1–2 minutes.

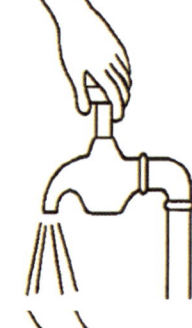

**c. Sterilize the tap**
Sterilize the tap for a minute with the flame from a gas burner, cigarette lighter, or an ignited alcohol-soaked cotton-wool swab.

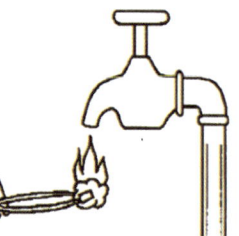

**d. Open the tap before sampling**
Carefully turn on the tap and allow the water to flow for 1–2 minutes at a medium flow rate. Do not adjust the flow after it has been set.

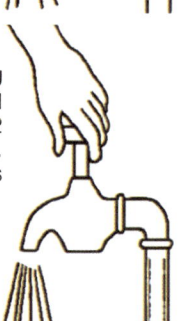

**e. Open the sterilized bottle**
Take out a borde and carefully unscrew the cap or pull out the stopper.

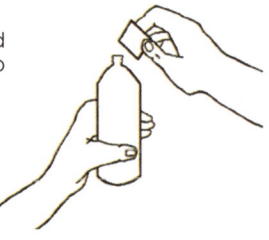

**f. Fill the bottle**
While holding the cap and protective cover face downwards (to prevent entry of dust, which may contaminate the sample), immedia-tely hold the bottle under the water jet, and fill.

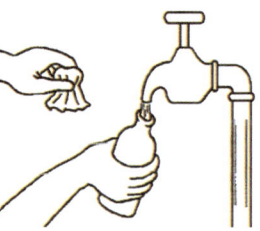

A small air space should be left to make before analysis easier.

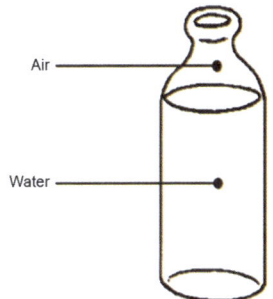

Air

Water

## G. Stopper or cap the bottle

Place the stopper in the bottle or screw on the cap and fix the brown paper protective cover in place with the string.

---

## Sampling from Surface Water

### Fill the bottle

Holding the bottle by the lower part, submerge it to a depth of about 20 cm, with the mouth facing slightly upwards, mouth should face towards the current. The bottle should then be capped or stoppered as described previously.

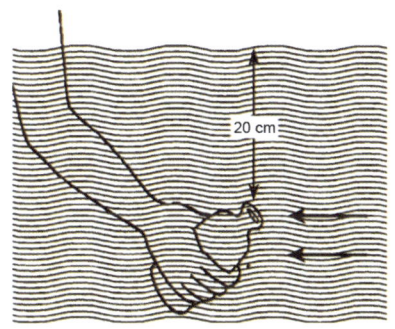

20 cm

---

## Sampling from a Open Dug Well

### a. Prepare the bottle

With a piece of string, attach a clean weight to the sampling bottle.

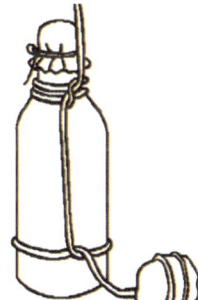

### b. Attach the bottle to the string

Take a 20 m length of clean string rolled around a stick and tie it to the bottel string.

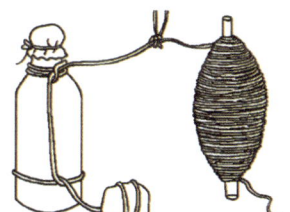

### c. Lower the bottle

Lower the bottle, weighed down by the weight, into the well, unwinding the well, unwinding the string slowly. Do not allow the bottle to touch the sides of the well.

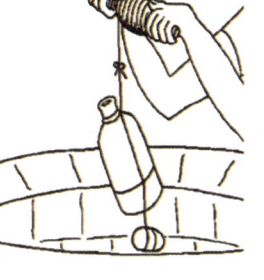

### d. Fill the bottle

Immerse the bottle completely in the water and lower it well below the surface without hitting the bottom or disturbing any sediment.

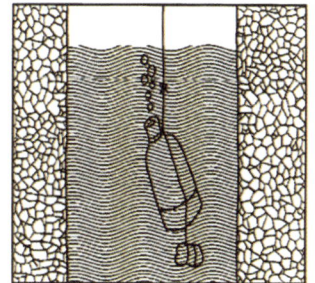

### e. Raise the bottle

Once the bottle is judged to be filled, rewind the string on the stick to bring up the bottle. If the bottle is completely full, discard some water to provide an air space. Stopper or cap the bottle as described previously.

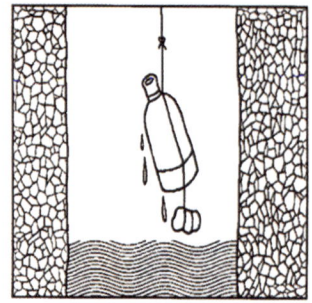

## Sampling of Water

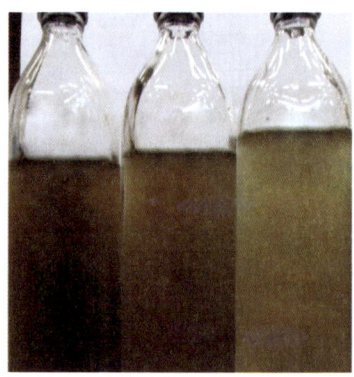

| Packing, Labelling and Dispatch Water Sample |
|---|
| **Frazile**      **This side up** |
| **Date:**      **Time:** |
| **Place:** |
| Authorized person's name with signature: |
| Urgent-send to laboratory ideally within 6 hrs. |

## Format of Sending Water Sample for Bacteriological Analysis

संस्थान का नाम ...............................................................

क्रमांक ........      दिनांक .

कनिष्ठ रसायनज्ञ
जनस्वा0 अभि0 विभाग ( प्रयोगशाला )
बून्दी

विषय :— जीवाणु जल नमूने भिजवाने बाबत ।

| क्र0 सं0 | ग्राम पंचायत | ग्राम का नाम | स्रोत | स्रोत का स्थान | संग्रह दिनांक | संग्रह समय | सेम्पल लेने वाले का नाम |
|---|---|---|---|---|---|---|---|
| | | | | | | | |
| | | | | | | | |
| | | | | | | | |
| | | | | | | | |
| | | | | | | | |
| | | | | | | | |
| | | | | | | | |

खण्ड चिकित्सा अधिकारी
सामु0 / प्राथ0 स्वास्थ्य केन्द्र

क्रमांक ........      दिनांक

प्रतिलिपि —

1. श्रीमान् मुख्य चिकित्सा एवं स्वास्थ्य अधिकारी, बून्दी ।

खण्ड चिकित्सा अधिकारी
सामु0 / प्राथ0 स्वास्थ्य केन्द्र

## Protocol for Result of Bacteriological Analysis

WATER-QUALITY
CONTROL
PROGRAMME

[.......................... Authority]

BACTERIOLOGICAL
WATER
ANALYSIS

COMMUNITY:
SAMPLE SITE:

SAMPLE NO. ........

PLACE:
SOURCE:
SENDER:
DATE OF SAMPLING ____/____/____       TIME:
DATE OF ANALYSIS ____/____/____        TIME:

RESIDUAL FREE CHLORINE [          ]  mg/litre

RESULTS

TOTAL COLIFORMS . . . . . . . . . . .        /100 ml

FAECAL COLIFORMS . . . . . . . . . . .       /100 ml

WATER BACTERIOLOGICALLY
     GOOD — BAD

.................................
Laboratory Technician

.................................
Chief (Signed)

## Frequency of Sampling

| Type of water | Residual chlorine test | Micro. Lab Exam. |
|---|---|---|
| Open well<br>Covered well with hand pump<br>Deep tube well with hand pump | Once/month | Once initially then·<br>• Changing environment<br>• Out-breaks<br>• Increase in water diseases |
| Piped supply from surface water | Once/day | Daily |

## No. of water sample to be collected as per population

| Population | Criteria | No. of sample per month |
|---|---|---|
| < 5000 population | Minimum one/month | 1 |
| 5000–1 lakh population | Minimum one/5000 pop./month | 1–20 |
| > 1 lakh population | Minimum one/10000 pop./month | 10 and above |

**Handling and transport of water sample:** Sample should reach to the assigned laboratory at earliest in the position as it was sampled.

# Water Sample Examination

## Measurement of Turbidity

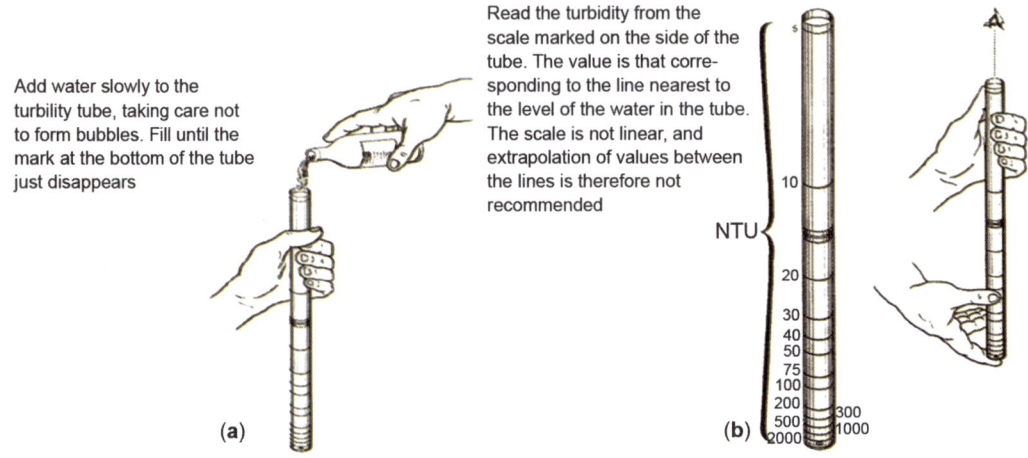

Add water slowly to the turbidity tube, taking care not to form bubbles. Fill until the mark at the bottom of the tube just disappears

Read the turbidity from the scale marked on the side of the tube. The value is that corresponding to the line nearest to the level of the water in the tube. The scale is not linear, and extrapolation of values between the lines is therefore not recommended

NTU

(a)     (b)

**Measurement of pH: Comparator disk method:** A comparator has following colour disc depending upon the range required by the reagent like:

- Bromothymol purple      pH 5.2–6.8
- Bromothymol blue        pH 6.0–7.6
- Phenol                  pH 6.8–8.4
- Thymol blue             pH 8.0–9.6

## Multiple-tube Method of Coliforms Test (for Faecal Contamination)

- A series of tubes containing a suitable selective broth culture medium is inoculated with test portions of a water sample.
- Each tube showing gas formation is regarded as "presumptive positive" since the gas indicates the possible presence of coliforms.
- A subsequent confirmatory test is essential—*confirmatory test.*

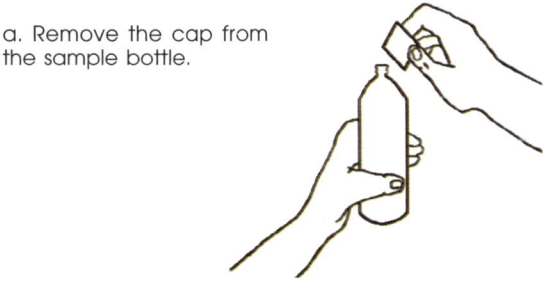

a. Remove the cap from the sample bottle.

b. With the stopper in position, shake the bottle vigorously to achieve a homogeneous dispersion of bacteria. (If the bottle is completely full, remove the stopper and discard about 20–30 ml of water; then replace the stopper and shake. This ensures thorough mixing.)

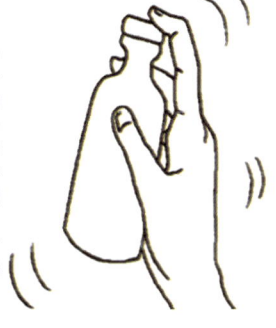

c. With a sterile 10 ml pipette, inoculate 10 ml of the sample into each of five tubes containing 10 ml of presumptive broth (double strength). Add 50 ml of presumptive broth. It is advisable to shake the tubes gently to distribute the sample uniformly throughout the medium.

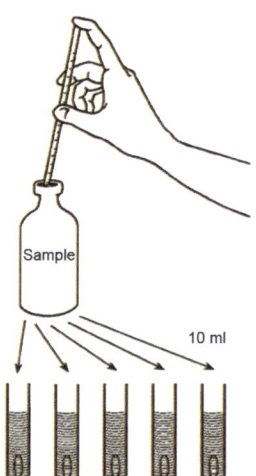

d. Incubate the tubes at 35°C or 37°C for 24 hours.

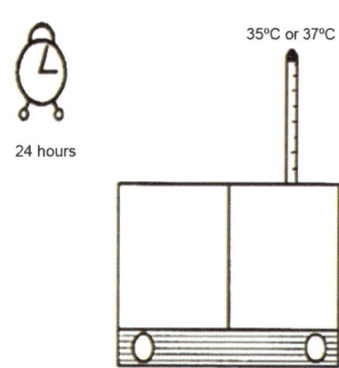

e. At the end of the 24 hours incubation period, examine each tube for the presence of gas. If present, gas can be seen in the Durham tube. If none is visible, gently shake the tube, if any effervescence (streams of tiny bubbles) is observed, the tube should be considered positive.

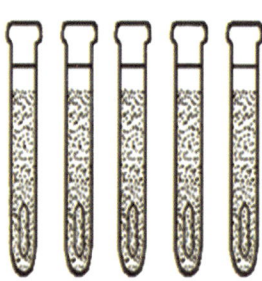

f. Using a table like the one shown here, record the number of positive tubes after 24 hours.

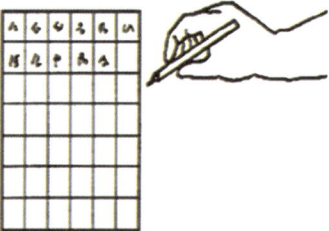

Presumptive results for 24-hour incubation

g. Reincubate negative tubes for a further 24-hour period. At the end of this period, check the tubes again for gas production in E above. Gas production at the end of either 24 or 48 hours incubation is presumed to be due to the presence of coliforms in the sample.

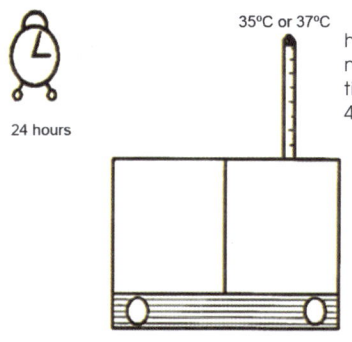

h. Record the number of positive tubes after 48 hours.

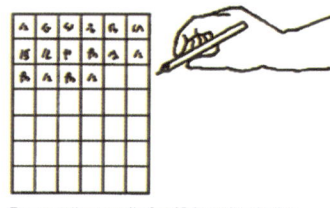

Presumptive results for 48-hour incubation

i. The confirmatory test should be carried out at the end of both the 24-hour and the 48-hour incubation. Using a sterile loop, transfer one or two drops from each presumptive positive tube into two tubes containing respectively confirmatory broth and tryptone water. (Sterilize the inoculation loop before each transfer by flaming and allow to cool.)

j. To confirm the presence of thermotolerant coliforms, incubate the subculture tubes from each presumptive positive tube for 24 hours at 44 ± 0.5°C.

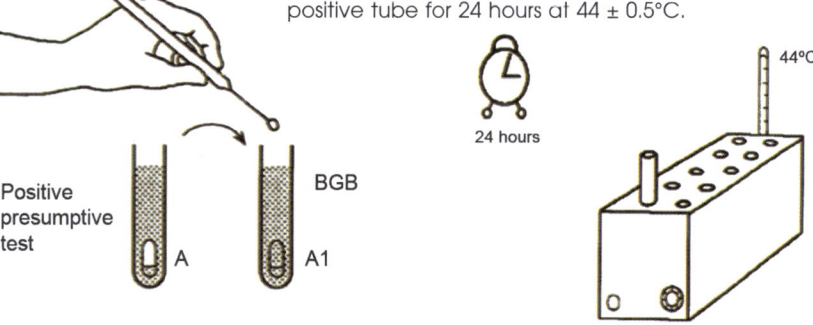

k. At the end of 24 hours' incubation, examine each broth tube for growth and the presence of gas in the Durham tube. Enter the results on the table as shown.

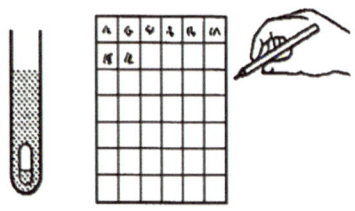

Results of confirmatory test

l. To each tube of tryptone water, add approximately 0.1 ml of Kovacs reagent and mix gently. The presence of indole is indicated by a red colour in the Kovacs reagent, forming a film over the aqueous phase of the medium.

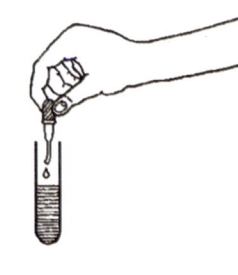

0.1 ml

m. Confirmatory tests positive for indole, growth, and gas production show the presence of *E. coli.* Growth and gas production in the absence of indole confirms thermotolerant coliforms.

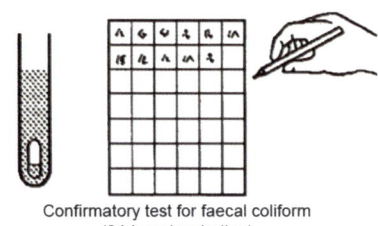

Confirmatory test for faecal coliform
(24-hour incubation)

**Media** often used for water sampling are MacConckey broth and peptone water.

**When water seems to be more polluted then following precaution will be taken.**

- 10 ml of sample to each of the 5 tubes containing 10 ml of double strength medium.
- 1 ml of sample to each of the 5 tubes containing 10 ml of single strength medium.
- 1 ml of 1:10 ml sample dilution (0.1 ml of sample) to each of the 5 tubes containing 10 ml of single strength medium.

## Residual free Chlorine Test

a. Rinse a comparator cell two or three times, and then fill it up to the mark with the water sample

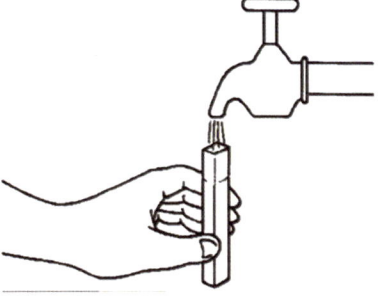

b. Place the cell in the cell carrier of the comparator, which is in line with the coloured standards (B).

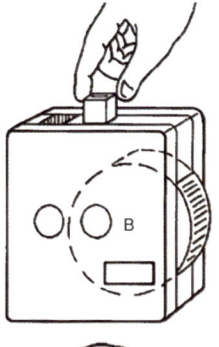

c. Rinse the second cell and fill it with the same water.

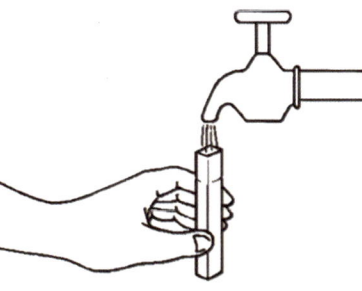

d. Add reagent to the second cell, in accordance with the manufacturer's instructions.

e. Shake the cell (for not more than 3–5 seconds) to mix the reagent.

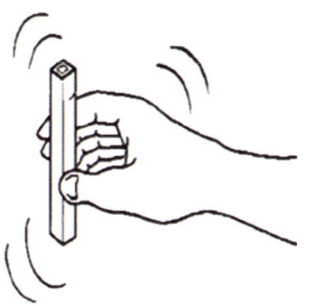

f. Place the cell in the comparator (A).

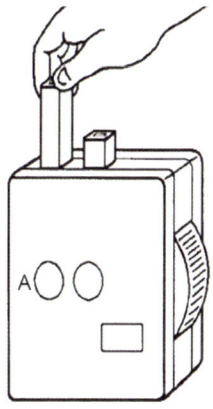

g. While holding the comparator facing good natural light, rotate the disc until the colour of a standard (B) is the same as that developed by the reagent (A). Immediately (i.e. in less than 20 seconds) read at C the value of free chlorine in mg/litre.

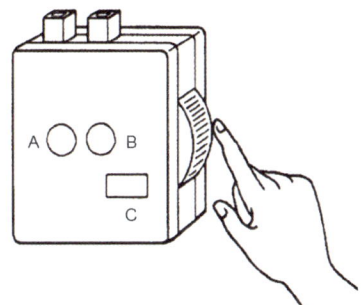

Result regarding chlorine in water will be directly read in 'C' as chlorine ____ mg/litre of water.

Chlorine in sample water can also be known by Horrock's apparatus which is detailed in chapter 'Water Chemistry'.

## Water Quality Standard

1. Acceptability aspects
2. Microbiological aspects
3. Chemical aspects
4. Radiological aspects.

### 1. Acceptability Aspects

| S. no. | Quality | Maximum permissible limit |
|---|---|---|
| 1. | Colour | < 15 true colour units (TCU) |
| 2. | Taste and odour | Acceptable |
| 3. | Turbidity | < 5 NTU |
| 4. | Total dissolved solids (TDS) | < 1000 mg/l of water |
| 5. | pH | 6.5 to 8.5 |
| 6. | Hardness | Up to 300 ppm |
| 7. | Chlorides | Up to 600 mg/litre of water |
| 8. | Iron | Up to 0.3 mg/l is acceptable |

## 2. Microbiological Aspects

| S. no. | Organism | Maximum permissible limit |
|---|---|---|
| 1. | *E. coli* | Zero, i.e. must not be detectable in any 100 ml sample |
| 2. | Total coliform bacteria | Zero, i.e. must not be detectable in any 100 ml sample at least 95% sample taken throughout the year should be free from coliform bacteria |

So, practically drinking water should be free from any bacteria.

## 3. Chemical Aspects: Inorganic chemicals of public health important in drinking water

| Type of chemical | Chemical name | Maximum limit permitted (mg/l) | Chemical name | Maximum limit permitted (mg/l) |
|---|---|---|---|---|
| Inorganic | Antimony | 0.005 | Arsenic | 0.01 |
| | Barium | 0.7 | Boron | 0.03 |
| | Cadmium | 0.003 | Cromium | 0.05 |
| | Cyanide | 0.07 | Copper | 2 |
| | Lead | 0.01 | Floride | 1.5 |
| | Murcury | 0.001 | Manganese | 0.5 |
| | Molybdenum | 0.07 | Nickel | 0.02 |
| | Nitrite | 3 | Nitrate | 50 |
| | Selenium | 0.01 | | |
| Organic | Aldrin/dieldrin | 0.03 | Chlordane | 0.2 |
| | Hexachlorobenzene | 1 | DDT | 2 |

**4. Radiological aspects:** WHO has proposed the following limits of radioactivity as acceptable
- Gross alpha activity 3 pCi/l (Picocuries per litre).
- Gross beta activity 30 pCi/l

## Household Water Storage and Treatment

**Household water containers for safe storage:** It should be easy to clean, lightweight, durable, heat and oxidation-resistant. It should be covered.

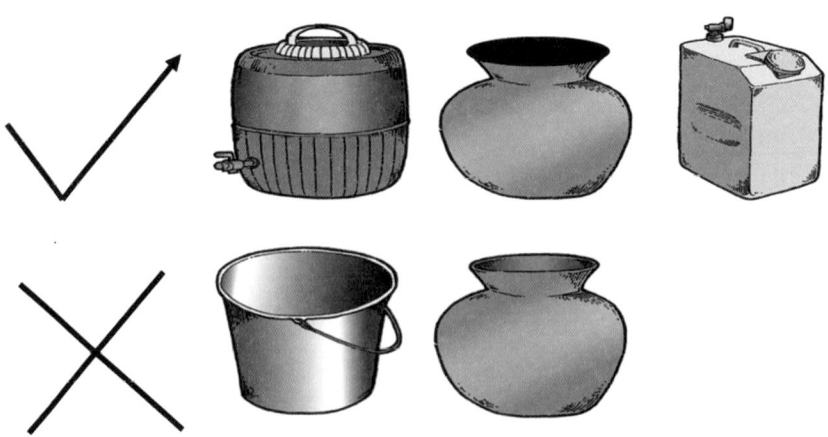

## Methods for Water Treatment

| Type of method | Method | Microbial efficiency |
|---|---|---|
| Physical | Boiling | High (> 95%) |
| | Exposed to sunlight | Moderate (90–95%) |
| | Plain sedimentation | Low (< 90%) |
| | Filtration | High (> 95%) |
| | Rapid sand filter | High (> 95%) |
| | Slow sand filter | Moderate (90–95%) |
| | Ceramic filter | Moderate (90–95%) |
| | Membrane filter | High (> 95%) |
| Chemical | Chlorination | High (> 95%) |
| | Ionization | High (> 95%) |
| | Ozonation | High (> 95%) |
| | Coagulation-flocculation and precipitation | Moderate (90–95%) |

Effectiveness of combined coagulation-flocculation and sedimentation-filtration systems:

• Effective (> 99.9%) reductions of viruses, bacteria and parasites
• Effective (> 99%) reductions in indicator bacteria reductions.

# Specimen Sampling

## SPECIMEN SAMPLING

Blood
Sputum
Nasopharyngeal swabs
Urine
Stool
Food

### General Precautions for Collection of Laboratory Samples

- All specimens from patients should be considered infectious.
- Wear appropriate protective barriers for the laboratory procedure.
- Syringes should not be recapped with needles.
- Samples must be processed as soon as possible.
- All specimens must be accompanied by a correctly filled order form, containing the relevant information.
- All specimens must be well labelled.
- Information on the specimen container must agree with that of the order form each sample must be registered at the laboratory reception and be given a code number, prior to processing.
- All samples must be processed in line with sop designed for the test.
- Results must be recorded immediately.
- In-patients' results must be despatched immediately and outpatients' results kept in a cabinet very well secured.
- Never leave results register on table when not in use.

### BLOOD SAMPLING

### Blood for Smears

**Collection:** Capillary blood from finger prick
- Make smear
- Fix with methanol or other fixative

## Handling and Transport

- Transport slides within 24 hours.
- Do not refrigerate (can alter cell morphology).

## Blood for Culture

**Collection:** Venous blood with aseptic technique

- Infants: 0.5 – 2 ml
- Children: 2 – 5 ml
- Adults: 5 – 10 ml

## Handling and Transport

- Collect into bottles with infusion broth
- Change needle to inoculate the broth
- Transport upright with cushion
- Prevents haemolytic
- Wrap tubes with absorbent cotton
- Travel at ambient temperature
- Store at 4ºC, if cannot reach laboratory in 24 hrs.

## Blood Collection for Serum

**Collection:** Venous blood in sterile test tube

- Let clot for 30 minutes at ambient temperature
- Glass tube is better than plastic.

## Handling

- Place at 4–8ºC for clot retraction for at least 1–2 hours
- Centrifuge at 1500 RPM for 5–10 min
- Separate serum from the clot

## Transport

- 4–8ºC if transport within 10 days
- Avoid haemolysis
- Freeze at –20ºC, if storage for weeks or months before processing and shipment to reference laboratory
- Avoid repeated freeze-thaw cycles

**Blood collection:** Blood may be collected from:

- Venepuncture (usually from cephalic, median, basilica, metacarpal plexus and dorsal venous arch)
- Fingerstick/finger prick

## Venepuncture Blood Collection

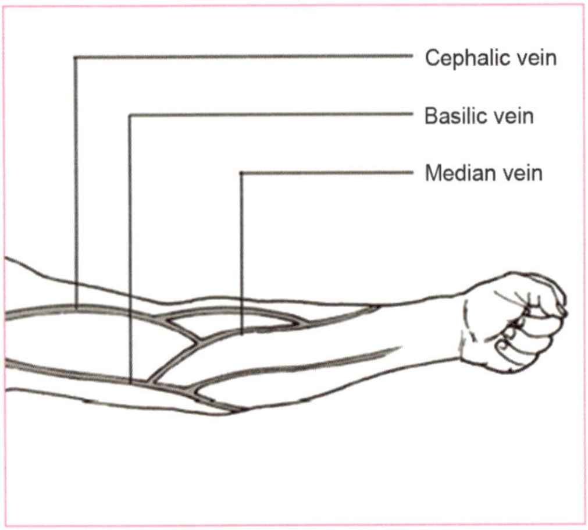

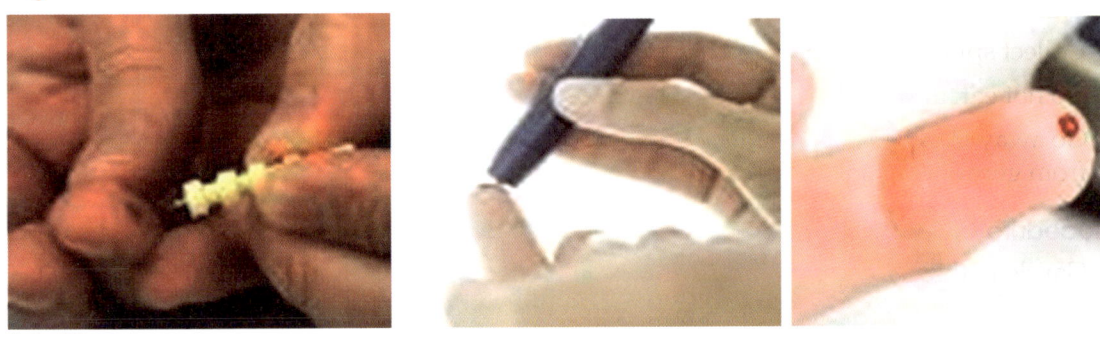

Cephalic vein

Basilic vein

Median vein

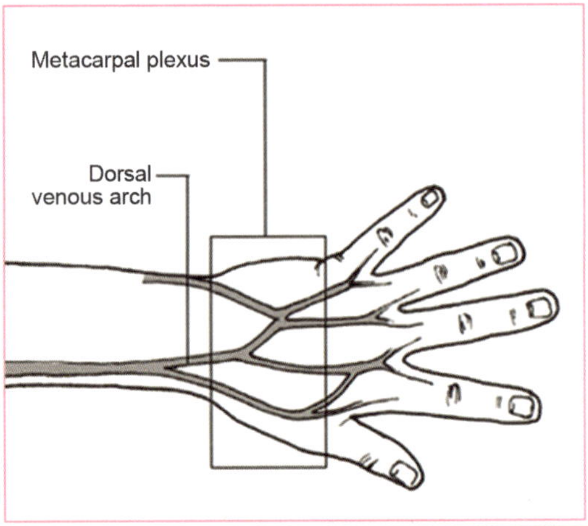

Metacarpal plexus

Dorsal venous arch

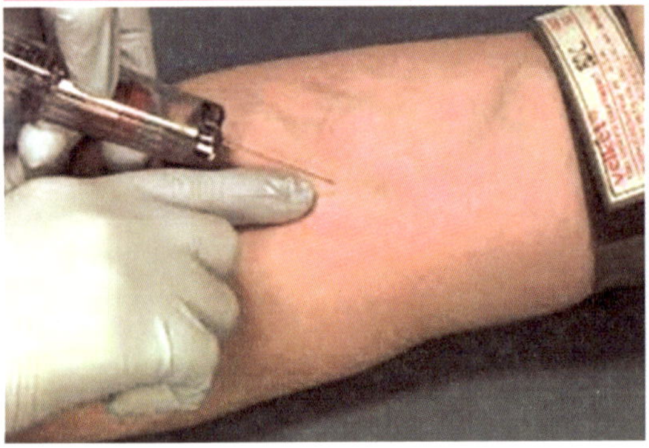

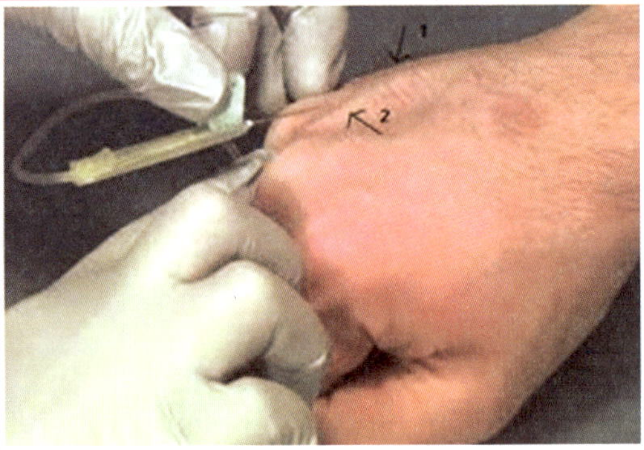

## Finger Prick Method

## Precaution during Sample Collection of Blood

1. Blood should be collected aseptically.
2. EDTA container must be used for whole blood and plasma specimens.
3. Use plain and dry containers for serum specimen; allow sample to clot, retract before spinning to recover the serum.

4. Blood samples should be stored at 2–8°C, if the test is to be run within 7 days.

5. Serum and plasma samples may be frozen at 20°C, if test is to be carried out after 7 days of collection.

6. Do not freeze whole blood.

7. Finger stick collection should be tested immediately.

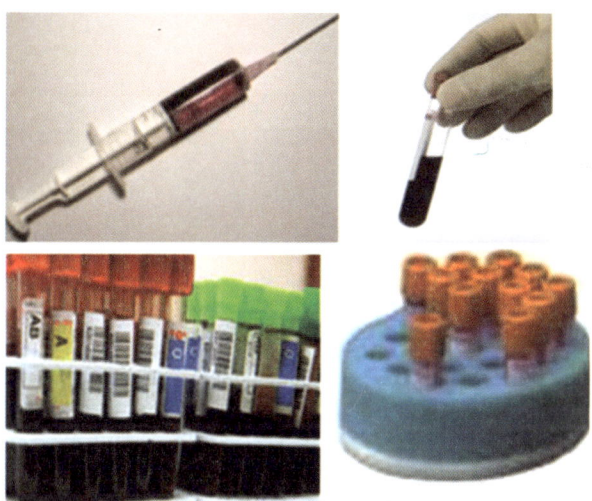

## SPUTUM SAMPLES FOR AFB EXAMINATION

**Sputum** is mucous that is coughed up from the lower airways. **It is not saliva** or mucous from the back of the throat. Sputum examination is done to study bronchial and pulmonary secretions.

### Sputum Collection

• Collect sputum specimen as soon as possible after waking in the morning.

• Do not eat, drink, smoke or brush your teeth before collecting the sputum.

• Go away from other people before collecting the specimen. This helps protect other people from germs when you cough.

### Procedure of Sputum Collection

1. Gargle with water immediately prior to obtaining a sputum specimen to reduce the number of oral bacteria. Do not use a mouthwash or any other gargle.

2. Take deep breaths through your mouth. Try and cough up mucous from deep in your chest.

3. Take the clean wide-mouth open sterile specimen cup (container) with you. Do not open it until you are ready to use it.

4. Open the container and hold it close to your under the lower lip to catch all of the expectorated sputum.

5. Cough deeply and expectorate sputum (not saliva) into the cup.

6. About a tablespoon of sputum is the amount that is needed.

7. Screw the lid tightly, so it does not leak.

8. For acid-fast culture, three specimens collected at a minimal interval of 8 to 24 hours.

9. Transport the specimen to the microbiology laboratory at room temperature within 24 hours of collection. If greater than 24 hours, refrigerate at 4°C.

1. Clean your mouth

2. Breath in and out 3–4 times

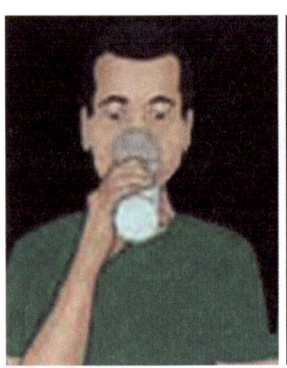
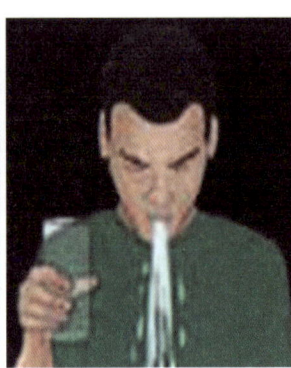
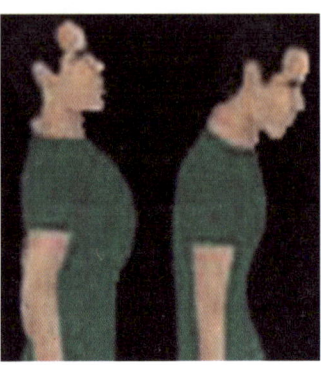

3. Cough

4. Spit in container

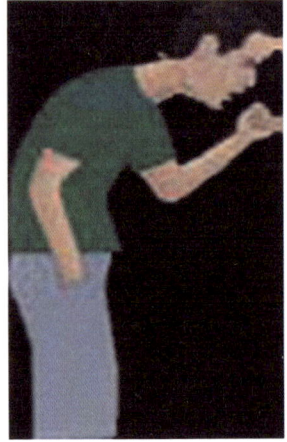
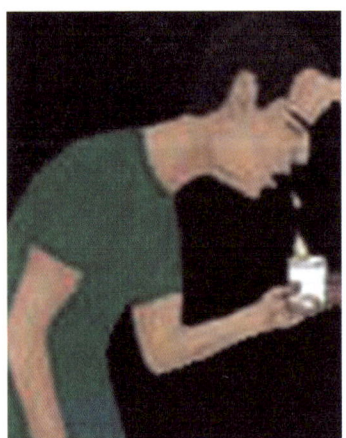

## Qualities of a good Sputum Sample

- Purulent
- Mucopurulent
- Mucoid

**Note:** Reject salivary samples and advise the patient to expectorate from the lower respiratory tract.

## Throat Swab
## (Posterior Pharyngeal Swab)

### Throat Swab

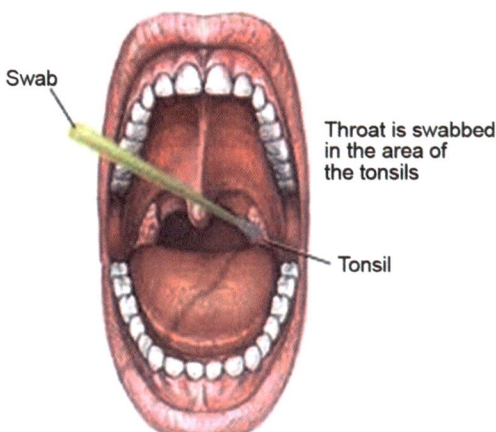

Swab

Throat is swabbed in the area of the tonsils

Tonsil

**Throat swab** is taken to find out infection in throat, e.g. diphtheria and streptococcal pharyngitis.

### Procedure

- Ask patient to open mouth and stick their tongue out.
- Use tongue spatula to press the tongue downward or hold tongue with tongue depressor.
- Locate areas of inflammation and exudate in posterior pharynx, tonsillar region of throat behind uvula.
- Use sterile cotton swab to swab both of the tonsillar arches and the posterior nasopharynx, without touching the sides of the mouth.
- Avoid swabbing soft palate; do not touch tongue.
- Rub area back and forth with cotton or Dacron swab.
- Insert swab into same transport tube containing nose swabs, break off shaft and recap tube firmly.
- Label the transport tube with the patient's initials, date of birth, case number and date of collection.
- Transport to laboratory.

### Nasal Swab

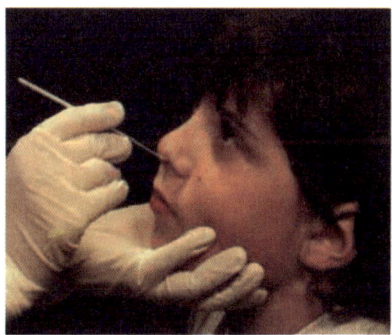

**Nasal swabs** and **nasopharyngeal** is done to find out infection in nasopharynx.

## Method for Nasal Swab

- Ensure that the patient does not blow his/her nose prior to taking the nasal swabs.
- Tilt patients head back gently and steady the chin.
- Insert cotton bud end of dry sterile swab into right nostril and rub firmly against the turbinate (to ensure swab contains cells as well as mucus).
- Withdraw slowly.
- Insert swab into tube of transport medium, break off shaft of swab and recap tube.
- Repeat procedure for left nostril using new sterile swab and insert into same tube of transport medium.

**Transport medium:** Allows organisms (pathogens) to survive and should be non-nutritive—does not allow organisms to proliferate.

- For bacteria, i.e. Cary-Blair
- For viruses—virus transport media (VTM).

**Nasopharyngeal swab**

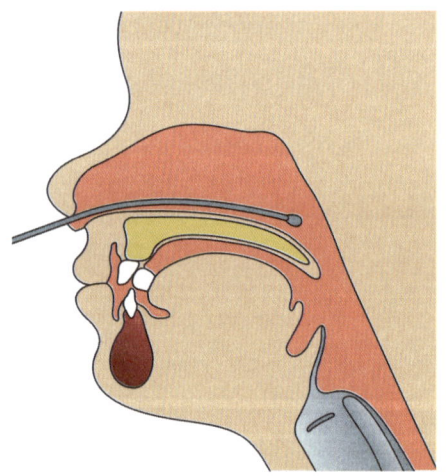

**Nasopharyngeal aspirate**

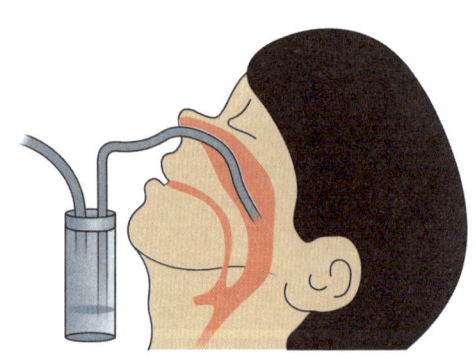

## Nasopharyngeal Swab Procedure

- Collect specimens after wearing gloves and a mask. Change gloves and wash your hands between each patient.
- Ensure that patient should not have a lot of mucus in the nose.
- Estimate the distance to the nasopharynx: Prior to insertion, measure the distance from the corner of the nose to the front of the ear and insert the shaft only half this length.
- Seat the patient comfortably.
- Tilt the patient's head back slightly to straighten the passage from the front of the nose to the nasopharynx to make insertion of the swab easier.
- Insert the swab provided along the medial part of the septum, along the floor of the nose, until it reaches the posterior nares; gentle rotation of the swab may be helpful. (If resistance is encountered, try the other nostril; the patient may have a deviated septum.)
- Allow the swab to sit in place for 5–10 seconds.
- Rotate the swab several times to dislodge the columnar epithelial cells. (Insertion of the swab usually induces a cough.)

- Withdraw the swab and place it in the collection tube.
- Refrigerate immediately.
- Remove gloves.
- Wash hands.
- Attach completed requisition.
- Transport specimen to the laboratory.

## Nasopharyngeal Aspirate Procedure

- Tilt head slightly backward.
- For aspirate after tilting head, instill 1–1.5 ml of VTM/sterile normal saline into one nostril.
- Use aspiration trap.
- Insert silicone catheter in nostril and aspirate the secretion gently by suction in each nostril

## URINE SAMPLING

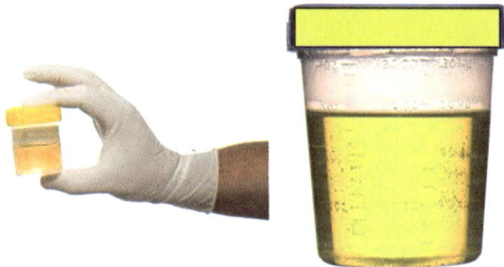

**Urine sample** is done to know if it contains anything unusual, this may indicate an underlying health problem, e.g. sugar, albumin, red cells and pathogens. Pregnancy test kit also uses urine.

## Collecting a Urine Sample

- Urine sample may be collected at any time of day but for pregnancy test first morning specimen is best.
- Take a sterile container to collect urine
- Label the container with your name, date of birth and the date.
- Wash your hands.
- Men should wash their penis and women should wash their genitals, including between the labia (lips around the entrance to the vagina).
- Start to urinate but don't collect the first part of urine that comes out.
- Collect a sample of urine 'mid-stream' (see below) in a sterile screw-top container.
- Screw the lid of the container shut.
- Wash your hands thoroughly.
- Hand it over the sample to laboratory at early as possible.
- Store a urine sample if it is not send to laboratory within one hour, in the fridge at around 4°C (39°F) for no longer than 24 hours.

**Midstream urine sample:** A midstream urine sample means that you don't collect the first part or the last part of urine that comes out, whereas collect mid-part of urine. This reduces the risk of the sample being contaminated with bacteria from:

- Your hands
- Skin around the urethra (tube that carries urine out of the body).

### STOOL SAMPLING

**Stool collection** is to find out the type of infection in gastrointestinal tract.

### Patient Instructions for Collection of Stool Sample

- Urinate before collecting the stool and do not to urinate while passing the stool, so that you do not get any urine in the stool sample.
- Wash your hands before and after you collect the specimen.
- Pass stool (but no urine) directly into the provided sterile cup or use the plastic wrap method.
- Place one teaspoonful of faeces into the bottle provided. Do not overfill the bottle. Do not pour the liquid out of the bottle.
- If you have diarrhoea, a plastic wrap method is used or plastic bag taped to the toilet seat may make the collection process easier. Do not collect the sample from the toilet bowl.
- Place the lid on the cup or bottle.
- Make sure the patient's name and the date of collection is on the cup/bottle.
- Deliver your stool specimen as soon as possible to laboratory for testing.

### Instructions for using a Plastic Wrap to Collect Stool

- Lift the toilet seat.
- Cover the toilet bowl with a large sheet of plastic wrap.
- Let a bowl depression be formed in the plastic wrap.
- Sit down to pass specimen onto plastic wrap.
- After passing the specimen, use a plastic spoon to put stool into the cup or the plastic bag as such can be placed in a sterile cup.

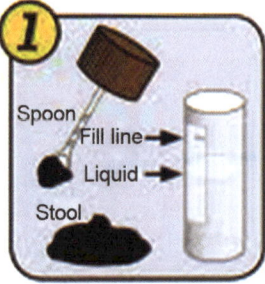 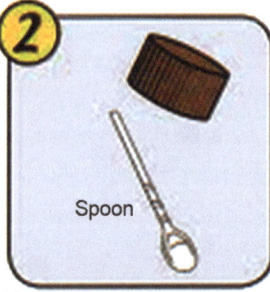 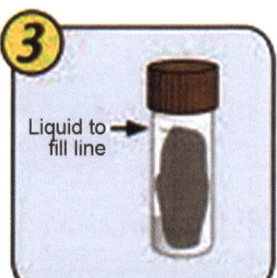

| Collect on plastic wrap and transfer to vial until liquid reaches fill line. | Remove spoon from lid and discard. | Replace cap on vial tightly and shake for a minute. Place vial in refrigerator until ready to ship. |

## Rectal Swab

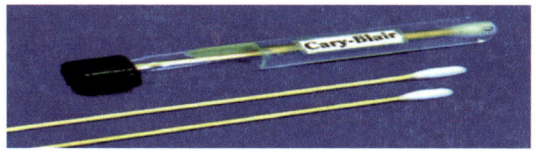

### Procedure

Insert swab 1–1.5 inches into rectum and gently rotate. Place both swabs into the same tube deep enough that Cary-Blair medium covers the cotton tips. Break off top portion of sticks and discard.

**Advantage:** Convenient and adapted to small children, debilitated patients and other situations where voided stool sample not feasible.

### Drawbacks

- No macroscopic assessment possible
- Less material available
- Not recommended for viruses.

### Stool Sample Collection for Various Purposes

| Purpose | Bacterial | Parasitic | Viral | Chemical |
|---|---|---|---|---|
| Timing of collection | During period of active diarrhoea | Anytime after onset of illness | Within 48–72 hours of illness | Within 48–72 hours of contaminant |
| Number of samples | 5–10 ml fresh stool 3 samples from each 10 ill persons and 10 controls | | | Uurine, vomitus and blood sample also |
| Method for collection | For rectal swabs, moisten 2 swabs in an appropriate transport (Cary-Blair) medium | Stool sample into 10% formalin and PVA at a ratio of 1 stool: 3 preservative | Fresh stool specimens (preferably liquid) | Fresh stool specimens. Whole blood collected in EDTA |
| Storage of specimens | Refrigerate swabs in transport media after collection at 4°C and test within 48 hours after collection. Store portion of each stool sample frozen at less than –15°C for antigen or PCR testing. For Ag detection and PCR testing, no transport medium is required | | | |
| Transportation | Refrigerate at 4°C, if testing within 48 hours, –70°C, if longer; store at –15°C for Ag detection and PCR<br>For frozen samples: Place bagged and sealed samples on dry ice. Mail in insulated box by overnight mail | | | |

### Reasons for False Positive Results of Stool Sample Examination

- Recent use of antibiotics, medicine to control diarrhoea, enemas, or laxatives.
- Recent X-ray tests using a contrast material containing barium.
- Stool sample mixed with urine or blood.
- Not collecting a large enough sample.
- Not getting the stool sample to the lab for testing in time.

## Qualities of Good Stool Sampling

- It has been also sampled from areas containing blood, mucous and areas of loose or watery consistency whereas a solid stool should be sampled from both ends and the middle.
- The stool sample amount should be enough.
- Mixing of stool with fixative is to preserve the morphology of the parasites. Fixative therefore, must come into contact with the organism and proper mixing will achieve this.
- All specimens must be properly labelled with patient's name, age, sex, and date of collection.
- Do not keep the specimen at warm temperatures. Try to keep it in cool, shady places.
- Prevent the drying of the specimen.
- Prevent contamination with urine or dirt particles.
- The specimen must reach the laboratory within 30 minutes of passing of the stool, since amoebic trophozoites die and become unrecognizable after that.
- Multiple stool examinations are required before the presence of parasitic infections is ruled out.

## Examination of Stool Sample

**Macroscopic examination:** Various points to be noted are:

- Consistency: The consistency of the stool could be formed, soft, loose or watery. The cysts are found maximum in the formed stool while trophozoites are most abundant in watery stool.
- Presence of blood and mucus.
- Presence of round worms, thread worms or tapeworm proglottids.
- Colour and smell of the stool.

**Microscopic examination:** A wet mount can be prepared directly from faecal material or from the concentrated specimens. The basic types of wet mounts that should be made from each sample include:

- Saline wet mount: It is used to detect worm eggs or larvae protozoan trophozoites and cysts. In addition it can reveal the presence of RBCs and WBCs.
- Iodine wet mount: It is used to stain glycogen and nuclei of the cysts.

**Preservation:** If the specimen cannot be examined within 1 hour, it should be placed in fixative.

To make up 100 ml of SAF:

- Sodium acetate – 1.5 grams
- Glacial acetic acid – 2.0 ml
- Formaldehyde – 40% to 4.0 ml
- Distilled water – 92.0 ml

## FOOD SAMPLES

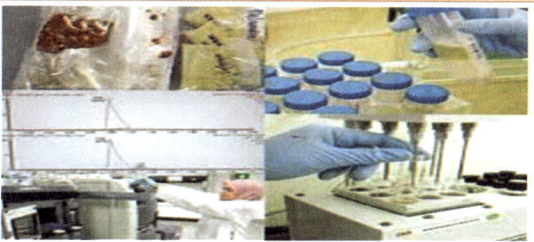

**Food sampling** is a process used to check that a food does not contain harmful contaminants or that it contains only permitted additives at acceptable levels, or that it contains the right levels of key ingredients or that its label declarations are correct or to know the present nutrients.

### Collection of Food Sample

- Collect suspect food earliest
- Collect aseptically—sterile tools, containers.
- For regulatory purposes, a minimum of 5 sample units from a lot is generally specified for examination.
- The size of the samples taken should also be adequate, i.e. a minimum sample size of 100, g or ml is commonly required.
- Cut 100 – 200 grams solid food from centre with sterile knife.
- Raw meat or poultry-refrigerate in a sterile plastic jar.
- For contact surfaces (utensils and/or equipment) for food processing a moisten swab with sterile 0.1% peptone water or buffered distilled water; put the swab in an enrichment broth.

### Handling and Transportation

- As fast as possible
- Keep perishable food at 2–8°C
- Cool hot food rapidly
- Pack samples to prevent spillage
- Contact the laboratory regarding method of transport and anticipated time of receipt.

### Labelling on Food Sample

- Patient's name
- Clinical specimen
- Unique ID number (research/outbreak)
- Specimen type
- Date, time and place of collection
- Name/initials of collector

### Glass Slides for Microscopy
### Label Slides Individually

- Use glass marking pencil
- Ensure markings do not interfere with staining process.

Each slide should bear:
- Patient name
- Unique identification number
- Date of collection

**Tests for food safety and quality:** Food samples are undergone certain tests and analyses like:
- Nutritional analysis and testing
- Food contact tests
- Food allergen testing
- Food chemical analysis
- Food contaminant testing
- Microbiological tests
- Pesticide residue testing
- Veterinary drug residue testing

## CATEGORIES OF MICROBIOLOGICAL QUALITY

**Satisfactory [S]:** Results indicate good microbiological quality, no action is required.

**Marginal [M]:** Results are borderline in that they are within limits of acceptable microbiological quality but may indicate possible hygiene problems in the preparation of the food.

Action: Re-sampling may be appropriate. Premises that regularly yield borderline results should have their food handling controls investigated.

**Unsatisfactory [US]:** results are beyond the acceptable microbiological limits and are indicative of poor food hygiene or food handling practices.

**Action:** Further sampling, including the sampling of other foods from the food premise may be required and an investigation undertaken to determine whether food handling controls and hygiene practices are adequate.

**Potentially hazardous [PH]:** The levels in this range may cause food-borne illness and immediate remedial action should be initiated.

**Microbiological Quality (CFU per gram)**

| Test | S | M | US | PH |
|---|---|---|---|---|
| *Enterobacteriaceae | < 102 | 102–104 | < 104 | |
| **Escherichia coli* | < 3 | 3–100 | Greater than 100 | |
| Coagulase +ve staphylococci | < 102 | 102–103 | 103–104 | Greater than 104 |
| *Clostridium perfringens* *Bacillus cereus* and other | < 102 | 102–103 | 103–104 | Greater than 104 |
| pathogenic *Bacillus* spp | < 102 | 102–103 | 103–104 | Greater than 104 |
| *Vibrio parahaemolyticus* | < 3 | 3–102 | 102–104 | Greater than 104 |
| *Salmonella* spp Action required | not detected in 25 g | – | – | Detected in 25 g |

*Enterobacteriaceae testing is not applicable to fresh fruits and vegetables or foods containing these.
**Pathogenic strains of *E. coli* should be absent.

# Research Methodology and Biostatistics

**8**

**Research** is systematized efforts to gain new knowledge.
**Research methodology** is a methodology adopted for research.

## Steps in Research Methodology

### 1. Process of planning:

  a. Define research problem
  b. Review of literature
  c. Planning for methodology

### 2. Process of execution:

  a. Data collection for pilot study (if proforma is not well established or it is a pioneer work)
  b. Correction in proforma, if needed
  c. Data collection for study

### 3. Process of concluding:

  a. Analysis of data
  b. Getting inference
  c. Report writing

### 4. Dissemination of reports

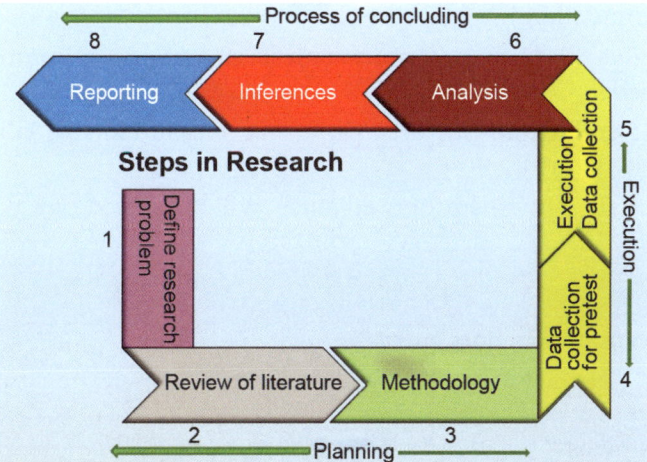

## Define Research Problem

**Research problem** is gap between ideal and present status; it refers to some problem which a researcher experiences and wants to obtain a solution for the same, i.e. a question or issue to be examined.

- Problem definition or problem statement should be clear, precise, self-explanatory and should include:
  - What
  - How
  - When
  - Where
- Transform the selected research problem into a scientifically **researchable statement**.

**Research objectives** are the statement of the questions that is to be investigated with the goal of answering the overall research problem.

## Review of Literature

**Literature review** is the documentation of a published work in the areas of specific interest to the researcher.

## Literature Review

- To find out already investigated problems and those that need further investigation.
- To formulate researchable hypothesis.
- To gain a background knowledge
- To identify data sources
- To learn how others structured their reports

## Methodology

**Study area:** Location where proposed study will be carried out, e.g. hospital and community.

**Study period:** Duration from start to end of study (maximum period available for study should be defined).

Selection of study design

Selection of study population

**Prerequisites of study:** Study tools, terminologies, criteria, orientation trainings, etc. should also be clearly defined.

**Study tools for data collection:** Subjects, proforma, measurements, lab investigations, etc. should also be clearly defined.

**Plan for action:** Actually how the proposed study will be carried out, which may be shown by flow chart.

## Planning

- Data collection, compilation, data entry
- Data cleaning
- Outcome variables
- Outcome analysis plans

**Confidentiality:** Confidentiality of gathered data/information should be maintained.

## Ethical Clearance: Consent from

- Institutional Review Board
- CTRI: In case of interventional study/drug trials.
- Observational units/subjects: Inform written consent.

## Study Design

***Study design** is a specific plan or protocol for conducting the study, which allows the investigator to translate the conceptual hypothesis into an operational one.

## Direction Wise Study Design

- Cross-sectional: At a point of time
- Retrospective: Backward direction
- Prospective: Forward direction
- Ambidirectional: From backward to forward direction.

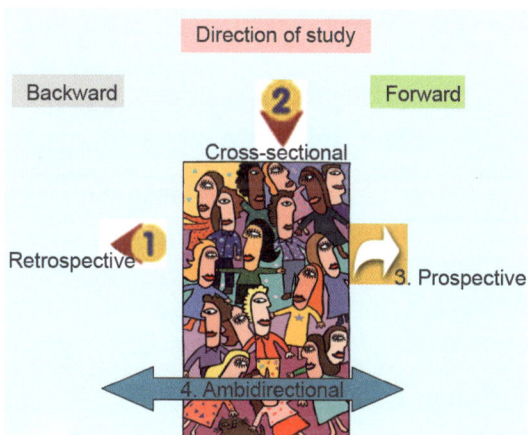

## Type of Study Design

*1. Observational Studies*

- Descriptive studies
- Analytical
  - Cross-sectional
  - Case-control
  - Cohort

*2. Experimental/Interventional Studies*

- As per control: RCT/NRCT
- As per design: Simple/cross-over

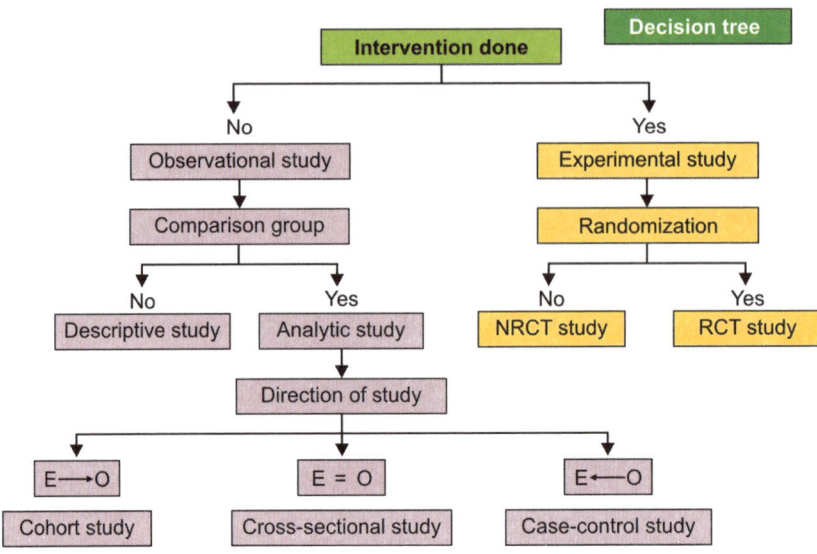

**Appropriate study design as per study question**

| Type of study question | Appropriate study design |
|---|---|
| Burden of illness | Field surveys |
| Prevalence | Cross-sectional survey |
| Incidence | Longitudinal survey |
| Causation, risk and prognosis | Case control study, cohort study, RCT |
| Treatment efficacy | RCT |
| Diagnostic test evaluation | RCT |

## Descriptive Study Design

- Other name — Case-series/population
- Unit of study — Case/individuals
- Study question — What is happening?
- Direction of inquiry — Cross-sectional/snap shot
- Study design
    Desired information
    about cases/individuals is collected

## Cross-sectional Study Design

Data collection is done at a single point of time, so also called snapshot study. It describes associations. Prevalence can be found with this design, if conducted in geographically defined area.

- Other name
- Unit study
- Study question
- Direction of inquiry
- Study design

Prevalence study
individual

What is happening?

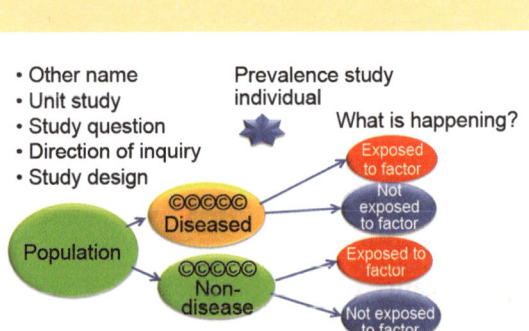

## Case-control Study

Start with people who have disease. These cases are matched with other individuals who do not have diseases otherwise they are same as cases in all other respects except the factor/disease under study. These matched individuals are known as 'Controls'. Now look backward to find out proportion of cases and controls positive for risk factor under consideration. Compare degree of exposure to possible risk factor in both the groups.

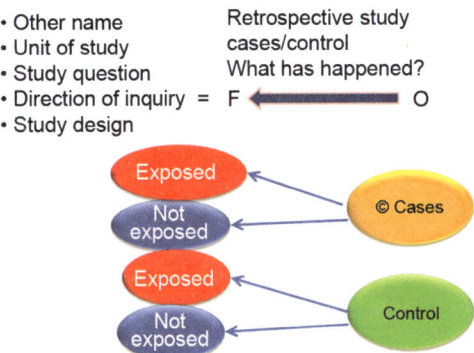

## Cohort Study

Begins with disease-free individuals known as cohort. They are classified as exposed/unexposed to factor under consideration. Both groups are followed for a specific period (> 1 year in case to find out incidence). Record and compare outcomes in the form of diseased/non-diseased in both groups.

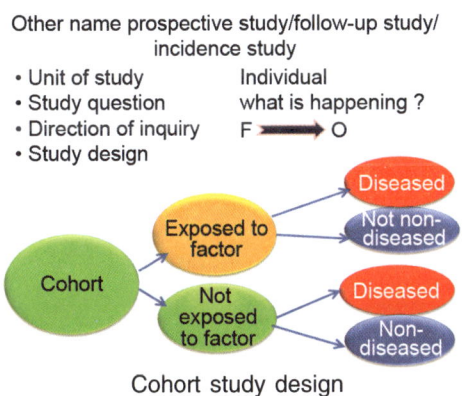

Cohort study design

## Measures of Association

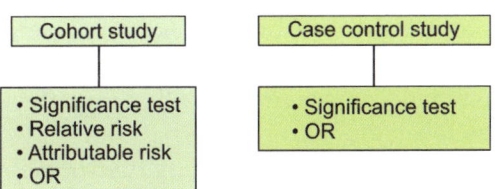

**Significance test** is to test significance of difference in exposure between control and cases.

**Odds ratio** is ratio of the odds among exposed to non-exposed.

**Relative risk** is ratio between incidence among exposed and incidence among non-exposed.

**Attributed risk** is percentage of difference between incidence among exposed and non-exposed with incidence among exposed.

## RR or OR of 1 Indicate no Effect of Exposure (Equal Odds)

**Experimental studies** are "gold standard" of determining the relationship between factor and the event.

## Type of Experimental Studies
## A. As per Randomization

1. **Randomized Control Trials (RCT)**
   i. Concurrent parallel design
   ii. Sequential RCT design
   iii. RCT with external control

2. **Non-randomized Trials**

## B. As per Design
- **Simple**
  - Before and after
  - Quincy experiment
  - Comparison with placebo
  - Comparison of two medicines/procedures/tests
  - Comparison of > two medicines/procedures/tests (block experiment)

- **Cross-over Study Design**

## C. As per Study Area
- Field trials
- Clinical trials
- Lab. trials

## Quality of Experimental Study
- Randomization
- Blinding
- Control
- Cross-over

**Randomization** can be done by chit box method (simple random technique) or alternate (systemic R.T.) to avoid personal biases.

**Blinding** is a good practice where subjective factors that can affect the evaluation of outcome are not allowed to influence the evaluation process.

- **Single-blind:** Patient or evaluator (one out of them) is blinded about the type of intervention given.

- **Double-blind design:** Neither patient nor the outcome evaluator knows about which intervention is given to which patient.
- **Triple-blind:** When research evaluator is a third party/agency, in that case that evaluator along with patient and doctor does not know about which intervention is given to which patient.

**Controls** are used for comparison of effects of medicine, procedure, etc. They can be:

i.  **Concurrent parallel RCT design:**
    a.  Placebo control
    b.  Out of two medicine, procedure, etc. comparison, one may act as control for other.

ii. **Sequential RCT design:** Patient him/herself can serve as control in before and after comparison.

iii. **RCT with external control:** Results obtained from other studies can be used for comparison as controls. These types of controls are also known as historical controls. External/historical controls are better than no control.

### Experimental Study Design 1 (RCT with Placebo)

- Other name — Intervention study
- Objective — To know the effect of intervention
- Unit of study — Individual meeting entry criteria
- Study question both — What is happening after intervention in group?
- Direction of inquiry — I ⟹ E
- Study design — 1 (intervention with placebo)

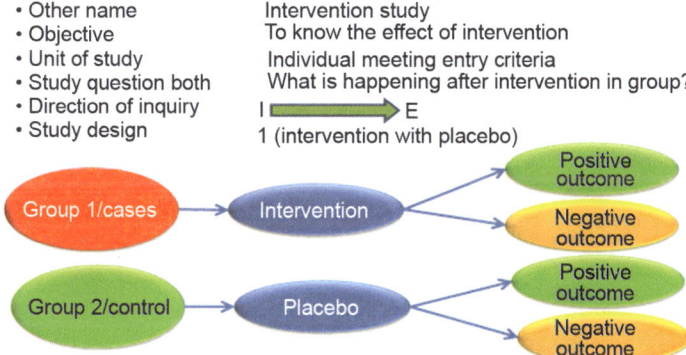

### Intervention Study Design 2 (Comparison of Effect of Two Interventions)

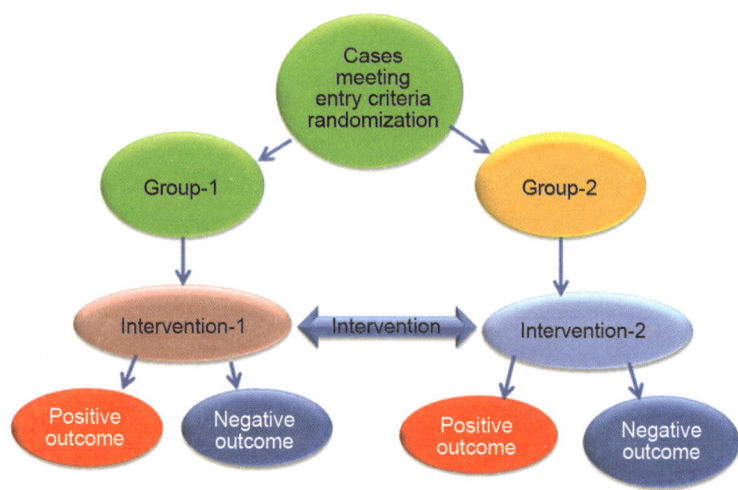

## Experimental Design of before and after Comparison of Quantitative Data

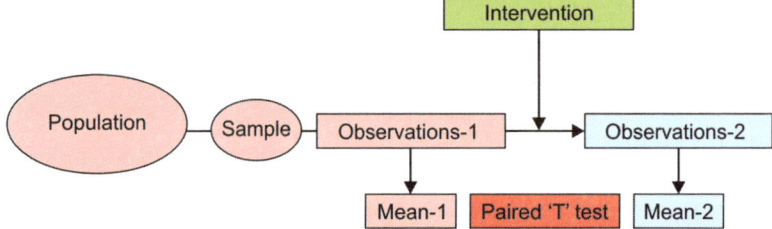

## Quincy Experimental Study Design

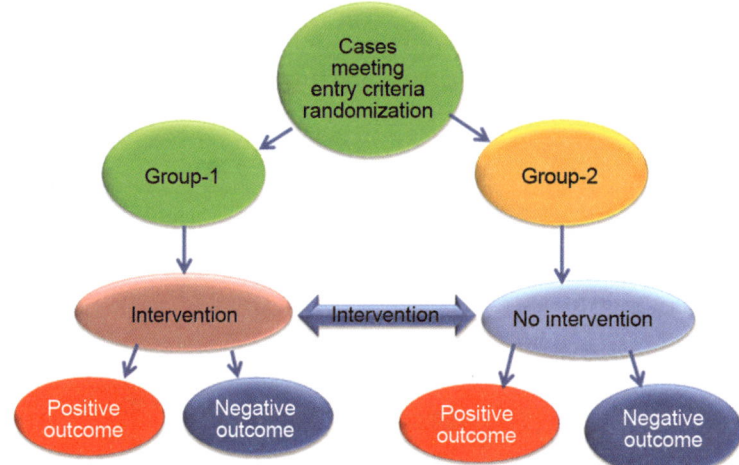

## Block Experimental Study Design

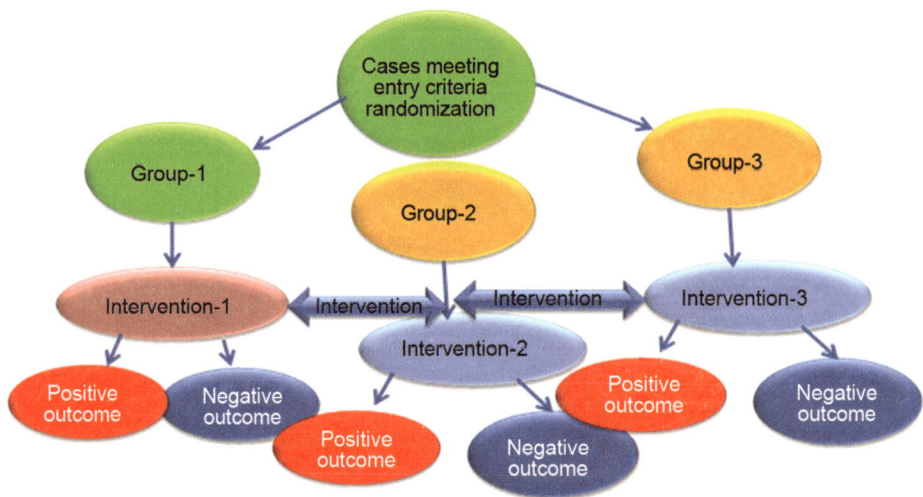

## Cross-over Study Design: Cross-over after Washout Period

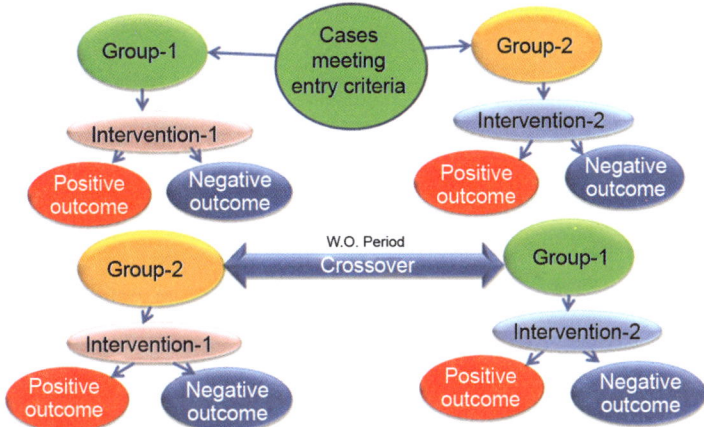

## Steps of Experimental Design

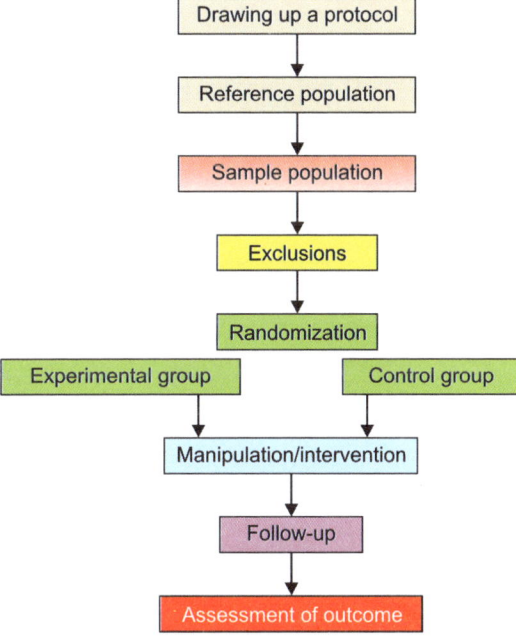

## Hierarchy of Epidemiological Study Design

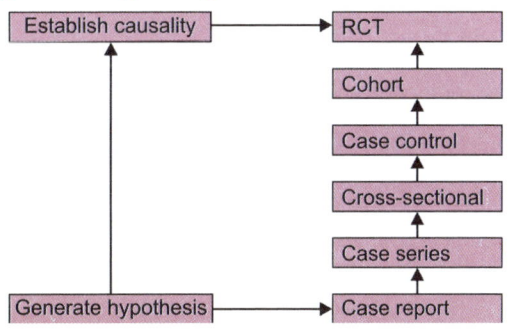

## Study Population

**Study population** is population included in study—may be whole population of interest or sample may be selected.

**Sample** is a small true representative segment of a population so inferences drawn from a sample are expected to be applicable for the source population.

### Qualities of a sample

- Adequate size
- Appropriate sampling technique

**Sample size** is adequate number of observation units by which inferences drawn are expected to be applicable for the source population with minimum resources.

**Sample size depend upon:**

- **Population factors**
  - Type of information available
- **Type of study**
  - Type of data
  - Type of study design
  - Type of sampling and design effect
  - Type of statistical analysis for outcome needed
- **Determined values of research by researcher**
  - Power
  - Significance level

|  | Test results | |
|---|---|---|
|  | $H_0$ **is true** | $H_0$ **is false** |
| $H_0$ **is accepted** | Correct conclusion | Type II error ($\beta$ error) |
| $H_0$ **is rejected** | Type I error ($\alpha$ error) | Correct conclusion |

$1-\beta$ is called statistical power of the test; $\alpha$ is called significance level of the test

**Power:** Ability to detect correct answer, i.e. true positives or true differences if it was really present.

**Alpha error:** Chance to miss correct answer.

### Type I error ($\alpha$)

- The probability of mistakenly concluding a 'difference' when actually there is 'no difference'.
- This probability is termed 'symbol $\alpha$ (alpha)' error.
- Conventionally this is set at 5% on $\alpha = 0.05$ or lower.

### Type II error ($\beta$)

- The probability of mistakenly concluding 'no difference' when actually there is 'difference'
- This probability is termed '$\beta$ (beta)' error.
- Conventionally this is set at 0.1 to 0.2.

- **1-beta** is known as **power** of the study.
- Thus, conventionally power is set at 80 to 90%.

**Design effect** is to adjust sample size according to type of sampling technique used to conduct the study.

Design effect = Variance of specific sampling technique/Variance of simple random sampling

| Type of technique | Design effect |
|---|---|
| Simple random technique | 1 |
| Systemic random technique | 1.2 |
| Stratified random technique | 0.8 |
| Cluster random technique | 2 |

**Contingency addition** is to adjust dropouts of study in sample size.

## SAMPLE SIZE CALCULATION

### For Descriptive Study

**For qualitative data (having prevalence)**

$$\text{Sample size} = Z^2PQ/L^2 = 4PQ/L^2$$

Here,     $Z = 1.96$ at 95% confidence limit $\approx 2$ at 95% confidence limit

         $P$ = Prevalence of disease/event

         $Q = 100 - P$

         $L$ = Allowable error (conventionally allowed up to 20% of P)

**For quantitative data (having mean and standard deviation)**

$$\text{Sample size} = Z^2SD^2/L^2 = 4SD^2/L^2$$

Here,     $Z = 1.96$ at 95% confidence limit $\approx 2$ at 95% confidence limit

         $SD$ = Standard deviation of disease/event

         $L$ = Allowable error (allowable difference of means to be detected)

### For Analytic Study

**For comparison of two proportions**

$$\text{Sample size} = \left(Z_\alpha \sqrt{P_1\,(1-P_2)} - Z_\beta \sqrt{2P_1\,(1-P_1) + P_2\,(1-P_2)}\right)$$

**For comparison of two means**

$$\text{Sample size} = 2\left((Z_\alpha - Z_\beta)SD/(M_1 - M_2))^2\right)$$

Here, $Z_\alpha$ = Z value related with 2 tailed value of Z score to particular $\alpha$ (conventionally + 1.96).

      $Z_\beta$ = Z value related with one tailed value of Z score to particular $\beta$ (coventionally – 0.8)

      $P_1$ = Prevalence of disease/event in 1st group

      $P_2$ = Prevalence of disease/event in 2nd group

      $M_1$ = Mean of 1st group

      $M_2$ = Mean of 2nd group

**For odds ratio**

$$n = \left(\frac{r+1}{r}\right)\frac{(\bar{p})(1-\bar{p})(Z_\beta + Z_{\alpha/2})^2}{(p_1 - p_2)^2}$$

Here, **n = Sample size** in the case group

**r = ratio** of controls to cases

$Z_\beta$ = Represents the **desired power** (conventionally 0.84 for 80% power)

$Z_\alpha$ = Represents the desired **level of statistical significance** (conventionally 1.96).

$p_1 - p_2$ = **Effect size** (the difference in proportions)

$p$ = Average proportion exposed

For 80% power, $Z_\beta$ = .84

For 0.05 significance level, $Z_\alpha$ = 1.96

$r = 1$ (equal number of cases and controls)

The proportion exposed in the control group is 20%.

To get proportion of cases exposed:

$$p_{case\ exp} = \frac{OR p_{controls\,exp}}{p_{controls\,exp}\,(OR - 1) + 1}$$

For correlation coefficient ($r$)

$$N = \frac{(Z_\alpha + Z_\beta)}{\dfrac{1}{4}\{\log e\,(1+r)/(1-r)\}2} + 3$$

$r$ = accepted correlation

$Z_\beta$ = Represents the *desired power* (conventionally 0.84 for 80% power).

$Z_\alpha$ = Represents the desired level of statistical significane (conventionally 1.96).

## Steps of Sample Size Calculation

1. Stage 1 – *Base sample size calculation ($n$)
2. Stage 2 – Sample size with design effect ($d$) = $n \times d$
3. Stage 3 – Contingency addition (5 – 20%)
4. Stage 4 – Sample size estimation for study population = ($n \times d$) + 5% of $n$

*Use appropriate equation for sample size calculation (http://stat.ubc.ca/~rollin/stats/ssize)

Sample size **finite population correction** is done where the population is less than 50,000 or calculated sample size is < 5% of population from which it was drawn

New sample size = SS (1 + SS/P)

here,     SS = sample size;

P = Population

## Sampling Technique

Appropriate sampling technique as per study question and design should be chosen. These techniques are:

I. Random sampling technique

1. Simple random technique
2. Systemic random technique
3. Stratified random technique
4. Multiphase random technique
5. Multistage random technique
6. Cluster random technique

II. Non-random sampling technique

1. Convenience
2. Purposive
3. Quota/judgmental
4. Snow ball study

## 1. Simple Random Sampling Technique (SRS)
### Lottery Method

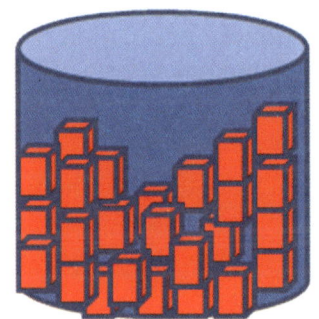 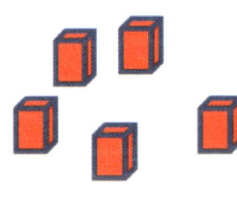

### Random Table Method

- Stage 1– Give number to each member of population
- Stage 2 – Determine total population size (N)
- Stage 3 – Determine sample size (S)
- Stage 4 – Drop one finger on random table with eyes closed
- Stage 5 – Drop one finger with eyes closed on direction to be chosen – Up/Down/Rt/Lt
- Stage 6 – Determine first number within 0 to N
- Stage 7 – *Determine other numbers till sample size (S)

 * Once a number is chosen do not repeat it again

## 2. Systemic Random Technique

Selection of sample follows a systemic interval (K) of selection.

Steps are as follows:
- Find serial interval (K) = Total population/sample size.
- First observation select from 1 to Kth through simple random technique.
- Next observation will be (1st + K)th observation.
- Next observation will be (2nd + K)th observation.
- Repeat till equal to sample size number observations are selected.

| Systemic Random Technique | *Population* | | | |
|---|---|---|---|---|

| | | | | |
|---|---|---|---|---|
| | 1 | 21 | 41 | 61 | 81 |
| | 2 | 22 | 42 | 62 | 82 |

**Systemic Random Technique**

➤ N = 1100 (given)

➤ S = 20 (estimated)

➤ K = N/S = 100/20 = 5

➤ 1st observation between 1 to 5 though SRS, e.g. 3

➤ Every 5th observation from 3rd observation will be included in sample population

➤ So, sample population will be – 3rd 8th, 13th, 18th, 23rd, 28th, 33rd, 38th, 43rd, 48th, 53rd, 58th, 63rd, 68th, 73rd, 78th, 83rd, 88th, 93rd, and 98th observation

*Population*

| | | | |
|---|---|---|---|
| 1 | 21 | 41 | 61 | 81 |
| 2 | 22 | 42 | 62 | 82 |
| 3 | 23 | 43 | 63 | 83 |
| 4 | 24 | 44 | 64 | 84 |
| 5 | 25 | 45 | 65 | 85 |
| 6 | 26 | 46 | 66 | 86 |
| 7 | 27 | 47 | 67 | 87 |
| 8 | 28 | 48 | 68 | 88 |
| 9 | 29 | 49 | 69 | 89 |
| 10 | 30 | 50 | 70 | 90 |
| 11 | 31 | 51 | 71 | 91 |
| 12 | 32 | 52 | 72 | 92 |
| 13 | 33 | 53 | 73 | 93 |
| 14 | 34 | 54 | 74 | 94 |
| 15 | 35 | 55 | 75 | 95 |
| 16 | 36 | 56 | 76 | 96 |
| 17 | 37 | 57 | 77 | 97 |
| 18 | 38 | 58 | 78 | 98 |
| 19 | 39 | 59 | 79 | 99 |
| 20 | 40 | 60 | 80 | 100 |

## Stratified Random Technique

**Stratified random** technique is good for heterogeneous population. In this, homogeneous strata are made before selecting sample and then sample population is selected from each stratum as per simple random/systemic random technique. If selected sample population size in each stratum is as per population proportion of strata, then it is called **'population proportion to size (PPS)'**.

## 4. Multiphase Random Technique

**Multiphase random technique** is used when diagnostic test to identify cases is quite expensive. In this situation, suspected cases are first isolated with the help of some less expensive test in first phase then diagnostic tests are used to diagnose cases from suspected ones in second phase. This technique is done more than one phase so called multiphase.

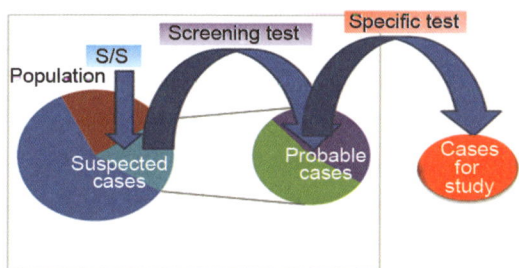

## 5. Multistage Random Technique

**Multistage random technique** is used when large population is to cover in less time, e.g. for evaluation of national programmes. In this situation, whole population is divided into block, out of these blocks, numbers of blocks are chosen as per sample size through SRS. Again these chosen blocks are divided into smaller blocks out of these smaller blocks, numbers of blocks, are chosen as per sample size through SRS. This technique is repeated again and again till it satisfies needs. As this technique passes through various stages so it is called multistage.

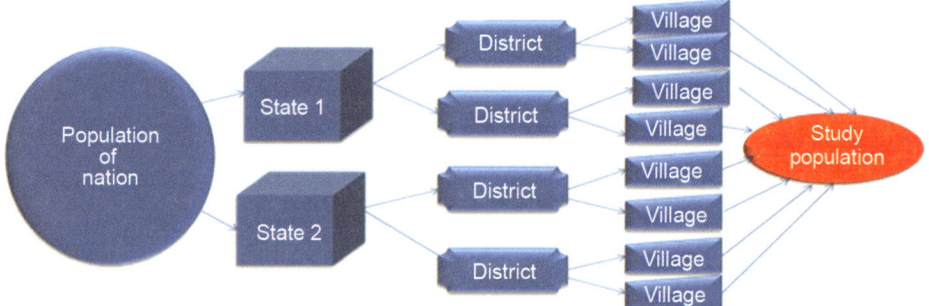

## 6. Cluster Random Technique

**Cluster random technique** is also used when large population is to cover in less time, e.g. for vaccination coverage. In this situation, whole population is divided into 30 blocks (30 cluster technique) known as 'Clusters', out of these 30 clusters, sample population is chosen either through simple random or systemic random technique.

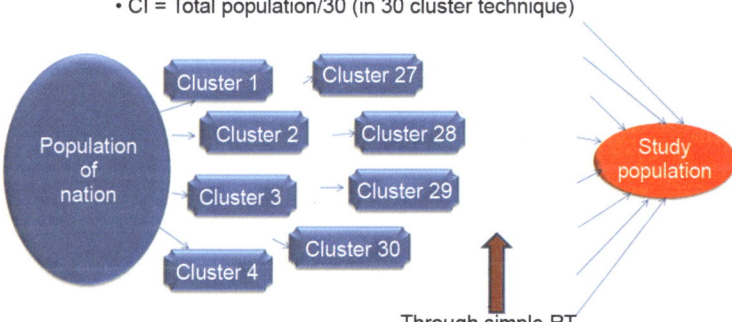

### Steps of Cluster Technique
- Find out total population to be surveyed.
- Estimate total sample size needed for study.
- Divide the total population with 30 to get 'Cluster interval.
- Estimate sample size needed from one cluster by dividing total sample size with 30.
- Choose any number randomly from 1st cluster.
- Survey that region where random number fall either by simple /systemic random technique till desired sample size is obtained from one sample.
- Add cluster interval for identified first random number to gent 2nd cluster for survey.
- Repeat the process for other dusters also.

## BIOSTATISTICS

**Statistics:** The collection of methods used in planning an experiment and analyzing data in order to draw accurate conclusions.

**Descriptive statistics** generally characterizes or describes a set of data elements by graphically displaying the information or describing its central tendencies and to know how it is distributed.

**Inferential statistics** tries to infer information about a population by using information gathered by data collection.

**Biostatistics** is application of statistics in biology, i.e. science of figure/data in medical science

$$\text{Biostatistics} = \text{Biology} + \text{Statistics}$$

**Data:** Set of information, facts or figures numerically coded and from which conclusions may be drawn is called data (singular—datum).

### Levels of Measurement of Data

The experimental (scientific) method depends on physically measuring things. Each level corresponds to how this measurement can be treated mathematically.

**Nominal:** Nominal data have no order and thus only gives **names** or labels to various categories. Gender is nominal data.

**Ordinal:** Ordinal data have **order**, but the interval between measurements is not meaningful. Data measured as poor, fair, good, better, best are example of ordinal data where a grade is given.

**Interval:** Interval data have meaningful intervals between measurements, but there is no true starting point (zero), i.e. no physical meaning of zero. Only interval is meaningful. Temperatures measured in Celsius degree, time measured, etc. are example of interval data.

**Ratio:** Ratio data have the highest level of measurement. Ratios between measurements as well as intervals are meaningful because there is a true starting point (zero).

### Types of Data: Specific terms are used as follows

**Qualitative** data are non-numeric. They are also known as 'quality count facts'. They are expressed as how many (percentage and proportion) were with this specific quality.

Type of status {poor, fair, good, better, best}, colours (red, blue, black, etc.), etc. are examples of qualitative data.

Qualitative data are often termed **categorical data**.

**Quantitative** data are numeric. They are also known as 'measured facts' or 'numerical facts'. Quantitative data are further classified as discrete and continuous.

**Discrete data** are numeric data that have a finite number of possible values.

A classic example of discrete data is a finite subset of the counting numbers, {1, 2, 3, 4, 5} perhaps corresponding to {Strongly disagree... Strongly agree}.

When quantitative data represent **counts**, they are discrete. For example 'how many students were absent on a given day'.

**Continuous** data have infinite possibilities: 1.4, 1.41, 1.414, 1.4142, 1.141421... Physically measurable quantities of length, volume, time, mass, etc. are generally considered continuous. At the physical level (microscopically), especially for mass, this may not be true, but for normal life situations is a valid assumption.

## Data Collection

Data collection depends upon:
- Nature of study
- Aims and objectives
- Availability of resources (funds/manpower/time, etc.)
- Precision required

## Sources

- Primary – own collected data
- Secondary – already generated data published or non-published.

## Type of Data Collection Methods

- Interview
  - Personal
  - Telephonic
- Observation
- Experimental
- Interview and observation
- Observation and experimental
- Interview, observation and experimental.

## Tools for Data Collection

- Questionnaire
- Schedule
- Case study

**Questionnaire** is set of semi-structured/structured open/closed questions which are to be asked to collect data. It may be filled by respondent or interviewer.

**Schedule** is also set of semi-structured/structured open/closed questions are to be asked along with writing down the findings of observations during supervision to collect data. It is to be filled by investigator.

## Consideration in Formulating Questionnaire

- Use simple and everyday language.
- Do not use ambiguous questions.
- Do not ask leading questions.
- Order of questions should be logical.
- Establish the logical link between the questions and objectives.
- Items/questions cover the full range of issue/attitude being measured.
- Guideline for filling an instrument should be given.
- Pre-testing should be done before applying to the study for data collection or use already tested questionnaire/schedule for reliability and validity.

## Organization and Compilation

**Organization and compilation** of data in such a way (master chart ) to have **reliable, relevant, adequate and reasonably complete data with following requisites:**

- Simplicity
- Briefness
- Utility
- Distinctiveness
- Comparability
- Scientific arrangement
- Attractiveness
- Effectiveness

## Classification and Tabulation

### Type of Tables

- As per purpose
  - General tables–about socio-demographic profile
  - Specific tables–about aims and objectives
- As per originality
  - Original tables – from original data
  - Derived tables – from original tables
- As per construction
  - Simple tables (one way tables) – showing one variable at one time
  - Complex tables—showing > 1 variable at one time.

### Contents of Table

- **Table no.** – where it stands in series of tables.
- **Tile of table**–short, clear and self-explanatory to say about for what the table is?
- **Body of table**–consists of rows and columns
  - Rows – 1st row shows heading of stubs
  - 1st column shows serial number of captions
  - 2nd column shows type of variables
  - Rest of rows and columns are showing data
  - Number of rows and columns should be limited to maintained simplicity of table.
- **Foot note**–written just below the body of table, if there is any hidden information including source of collected data if it is other than the present study.
- **Inferences**–summary value of table.

### *Preparation of a Frequency Table

Steps are as follows:
1. Arrange scores in an ascending or descending manner.
2. Draw a table containing three columns
   - a. Class interval       b. Tally      c. Frequency
3. Define 'Class intervals' from the available scores. Class interval can be decided in either an arbitrary manner considering the nature of problem being studied or as per 'Sturges rule'. 'Sturges Rule' is      $k = 1 + 3.322 \log N$
   - a. Here, '$k$' is number of classes that need to be formed and '$N$' = total number of observations.
   - b. Now, a class interval (as far as possible of equal size) is decided as per the upper and the lower limit of the data set.

4. Write down the class intervals defined in the respective column of the table.

5. Against each interval or the variable, draw a vertical tally line for each score falling in the interval. Once the tally line reaches the count of 4, mark the 5th score by crossing the 4 lines, ⲎⲎⲎ.

6. Count the number of tally lines and put the total number in the 'Frequency column'.

7. Note that the total of the frequency column must be equal to the total number of observations of the given data set.

*Table can be prepared directly from master chart by insert 'Pivot-table' in MS Excel.

## Diagrammatic Presentation of Data

**Graphical representation of ungrouped data:** Data may be depictive as following graphical representation:

1. Bar graph or bar diagrams
2. Circle graph or pie diagram
3. Line graphs
4. Pictograms

## Bar Diagram

- Bar diagrams are the simplest graphs used for discrete data for both qualitative as well as quantitative.
- The bars should be of uniform width.
- The space between the bars should be equal.
- The length of the bar is proportional to the value it represents.
- The scale should be clearly indicated and baseline be clearly shown.
- The width of bars can be arbitrarily decided.
- Space between the bars should be about one-half of the width of a bar.

**Bar diagrams** are of four types:

1. Simple bar diagram

2. Multiple or grouped bar diagram: Shows >1 variable variation at a time.

3. Subdivided or component bar diagram: It shows components of variable variation.

4. Percentage subdivided bar diagram: It shows % components of variable variation.

For example, table is as follows:

**Comparison of blood groups variation in population of various countries**

| S. no. | Country | RH compatibility | O | A | B | AB |
|--------|---------|------------------|------|------|------|------|
| 1 | India | RH positive (in %) | 37 | 26 | 19 | 2 |
| | | RH negative (in %) | 8 | 5 | 2 | 1 |
| 2 | US | RH positive (in %) | 37.4 | 35.7 | 8.5 | 3.4 |
| | | RH negative (in %) | 6.6 | 6.3 | 1.5 | 0.6 |
| 3 | China | RH positive (in %) | 47.7 | 27.8 | 18.9 | 5 |
| | | RH negative (in %) | 0.3 | 0.2 | 0.1 | 0.03 |

## Simple Bar Diagram

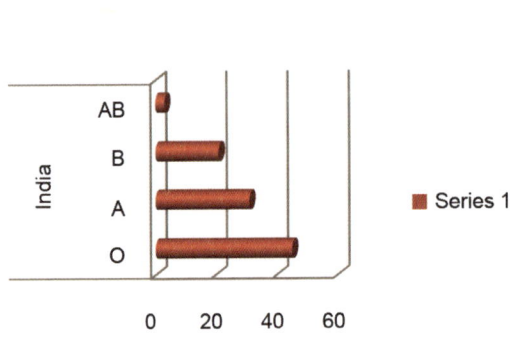

## Multiple Bar Diagram

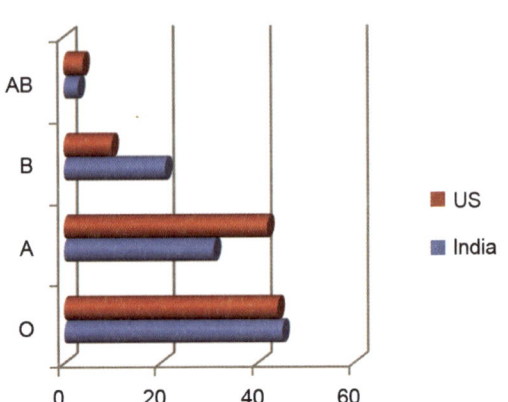

## % Component Bar Diagram

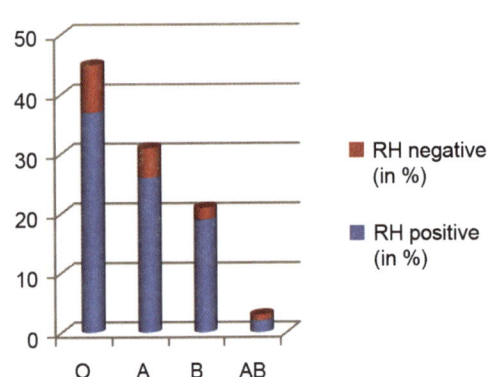

## Component Bar Diagram

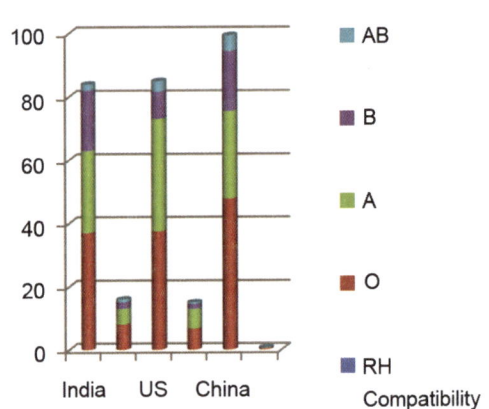

## Pie Diagram

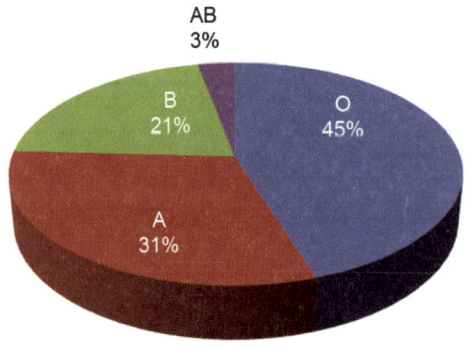

## Line Diagram

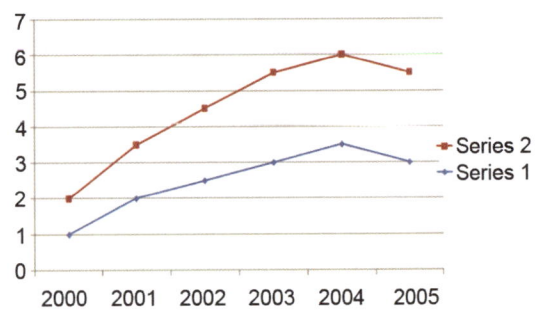

## Pie Chart

- A pie chart is also known as circular chart or sector chart.
- Pie chart is a circular graph used for representing the total value as components.
- The area of a circle is the total value while the different sectors of the circle are the different parts of the total value.

- The areas of the sectors are proportional to the angles at the centre.
- It is generally used for comparing the relation between various components of a value and between components and the total value.
- In pie chart, the data is expressed as percentage.

### Steps to make a Pie Chart

1. Plot a circle of appropriate size.
2. Convert the values of each component in percentages of the total value.
3. It is conventional and appealing to arrange the sectors according to size with the largest sector at the top and the others following in sequence in a clockwise manner.
4. 100% represents 360° angles at the centre of the circle, therefore, 1% value is equal to 3.6° angle.
5. Measure with protector the points on a circle representing the size of each sector and label each sector for identification.

### Line Graph

- In line graphs, one variable is plotted on the $x$-axis (horizontal axis) and the other variable is plotted on $y$-axis (vertical axis).
- This is used to see the effect of one variable on the other variable.

### Quantitative Data Presentation

- Histogram
- Frequency polygon
- Frequency curve
- Cumulative frequency curve
- Scatter diagram
- Radar
- Box and whisker
- Correlation diagram
- Proportional change diagram
- Ratio diagram or arithlog

### Histogram

- Histogram is a form of area diagram, containing a set of rectangles.
- Total area represents the total frequency and the proportionate frequency is represented by the area of each rectangle comprising the histogram.
- Size of the class interval is shown by the width of rectangle and the frequency by height.
- When the class-intervals are unequal, the heights of rectangles are made proportional not to the class frequencies, but to the frequency densities.
- This type of diagram is used exclusively for showing frequency distributions of quantitative data that are continuous in nature.

### Preparing a Histogram

1. Convert the data in the exclusive series, if it is given in the inclusive series.
2. Actual lower limits of all the class intervals (including the extra intervals) are taken and plot on the $x$-axis.

3. Lower limit of the lowest interval (one of the extra intervals) is taken at the intersecting point of $x$-axis and $y$-axis.
4. Each class or interval with its specific frequency is represented by a separate rectangle.
5. Base of each rectangle is the width of the class interval.
6. Height is the respective frequency of that class or interval.
7. Frequencies of the distribution are plotted on the $y$-axis.

### Frequency Polygon

- It is made by joining the mid-points of the apices of the rectangle of a histogram.
- It has many angles.

### Frequency Curve

- Frequency polygon when drawn by a free hand results in frequency curve.
- Area of the frequency polygon and the curve would essentially remain the same.
- Angulations of the frequency polygon are lost in a frequency curve.

### Histogram

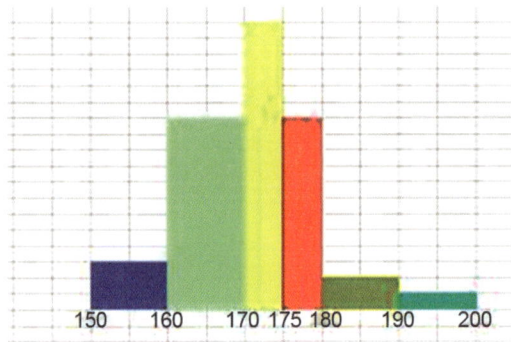
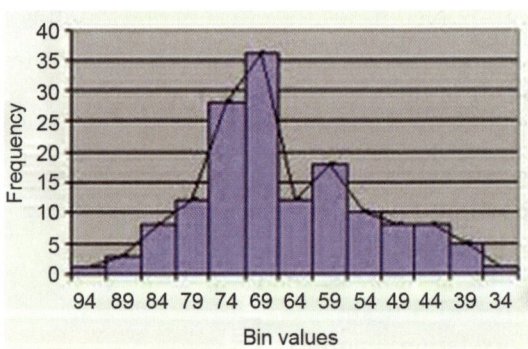

### Cumulative Frequency Curve or Ogive

- This represents a cumulative frequency distribution graphically.
- An Ogive takes the shape of a curve.
- Curve drawn from the data cumulated down ward is known as 'less than Ogive' and the curve drawn from the data cumulative upward as 'more than Ogive'.
- It helps in identifying the median, quartiles, deciles and percentiles, etc.
- Further it also helps to find the number of observations which are expected to lie between two given values.

### Steps for Drawing an Ogive

   i. The upper limits of the classes are plotted along $x$-axis.
  ii. The cumulative frequency of a particular class is plotted along the $y$-axis.
 iii. The points corresponding to cumulative frequency at each upper limit of the class are joined by a free hand curve. This curve is called a cumulative frequency curve or an Ogive. The main difference between the construction of a frequency graph and the Ogive is that in the case of former the frequencies must be plotted at the mid-points of the class but in the case of an Ogive, the cumulative frequency is plotted at the upper limit of the class.

## Analysis of Data

1. Descriptive analysis
2. Inferential analysis

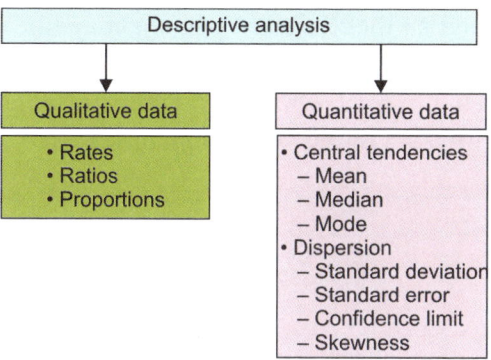

## Descriptive Analysis of Qualitative Data

**Rate:** It is proportion of specific events in a specific period from total events in a geographically defined area.

$$\text{Rate} = \frac{\text{No. of the events occurring in a specified period in a particular area}}{\text{No. of susceptibles in that area}} \times 10^N$$

**Ratio:** It is relative proportion of two events

$$\text{Ratio (A : B)} = \frac{\text{No. of the events event 'A'}}{\text{No. of the events event 'B'}}$$

**Proportion:** It is proportion of specific event of a specific categories from total such events in a defined geographical area.

$$\text{Proportion} = \frac{\text{No. of the events event 'A'}}{\text{Total no. of the events}} \times 10^N$$

**Percentage:** When proportion is expressed in percentage, i.e. proportion of specific event in a specific categories from total such 100 events in a defined geographical area.

$$\text{Percentage} = \frac{\text{No. of the events event 'A'}}{\text{Total no. of the events}} \times 100$$

## Descriptive Analysis of Quantitative Data

### Central Tendency or Average

- **Central tendency** is a measure of the values lying between the extremes and shared by most of the group members.
- This helps in conveying a fairly good idea about the whole group through a single value.
- In statistics, it is known as the average.
- **Averages** are central part of the distribution so they are also called the measures of central tendency.

**Most common measures of central tendency are:**

1. Arithmetic mean or mean
2. Median
3. Mode

## Characteristics of an Ideal Measure of Central Tendency

A good average must have the following characteristics:

1. It should be easy to understand and easy to calculate
2. It should be rigidly defined so that different persons may not interpret it differently.
3. It should be least affected by the fluctuations of the sampling.
4. It should be easily subjected to further mathematical calculations.
5. It should not be unduly affected by the extreme values.
6. It should be easy to interpret.

## Mean

### 1. For simple data

$$\text{Arithmetic mean} = \frac{\text{Sum of all observation}}{\text{No. of observation}}$$

**Example:** Find the arithmetic mean of the marks obtained by 10 students of a class in mathematics in a certain examination. The marks obtained are:

25, 30, 21, 55, 47, 10, 15, 17, 45, 35

**Solution:** Let be the average marks

∴ Sum of all the observations = 25 + 30 + 21 + 55 + 47 + 10 + 15 + 17 + 45 + 35 = 300

Number of students = 10

∴ Arithmetic mean = 300/10 = 30

### 2. For discrete series

$$\text{Arithmetic mean} = \frac{\Sigma fx}{N}$$

Here, $x$ = value of observation
$f$ = Frequencies
$\Sigma fx$ = Sum of all observation
$N$ = Total observation

### 3. For continuous series

$$\text{Arithmetic mean} = \frac{\Sigma fx}{N} \quad \text{here '}x\text{' is mid-value of class interval}$$

## Merits of Arithmetic Mean

1. Easiest average to calculate and also the simplest to understand.
2. No grouping of variables is required as in median/mode.
3. It is affected by the value of every item in the series.
4. Calculation is done through a rigid mathematical formula, ensuring that the same result is obtained by everyone.
5. It lends itself to subsequent algebraic treatment better than median and mode since it is calculated by a rigid formula.
6. Minimum sampling variations as compared to median/mode.
7. It is not a positional average.
8. Mean is typical in the sense that it is centre of gravity of the series.

## Limitations

1. When there are smaller numbers of observations, any extreme value in series would unduly affect the value of the average.
2. It might contain errors when calculated after making assumptions regarding the size of class interval of an open end class in a distribution with open end class.
3. Useful only when distribution is reasonably bell-shaped (normal).

## Geometric Mean

- Geometric mean of a set of observations is the nth root of their product.
- Calculation of the geometric mean requires all observations to be positive, i.e. greater than zero.
- A general formula for computing the geometric mean of the set of observations $x_1$, $x_2$ ... $x_n$ is $\sqrt[n]{x_1 x_2 \dots x_n}$ .
- An interesting property is that the logarithm of the geometric mean is the arithmetic mean of the logarithms of the individuals observations.
- This result is expressed by the formula
  $\log (GM) = \text{Log } x_1 + \text{Log } x_2 \dots \text{Log } x_n /n.$

## Harmonic Mean

- Harmonic mean of a set of observations is the reciprocal of the arithmetic mean of the reciprocals of the observations.
- That is, if the observations are $x_1$, $x_2$, ... $x_n$ then

$$\text{Harmonic mean} = \frac{n}{\dfrac{1}{x_1} + \dfrac{1}{x_2} \dots \dfrac{1}{x_n}}$$

## Median

**Median** is the observation which lies in the middle of the ordered observations.

## For Discrete Series

$$\text{Median} = \left(\frac{N+1}{2}\right)^{th} \text{observation}$$

## For Continuous Series

$$\text{Median} = L + \frac{(N/2 - cf)}{f} \times \text{C.I.}$$

- Here, '$L$' is lower limit of the median class
  - '$N$' is total no. of observations
  - '$c.f.$' is cumulative frequency of pre-median class
  - 'C.I.' is class interval
  - '$f$' is frequency of median class

## Merits of Median

1. Easily understood.
2. Not affected by extreme values.
3. Can be located graphically.
4. Can be determined even by inspection in many cases.
5. The best measure for qualitative data.
6. Can be easily located, even if the class intervals in the series are unequal.

## Demerits of Median

1. Cannot be subjected to algebraic treatments.
2. Cannot represent the irregular distribution series.

## Mode

**Mode** is the value which occurs with the greatest frequency, i.e. the most common value
For continuous series, it can be calculated with following formula:

$$\text{Mode} = L + \frac{\text{C.I.}(f_m - f_1)}{2f_m - f_1 - f_2}$$

- Here, '$l$' is lower limit of the modal class
  - 'C.I.' is class interval
  - '$f_m$' is frequency of modal class
  - '$f_1$' is frequency of pre-modal class
  - '$f_2$' is frequency of post-modal class

## Merits of Mode

1. Can be easily understood.
2. Can be located in some cases by inspection.
3. Capable for being ascertained graphically.
4. Not affected by extreme values.
5. Represents the most frequent value and therefore used more often.
6. Arrangement of data is not necessary, if the items are a few.

## Demerits of Mode

1. Calculation by different formulae gives different answers.
2. Mode is determinate. Some series have two or more than two modes.

**Example 1:** Find the central tendencies from the following frequency table.

| Marks | 52 | 58 | 60 | 65 | 68 | 70 | 75 |
|---|---|---|---|---|---|---|---|
| No. of students | 7 | 5 | 4 | 6 | 3 | 3 | 2 |

**Solution:** Let $x$ be the marked and $f$ be the frequency so that we have the following table:

| x | f | fx | c.f. |
|---|---|---|---|
| 2 | 7 | 364 | 7 |
| 58 | 5 | 290 | 12 |
| 60 | 4 | 240 | 16 |
| 65 | 6 | 390 | 22 |
| 68 | 3 | 204 | 25 |
| 70 | 3 | 210 | 28 |
| 75 | 2 | 150 | 30 |
| **Total** | **30** | **1848** | |

Here, $N = \sum f = 30$ and $\sum fx = 1848$

$\therefore$ Mean $= \bar{x} = \dfrac{1848}{30} = \dfrac{616}{10} = 61.6$

Median $= \left(\dfrac{N+1}{2}\right)^{th}$ observation's value $= \left(\dfrac{30+1}{2}\right)^{th}$ observation's value

$= \left(\dfrac{31}{2}\right)^{th}$ observation's value $=$ value of 16 c.f., i.e. 60

Mode $=$ Most frequent value $=$ Maximum frequency value $= 2$

**Example 2:** Calculate the arithmetic mean for the following data.

| Class interval | Frequency | Class interval | Frequency |
|---|---|---|---|
| 10 – 20 | 2 | 60 – 70 | 10 |
| 20 – 30 | 7 | 70 – 80 | 3 |
| 30 – 40 | 17 | 80 – 90 | 2 |
| 40 – 50 | 29 | 90 – 100 | 1 |
| 50 – 60 | 29 | | |

**Solutions:** While calculating the arithmetic mean for such a tabular data, it is assumed that all the observations in any particular class interval have the same value. This value is the middle value or midpoint of the class interval, i.e. we replace the classes by the mid-values and process as above:

| Class interval | Mid value (x) | Frequency (f) | fx | c.f. |
|---|---|---|---|---|
| 10 – 20 | 15 | 4 | 60 | 4 |
| 20 – 30 | 25 | 10 | 250 | 14 |
| 30 – 40 | 35 | 17 | 595 | 31 |
| 40 – 50 (median class) | 45 | 29 | 1305 | 60 |
| 50 – 60 (modal class) | 55 | 32 | 1760 | 92 |
| 70 – 80 | 75 | 5 | 375 | 97 |
| 80 – 90 | 85 | 2 | 170 | 99 |
| 90 – 100 | 95 | 1 | 95 | 100 |
| **Total** | | **100** | **4610** | |

Here, $N = \sum f = 100$, $\sum fx = 4610$

$$\text{Mean} = \frac{\sum fx}{\sum f}, = \frac{4610}{100} = 46.1$$

$$\text{Median} = \left(\frac{N+1}{2}\right)^{th} \text{observation} = \left(\frac{100+1}{2}\right)^{th} \text{observation} = (50 + 51)\text{th observation}$$

$$\text{Median} = L + \frac{\text{C.I.}\left(\frac{N}{2} - c.f\right)}{f} = 40 + \frac{5(50+31)}{29} = 43.28$$

$$\text{Mode} = L + \frac{\text{C.I.}(f_m - f_1)}{2f_m - f_1 - f_2} = 50 + \frac{5(32+31)}{(64-29-5)} = 50 + \left(\frac{25}{30}\right) = 50 + 0.8 = 50.8$$

## Non-central Tendency

$$\text{Percentile} = L + \frac{(p - c.f.)}{f} \times \text{C.I.}$$

- Here, '$L$' is lower limit of the percentile class
- '$P$' is percentile
- '$c.f.$' is cumulative frequency of pre-percentile class
- 'C.I.' is class interval
- '$f$' is frequency of percentile class

## Quartile

$$\text{1st quartile} = l + \frac{\left(\frac{N}{4} - c.f.\right)}{f} \times \text{C.I.}$$

- Here, '$L$' is lower limit of the quartile class, i.e. including $c.f.$ 25
- '$N$' is total no. of observations
- '$c.f.$' is cumulative frequency of pre-quartile class
- 'C.I.' is class interval
- '$f$' is frequency of quartile class

## Skewness

- **Skewness** is property of deviation of peak of normal curve from its standard normal curve symmetry.
- It can be positive skewness, i.e. when peak shifted towards positive side (right) or negative skewness, i.e. when peak shifted towards negative side (left).

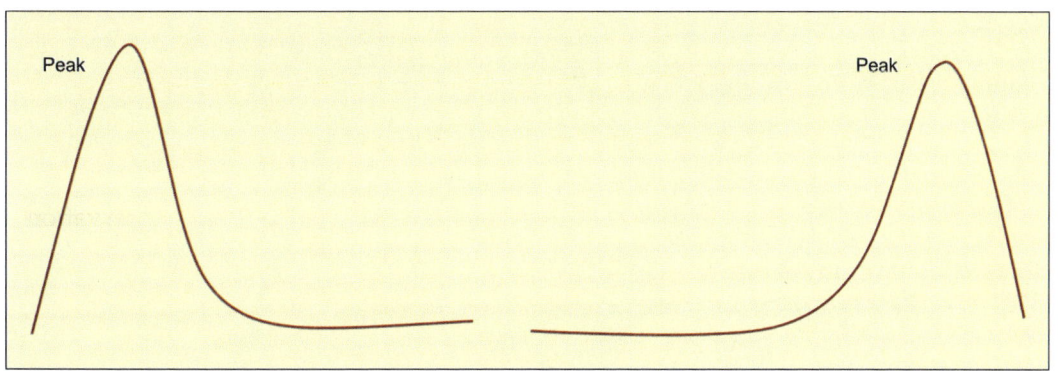

**Negative skewness: Median ≥ Mean**      **Positive skewness: Mean ≥ Median**

**Absolute skewness** = Mean – Mode
$$= Q_3 + Q_1 - 2 \text{ Median}$$

**Coefficient of skewness** $= \dfrac{(\text{Mean} - \text{Mode})}{\text{S.D.}} = \dfrac{3 \,(\text{Mean} - \text{Median})}{\text{S.D.}}$

## Kurtosis

- **Kurtosis** is sharpness of peak of curve obtained.
- When sharpness of peak of curve obtained is more, it is called 'Leptokurtosis'.
- When sharpness of peak of curve obtained is less, i.e. more or less flat, it is called 'Platykurtosis'.

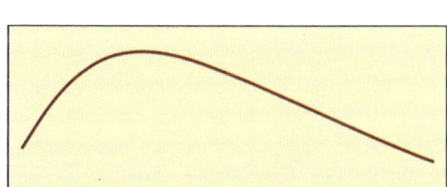

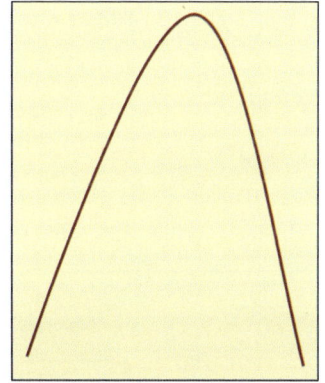

**Platykurtosis**      **Leptokurtosis**

**Range** = Highest – Lowest

**Semi-interquartile range** $- Q = \dfrac{(Q_1 - Q_2)}{2}$

**Coefficient of variance** (C.V.) $= \dfrac{\text{S.D.}}{\text{Mean}} \times 100$

**Variance** is standard deviation square

$$\text{Variance} = \text{S.D.}^2$$

**Standard deviation** is root mean square of deviation from mean

$$\text{Standard deviation} = \sqrt{\text{Variance}} = \sqrt{\frac{\sum(\text{Mean deviation})^2}{N}}$$

$$\text{Simple series} = \sqrt{\frac{\sum(X-\bar{X})^2}{N}} = \frac{\sum X^2 - \frac{(\sum X)^2}{N}}{N}$$

Discrete/continuous series

$$= \sqrt{\frac{\sum f(X-\bar{X})^2}{\sum f}} = \frac{\sum fX^2 - \frac{(\sum X)^2}{N}}{N}$$

here,

$X$ = Observation values

$\bar{X}$ = Mean

(If sample is < 30, then divided by 'N – 1' instead of 'N')

**Standard error:** It is a measure of variability among means/proportions of samples selected from certain population.

$$\text{Standard error for mean (SEM)} = \frac{\text{Standard deviation}}{\sqrt{n}}$$

$$\text{Standard error for proportion (SEP)} = \frac{\sqrt{pq}}{\sqrt{n}}$$

## Test of Significance

**Test of significance** is a group of tests used to infer the difference between two proportions/means/medians.

Test of significance depends upon:

- Type of data
- Type of study design
- Type of outcome variable to be compared

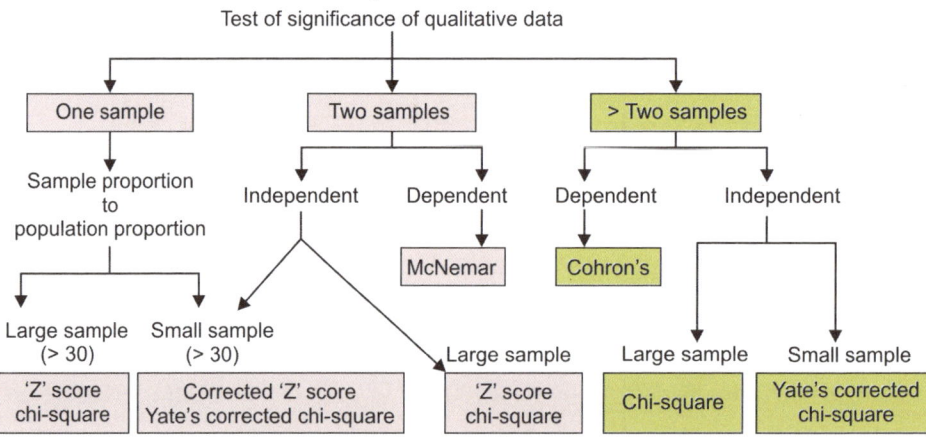

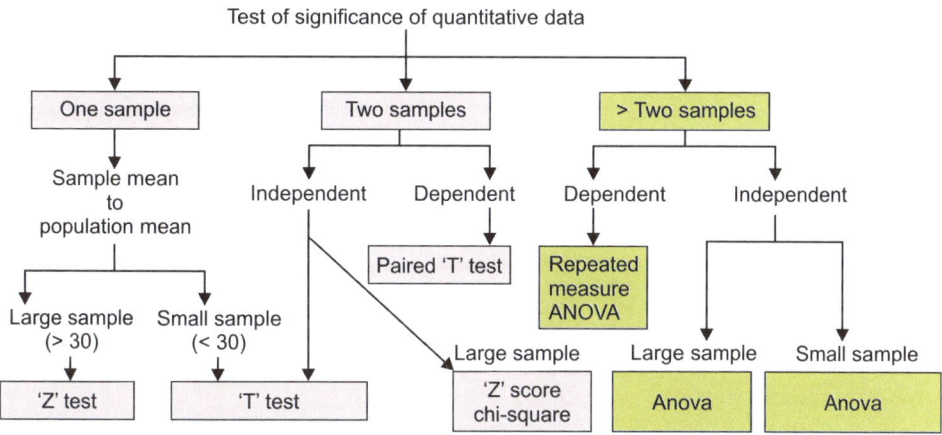

## Statistical test for significance as per type of data

| | Nominal | Numerical | Ordinal |
|---|---|---|---|
| Two groups | 'Z' Score test<br>Chi-square test | 'Z' test ($n > 30$)<br>'t' test ($n < 30$) | Mann-Whitney test |
| > Two groups | Chi-square test | ANOVA | Kruskal-Wallis test |
| Paired two | McNemar | Paired '$t$' test | Wilcoxon signed-rank test |
| Multiple observation in same individual (> 2) | Cohron's | Repeated measure ANOVA | Friedman |
| Association of two variable | Contingency coefficient | Correlation (Pearson) regression | Spearman correlation |

## Statistical tests for significance as per study design

| Type of study | Study design | Type of data | Test of significance |
|---|---|---|---|
| Analytic | Cross-sectional | Qualitative | 'Z' score test/Chi-square test |
| | | Quantitative | Z-test (if SS > 30)/t-test (if SS < 30) |
| | | Ordinal | Mann-Whitney test |
| | Case-control | Qualitative | OR and 'Z' score test/Chi-square test |
| | | Quantitative | OR and Z-test (if SS > 30)/t-test (if SS <30) |
| | | Ordinal | OR and Mann-Whitney test |
| | Cohort | Qualitative | OR, RR, AR and Chi-square test |
| | | Quantitative | OR, RR, AR and Z-test /t-test (if SS < 30) |
| | | Ordinal | OR, RR, AR and Mann-Whitney test |
| Experimental | Before and after | Qualitative | McNemar test |
| | | Quantitative | Paired t-test |
| | | Ordinal | Wilcoxon signed-rank test |

*Contd.*

*Contd.*

| Type of study | Study design | Type of data | Test of significance |
|---|---|---|---|
| | Repeated follow-ups | Qualitative | Conchron's test |
| | | Quantitative | Repeated measure ANOVA |
| | | Ordinal | Friedman test |
| | Two different groups | Qualitative | 'Z' Score test/ Chi-square test |
| | | Quantitative | Unpaired t-test |
| | | Ordinal | Mann-Whitney test |
| | More than two different groups | Qualitative | Chi-square test |
| | | Quantitative | ANOVA |
| | | Ordinal | Kruskal-Wallis test |

Descriptive study design describe the event usually no need of test of significance

## Statistical tests for significance as per study question

| Research question | Number and type of DV | Number and type of IV | Covariates | Test | Goal of analysis |
|---|---|---|---|---|---|
| Group differences | Nominal | 1 nominal | | Chi-square | Determine if significant difference between croups |
| | Continuous | 1 dichotomous | | t-test | Determine significance of mean group differences |
| | | 1 Categorical | 1 | One-way ANOVA | |
| | | | 1+ | One-way ANCOVA | |
| | | 2+ Categorical | 1 | Factorial ANOVA | |
| | | | 1+ | Factorial ANCOVA | |
| | 2+ Continuous | 1 Categorical | 1 | One-way MANOVA | Create linear combinations of dependent variables (DVs) to maximize mean group differences |
| | | | 1+ | One-way MANCOVA | |
| | | 2+ Categorical | 1 | Factorial MANOVA | |
| | | | 1+ | Factorial MANCOVA | |
| Degree of relationship | Continuous | 1 Continuous | | Bivariate correlation | Determine relationship/prediction |
| | | 2+ Continuous | | Multiple regression | Linear combination to predict the DV |

*Contd.*

*Contd.*

| Research question | Number and type of DV | Number and type of IV | Covariates | Test | Goal of analysis |
|---|---|---|---|---|---|
| | 1+ Continuous | 2+ Continuous | | Path analysis | Estimate causal relations among variables |
| Prediction of group membership | Dichotomous | 2+ Nominal | | Logistic regression | Create linear combination of independent variables (IVs) of the log odds of being in one group |

DV: Dependent variable
IV: Independent variable

## 'Z' Score

### Indications

- Qualitative data
- Comparing difference between:
  - Sample proportion to population proportion
  - Two sample proportions

## Comparing Difference between two Sample Proportions

### 'Z' Score Test

$$\text{'Z' score} = \frac{P_2 - P_1}{\text{SEDP}}$$

$$\text{SEDP} = \sqrt{\frac{P_1 Q_1}{N_1} + \frac{P_2 Q_2}{N_2}}$$

Here, $P_1$ – proportion of that event in 1st sample

$P_2$ – proportion of that event in 2nd sample

SEDP – Standard error of difference in proportion

$Q_1$ – proportion without that event in 1st sample, i.e. $Q_1 = 1 - P_1$

$Q_2$ – proportion without that event in 2nd sample, i.e. $1 - P_2$

$N_1$ – sample size of 1st sample

$N_2$ – sample size of 2nd sample

### Corrected 'Z' score for Small Sample ( N < 30)

$$\text{'Z' score} = \frac{(P_2 - P_1) - \frac{1}{2}\left(\frac{1}{N_1} + \frac{1}{N_2}\right)}{\text{SEDP}}$$

Here, $P_1$ – proportion of that event in 1st sample

$P_2$ – proportion of that event in 2nd sample

$Q_1$ – proportion without that event in 1st sample, i.e. $1 - P_1$

$Q_2$ – proportion without that event in 2nd sample, i.e. $1 - P_2$

## Inference of 'Z' Score

'Z' score > 2 = Difference is significant at 95% confidence limit.

'Z' score < 2 = Difference is not significant at 95% confidence limit.

'Z' score > 3 = Difference is highly significant at 95% confidence limit.

## Chi-square Test

### Indications

- Qualitative data
- Normal distribution
- Comparing difference between:
  - Two sample proportions
  - Multiple sample proportions

### Comparing Difference between > Two Sample Proportions Chi-square Test

$$\text{Chi-square } (\chi^2) = \sum_{\text{all cells}} \frac{(O-E)^2}{E} \qquad E = \frac{T_r \times T_c}{T}$$

$$\text{Chi-squire} = \frac{(Q_1 - E_1)^2}{E_1} + \frac{(Q_2 - E_2)^2}{E_2} + \frac{(Q_3 - E_4)^2}{E_3} + \cdots + \frac{(Q_3 - E_4)^2}{E_n}$$

Here, O – observed value of cell

E – expected value of cell,
considering null hypothesis

$T_r$ – total of that row

$T_c$ – total of that column

T – grand total, i.e. $a + b + c + d$

R = no. of rows

C = no. of column

### Inferences of Chi-square Test

Chi-square ($\chi^2$) value is seen at degree of feedom (DF) = (R – 1) (C – 1) in Chi-square table at desired level of significance (here R = no. of rows and C = no. of column)

   If Chi-square ($\chi^2$) test value is higher than table value = Difference in proportions is significant at that desired level of significance.

## 'Z' Test

### Prerequisites

- Quantitative data
- Homogeneous normally distributed random sample
- Sample size > 30

### Indications

- To see the significance of any observation in reference of mean value of that sample.
- Comparing difference between:
  - Sample mean to population mean
  - Means of two independent samples

## Comparing Difference between Two Sample Means (> 30)

### Z-test

$$Z\text{-test} = \frac{\bar{X}_2 - \bar{X}_1}{SEDM}$$

$$SEDM = \sqrt{\frac{S.D._1^2}{N_1} + \frac{S.D._2^2}{N_2}}$$

Here, $\bar{X}_1$—mean of that event in 1st sample

$\bar{X}_2$—mean of that event in 2nd sample

SEDM—standard error of difference in means

S.D.$_1$—standard error of 1st sample

S.D.$_2$—standard error of 2nd sample

$N_1$—sample size of 1st sample

$N_2$—sample size of 2nd sample

### Prerequisites

- Random sample
- Quantitative data
- Normally distributed
- Sample size <30

## Comparing Difference between Two Sample Means (< 30)

### t-test

$$t\text{-test} = \frac{\bar{X}_2 - \bar{X}_1}{SEDM}$$

$$SEDM = \sqrt{\frac{S.D._1^2}{N_1} + \frac{S.D._2^2}{N_2}}$$

Here, $\bar{X}_1$—mean of that event in 1st sample

$\bar{X}_2$—mean of that event in 2nd sample

SEDM—standard error of difference in means

S.D.$_1$—standard error of 1st sample

S.D.$_2$—standard error of 2nd sample

$N_1$—sample size of 1st sample

$N_2$—sample size of 2nd sample

Degree of freedom (DF) = $(N_2 - 1) + (N_2 - 1) = N_1 + N_2 - 2$

### Inferences of t-test

t-test value is matched at degree of freedom (DF) = $N_1 + N_2 - 2$ in the table of '*T*' at desired level of significance.

If t-test value is higher than table value = Difference in means is significant at that desired level of significance.

## ANALYSIS OF VARIANCE (ANOVA) TEST

### Prerequisites

- Quantitative data
- Homogeneous normally distributed random sample.

### Indications

Comparing difference between more than two means.

## Comparing Difference between > Two Sample Means

### 'ANOVA' Test

$$\text{ANOVA} = \frac{\text{MSOS}_1}{\text{MSOS}_2}$$  MSOS$_2$—mean sum of squares within classes = Total SOS – MSOS$_1$

$$\text{TSOS} = \sum X^2 - \frac{\left(\sum X\right)^2}{N}$$

MSOS$_1$—mean sum of squares between classes = $\dfrac{\text{SOS}_1}{K-1}$ here, K = number of classes

SOS$_1$—sum of squares between classes

$$= \frac{\left(\sum X_a\right)^2}{N_a} + \frac{\left(\sum X_b\right)^2}{N_b} + \frac{\left(\sum X_c\right)^2}{N_c} + \cdots + \frac{\left(\sum X_k\right)^2}{N_k} = \frac{\left(\sum X\right)^2}{N}$$

At degree of freedom (DF) = $(K - 1)$ horizontal S $(N - K)$ veritical.

### Inferences of ANOVA

Find out variance ratio value at degree of freedom (DF) = $(K - 1)$ horizontal and $(N - K)$ vertical from the variance ratio table at desired level of significance.

If test value is > table value = Difference in means is significant at that desired level of significance.

### Sign Test

Sign test is a non-parametric test based on sign.
- Simplest
- Based on direction $(-/+/0)$
- Signs as per the direction are counted
- Inference – if $S \leq K$ = Null hypothesis (HØ) is rejected
- Here 'S' is net sum of signs as per sign
- 'K' is constant

### Steps of Sign Test

**Sign K-test for small sample ($n < 30$)**
- Find out net sum of signs as per sign (S)
- $S = (\text{total} + \text{signs}) - (\text{total} - \text{signs})$
- $K = \dfrac{(n-1)}{2} - 0.98\sqrt{n}$

**Inference – if $S \leq K$ = Null hypothesis (HØ) is rejected**

**Sign Z-test for large sample ($n > 30$)**

- Find out no. of ties with less frequent sign ($X$)

- $Z = \dfrac{(X - np)}{\sqrt{np\,(1-p)}}$ here $X$= no. + sign

## Inference

**For small sample (*n* < 30)**

If $S \leq K$ = Null hypothesis (HØ) is rejected (difference, if significant).

**For large sample (*n* > 30)**

If $Z > 2$ = Null hypothesis is rejected (difference, if significant).

## Correlation

- It is used to quantify strength and direction of the relationship between two variables.
- Correlation is expressed in terms of correlation coefficient, denoted by '*r*'.
- Value of '*r*' varies from –1 to + 1.
- Strength of the relationship is indicated by the size of the coefficient.
- Its direction is indicated by the sign.
- Plus sign means that there is positive correlation between the two variables, i.e. high values of one variable (e.g. as salt intake) are associated with high values of the other variable (e.g. blood pressure).
- Minus sign means that there is a negative correlation between the two variables. High values of one variable (e.g. cigarette consumption) are associated with low value of other (e.g. life expectancy).

**Types of correlation coefficients are:**

**Pearson's correlation coefficient** is used for interval or ratio scale data such as the association between salt intake and blood pressure.

$$r = \frac{\sum xy}{\sqrt{\sum x^2 \times \sum y^2}}$$

Where $x = (X - \tilde{X})$ and $y = (Y - \tilde{Y})$

**Spearman's rank-order correlation coefficient** is used for ordinal scale data such as the association between birth order and the class position at school.

$$R = 1 - \frac{6 \sum D^2}{n(n^2 - 1)}$$

Where $D^2$ is the square of the difference of corresponding ranks and '*n*' is the number of pairs of observations.

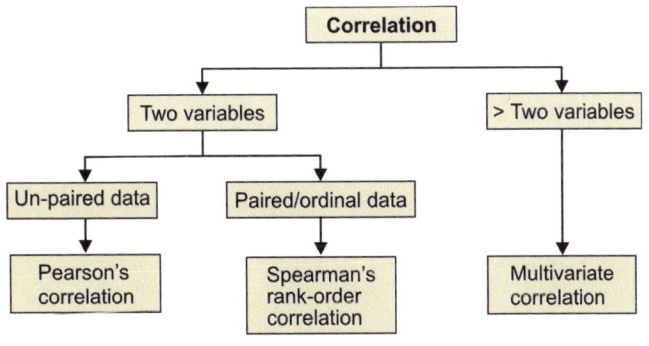

## Type of Correlation

Perfect +ve – both variables rise in same proportion.

Perfect –ve – if one variable rises, other falls in same proportion.

Moderately +ve – if one variable rises, other will also rise but not in same proportion.

Moderately –ve – if one variable rises, other will fall but not in same proportion.

No Correlation – no linear relationship at all between two variables.

### Inference of Correlation (r)

| Correlation | Inference | Correlation (r) | Inference |
|---|---|---|---|
| +1 | Perfect +ve correlation | – 1 | Perfect +ve correlation |
| > 0.95 | About perfect +ve correlation | > – 0.95 | About perfect +ve correlation |
| > 0.75 | V. Good correlation | > – 0.75 | V. good correlation |
| 0.75 – 0.5 | Moderate correlation | – 0.75 to – 0.5 | Moderate correlation |
| 0.5 – 0.25 | Fair correlation | – 0.5 to – 0.25 | Fair correlation |
| 0.25 – 0 | No correlation | < – 0.25 | No correlation |

## Significance Test for Correlation (r)

### A. Large Samples

$$\text{SE of correlation } (r) = \frac{\text{Correlation } (r)}{\sqrt{1/(n-1)}} = r\sqrt{n-1}$$

### Inference

If difference > 2SE of $r$ = Difference is significant at 95% level.

If difference < 2SE of $r$ = Difference is not significant at 95% level.

### B. Small Samples

$$\text{'}t\text{' test for correlation (r)} = \frac{r\sqrt{n-2}}{\sqrt{1-r^2}}$$

### Inference

If '$t$' test value is > table critical value = Difference is significant.

If '$t$' test value is < table critical value = Difference is not significant.

## Regression

Regression is to find out causal relationship between variables

Regression coefficient is a measure of change in one dependent variable (y) with one unit change in the other variable (x).

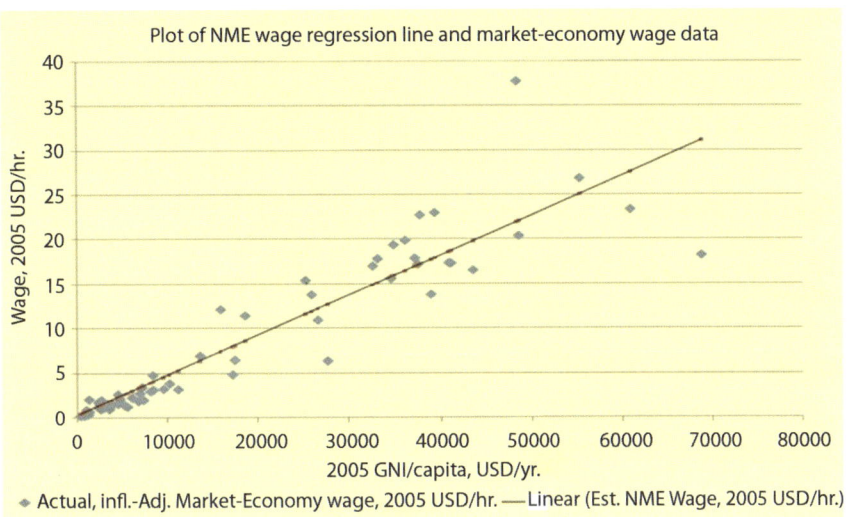

Plot of NME wage regression line and market-economy wage data

• Actual, infl.-Adj. Market-Economy wage, 2005 USD/hr. —Linear (Est. NME Wage, 2005 USD/hr.)

Regression line of Y on X is $Y = a + bX$ ...(1)

Regression line of X on Y is $X = a + bY$ ...(2)

- Here $Y$ = one variable
- $X$ = other variable
- $a$ = interceptor
- $b$ = slope of $X$ line on $Y$ line regression

## Regression equation of X on Y

Regression equation of X and Y = $r \dfrac{\text{SD of series } X}{\text{SD of series } Y}$

## Regression equation of Y on X

Regression equation of X and Y = $r \dfrac{\text{SD of series } Y}{\text{SD of series } X}$

## Regression coefficient of X on Y

$$b\,(xy) = r \dfrac{\text{SD of series } X}{\text{SD of series } Y}$$

## Regression coefficient of Y on X

$$b\,(yx) = r \dfrac{\text{SD of series } Y}{\text{SD of series } X}$$

Relation between correlation and regression: Correlation $(r) = \sqrt{b_{xy}\, b_{by}}$

## Characteristics of Performance of Diagnostic Tests

**Sensitivity:** It is an ability of a test to detect 'true positives'.

$$\text{Sensitivity} = \frac{\text{Diseased with positive test}}{\text{All diseased}}$$

**Specificity:** It is an ability of a test to detect 'true negatives'

$$\text{Specificity} = \frac{\text{Diseased with negative test}}{\text{All disease free}} \times 100$$

**Positive predictive value (PPV):** It is a proportion of true positives among total positives.

$$\text{PPV} = \frac{\text{Diseased with positive test}}{\text{All positives}} \times 100$$

**Negative predictive value (NPV):** It is a proportion of true negatives among total negatives

$$\text{NPV} = \frac{\text{Disease-free with negative test}}{\text{All negatives}} \times 100$$

**False negative rate (FNR):** It is a probability of negative test result in diseased individuals.

$$\text{FNR} = \frac{\text{Diseased with negative test}}{\text{All diseased}} \times 100$$

**False positive rate (FPR):** It is a probability of positive test result in disease-free individuals.

$$\text{FPR} = \frac{\text{Disease-free with positive test}}{\text{All disease-free}} \times 100$$

## Relationship between Test Performance Characteristics

### Sensitivity and FNR

Sensitivity in terms of FNR: Sensitivity = 1 – FNR

FNR in terms of sensitivity: FNR = 1 – sensitivity

A highly sensitive test will have low FNR.

### Specificity and FPR

Specificity in terms of FPR: Specificity = 1 – FPR

FPR in terms of specificity: FPR = 1 – specificity

A highly specific test will have a low FPR.

**General rules:** Sensitivity and specificity are independent of prevalence.

1. As prevalence decreases, PPV decreases and NPV increases.
2. As prevalence increases, PPV increases and NPV decreases.
3. The more sensitive a test, the better its NPV.
4. The more specific a test, the better its PVP.

## Comparison between Tests/Procedures

## Comparison with Gold Standard

- Sensitivity
- Specificity
- PPV
- NPV
- ROC

  **For agreement of association:** Kappa
  **For cut off value of diagnostic test:** ROC

## 2 × 2 Table for A New Diagnostic Test

|  |  | Status based on gold standard test | |
|---|---|---|---|
|  |  | Diseased | Normal |
| Observation in new test | Test positive | True positive<br>*a* | False positive<br>*b* |
|  | Test negative | False negative<br>*c* | True negative<br>*d* |

Sensitivity = $a/(a + c)$    Specificity = $d/(b + d)$

PPV = $a/(a + b)$    NPV = $d/(c + d)$

FNR = $c/(a + c)$    FPR = $b/(b + d)$

## Kappa

Kappa is to find out agreement of association between two tests/procedures/samples, etc.

## Inference of Kappa

| Test value | Inference |
|---|---|
| 0.93 – 1 | Excellent agreement |
| 0.81 – 0.92 | Very good agreement |
| 0.61 – 0.80 | Good agreement |
| 0.41 – 0.60 | Fair agreement |
| 0.21 – 0.40 | Slight agreement |
| 0.01 – 0.20 | Poor agreement |
| < 0.01 | No agreement |

## ROC

ROC is to decide the cut off value for a diagnostic test.

## Steps for ROC

1. Frame table of test value with positive and negative for disease.
2. Frame 2nd derived table of test value cut off with true and false positive.
3. Plot graph of 2nd table, i.e. between true and false positivity.

4. Find out sensitivity with specificity at every cut off value of test.
5. Chose desirable (> 80% for each) combination of sensitivity and specificity.
6. Select cut off test value at which desirable (> 80% for each) combination of sensitivity and specificity lies.

## ROC

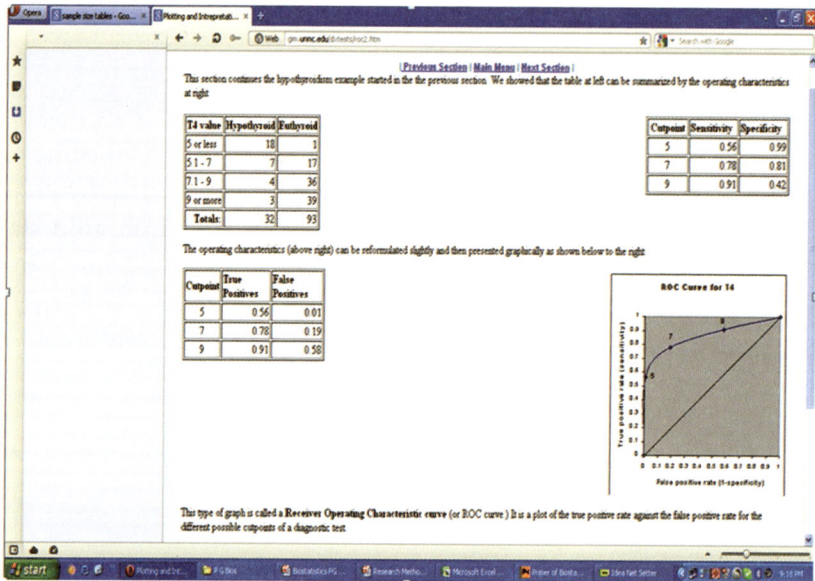

## Probability

**Probability** is a quantitative expression of the chance (likelihood) of occurrence of a certain event.

• It is used for making predictions.
• $p$ of the happening of an event is also known as probability of success.
• $q$ the non-happening of the event as the probability of failure.
• It ranges from 0 to 1.
• If P(A) = 1, E is called a certain event.
• If P(A) = 0, E is called an impossible event.
• The probability of an event 'A' is a number such that 0 d" P(E) d" 1, and the sum of the probability that an event will occur and an event will not occur is equal to 1, i.e. $p + q = 1$

The probability of the happening of 'A' when there are '$n$' mutually exclusive events in an experiment and out of which '$m$' are favourable to the happening of event 'A', is denoted by

$$P(A) = \frac{m}{n} = \frac{\text{Number of specific favourable cases}}{\text{Total number of equally likely cases}}$$

Here, experiment is known as a 'trial' whereas the outcomes are known as 'events or cases'. Events may be mutually exclusive or independent.

**Mutually exclusive:** Mutually exclusive is that either of one can occurs or not more than one can occurs simentaneouly, e.g. in a tossing of a coin either head or tail can come but both cannot come simultaneously.

**Independent events:** If the occurrence and non-occurrence of an event is not affected by each other, e.g. taking out the a 'Hukum card' and a 'Queen' may and may not come simultaneously.

## Probability Theorem

There are two probability theorems:

1. **Addition theorem of probability:** If the events are *mutually exclusive*, then the probability of any one of them is equal to the sum of the probabilities of the happening of the separate event. For example, if 2 events A and B are mutually exclusive then the probability of the occurrence of either A or B is:

   $P(A \text{ or } B)$ or $P(A \cup B) = P(A) + P(B)$

2. **Multiplication theorem of probability:** If the events are *independent*, then the probability of occurrence of both is equal to the product of the individual probability, e.g.

$$P(AB) = P(A).P(B)$$

Other examples are as follows:

### Probability in case of dependent events

| Case | Formula |
|---|---|
| Probability of occurrence of at least A or B, when events are mutually exclusive | $P(A \cup B) = P(A) + P(B)$ |
| Probability of occurrence of at least A or B, when events are not mutually exclusive | $P(A \cup B) = P(A) + P(B) - P(A \cap B)$ |
| Probability of occurrence of both A and B | $P(A \cap B) = P(A) + P(B) - P(A \cup B)$ |
| Probability of occurrence of A and not B | $P(A \cap \overline{B}) = P(A) - P(A \cap B)$ |
| Probability of occurrence of B and not A | $P(\overline{A} \cap B) = P(B) - P(A \cap B)$ |
| Probability of non-occurrence of both | $P(\overline{A} \cup \overline{B}) = 1 - P(A \cup B)$ |

### Probability in case of independent events

| Case | Formula |
|---|---|
| Probability of occurrence of both A and B | $P(A \cap B) = P(A) \times P(B)$ |
| Probability of occurrence of A and not B | $P(A \cap \overline{B}) = P(A) \times P(\overline{B})$ |
| Probability of occurrence of B and not A | $P(\overline{A} \cap B) = P(\overline{A}) \times P(B)$ |
| Probability of non-occurrence of both | $P(\overline{A} \cap \overline{B}) = P(\overline{A}) \times P(\overline{B})$ |
| Probability of occurrence of at least A or B | $P(\overline{A} \cup \overline{B}) = 1 - P(\overline{A} \cap \overline{B}) = 1 - [P(\overline{A}) \times P(\overline{B})]$ |
| Probability of non-occurrence of at least A or B | $P(\overline{A} \cup \overline{B}) = 1 - P(A \cap B) = 1 - [P(A) \times P(B)]$ |
| Probability of occurrence of only one event | $P(A \cap \overline{B}) + P(\overline{A} \cap B) = [P(A) \times P(\overline{B})] + [P(\overline{A}) \times P(B)]$ |

## Normal Distributions Curve

Normal distribution curve is often called the Gaussian distribution, after Carl Friedrich Gauss, who discovered many of its properties.

**Synonyms of normal distribution curve.** The Gaussian distribution, density curve, The 68-95-99.7 rule density curve, standard normal distribution, etc.

### Properties of Normal Distribution Curve

- Normal curves are symmetrical, unimodal and bell-shaped.
- Two halves of the curve are the same (mirror images).
- Mean, median, and mode all have the same value, i.e. mean of the curve = median = mode.
- It is symmetric around the mean.
- Tails of the curve are infinite.
- "Area under the curve" is measured in standard deviations from the mean
- Total area under the curve is 1 (or 100%).
- It links frequency distribution to probability distribution.
- Mean I1SD covers 68%, mean I2SD covers about 95% and mean I3SD covers 99.7% of observations.

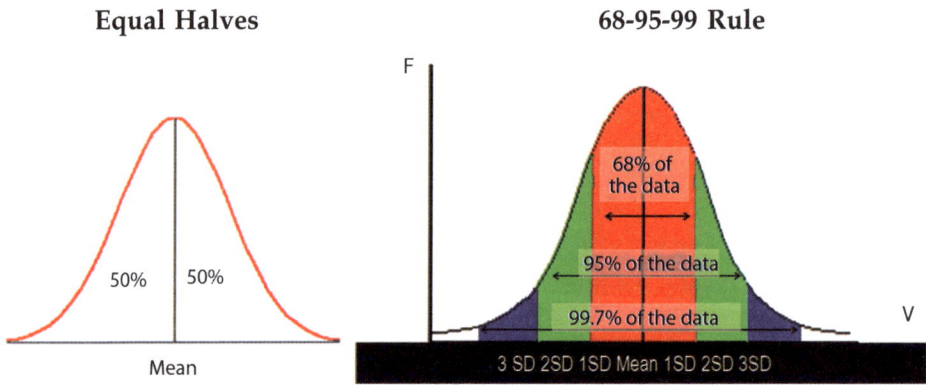

### Uses of Normal Curve

- Its application goes beyond describing distributions.
- To explore standard scores (e.g. Z score) for comparison.
- In making statistical inference.
- In hypothesis testing.
- It helps managers/management make decisions.

### Note

- Areas can never be negative.
- Z scores can be negative.
- 95% of values will lie within the limit of mean/proportion ± 1.96 S.E., therefore, it is only 5% likely that the population parameter will lie beyond this limit.

- This holds true only if the sample is truly representative of the population being studied.
- Population parameter (mean or proportion) = Sample mean/proportion ± 1.96S.E.

## Hypothesis Testing with Normal Curve

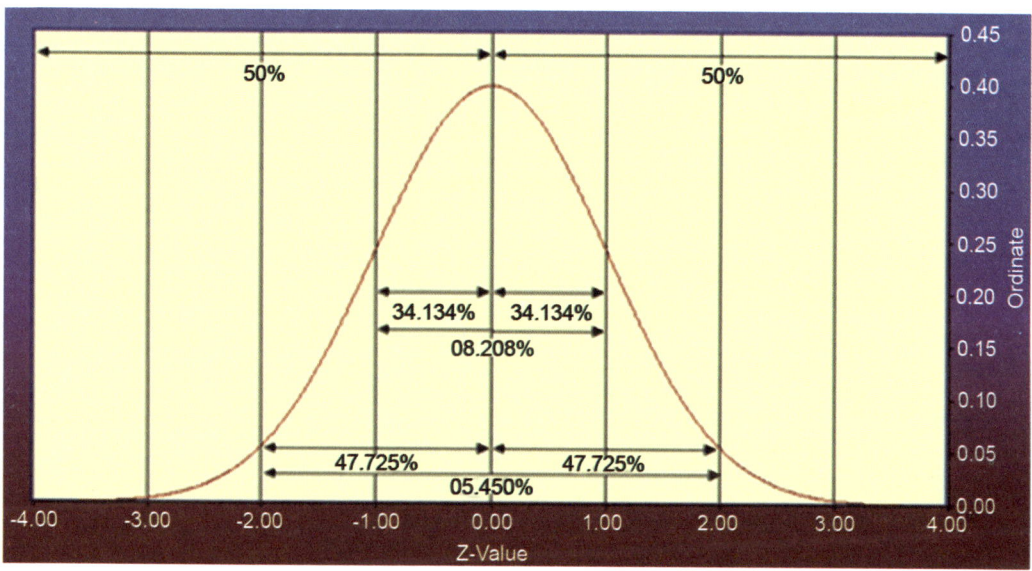

Normal curve, P value and inference

### Conventionally Accepted

- P value > 0.05      LS = Not significant
- P value < 0.05      LS = Significant
- P value < 0.001      LS = Highly significant

### Hypothesis

- $H_0$: No difference between two (by default).
- $H_a$: There is difference between two.

Acceptance zone (for $H_0$) at 95% CL: with in Mean ± 2 SD
Rejection zone (for $H_0$) at 95% CL: beyond Mean ± 2 SD and < Mean ± 2 SD

### Vital Statistics

Statistics related to vital events.

### Morbidity Statistics

**Prevalence:** Total number of cases in a defined geographical area at a point/period of time.

$$\text{Prevalence} = \frac{\text{Total number of cases at a point of time}}{\text{MYP of that region}} \times 10^n$$

**Incidence:** Number of new cases occurring in a defined year in a defined geographical area.

$$\text{Incidence} = \frac{\text{Total number of new cases occurring in a year}}{\text{MYP of that region}} \times 10^n$$

**Relation between prevelance and incidence:**

$P = D \times I$; here, P = Prevellence, I = Incidence, and D = Duration of illness

**Proportional case rate:**

$$PCR\ (CAD)\ =\ \frac{\text{Total number of cases of CAD}}{\text{Total cases due to all regions}} \times 100$$

**Attack rate:**

$$\text{Attack rate}\ =\ \frac{\text{Total number of new cases occurring}}{\text{Total population exposed}} \times 10^n$$

**Secondary attack rate:**

$$SAR\ =\ \frac{\text{Number of new cases occurring in incubation period}}{\text{Total cases already occurred}} \times 10^n$$

## Mortality Statistics

**Crude death rate:**

$$CDR\ =\ \frac{\text{Total number of deaths in a year}}{\text{MYP of that region}} \times 1000$$

**Specific death rate:**

$$SDR\ (CAD)\ =\ \frac{\text{Total number of deaths due to CAD in a year}}{\text{Total deaths due to all causes}} \times 100$$

**Proportional death rate:**

$$PCR\ (CAD)\ =\ \frac{\text{Total number of deaths due to CAD}}{\text{Total cases of CAD}} \times 100$$

**Case fatality rate:**

$$CFR\ (CAD)\ =\ \frac{\text{Total number of deaths due to CAD}}{\text{Total cases of CAD}} \times 100$$

**Maternal mortality rate:**

$$MMR\ =\ \frac{\text{Total no. of deaths during pregancy and post-partum period}}{\text{Total live births}} \times 1000$$

**Infant mortality rate (IMR):**

$$IMR\ =\ \frac{\text{Total no. of late foetal deaths + deaths within one year}}{\text{Total live births + late foetal deaths}} \times 1000$$

**Neonatal mortality rate:**

$$NMR\ =\ \frac{\text{Total no. of late foetal deaths + deaths within 4 weeks}}{\text{Total live births + late foetal deaths}} \times 1000$$

**Perinatal mortality rate:**

$$\text{Peri-NMR} = \frac{\text{Total no. late foetal deaths} + \text{deaths within 7 days}}{\text{Total live births} + \text{Late foetal deaths}} \times 1000$$

**Post-neonatal mortality rate:**

$$\text{Post-NMR} = \frac{\text{Deaths from 4 week to one year}}{\text{Total live births}} \times 1000$$

## Fertility Statistics

**Crude birth rate:**

$$\text{CBR} = \frac{\text{Total number of live births in a year}}{\text{MYP of that region}} \times 1000$$

**Crude marriage rate:**

$$\text{C Mar. R} = \frac{\text{Total number of marriages in year}}{\text{Total MYP of that region}} \times 1000$$

**General fertility rate:**

$$\text{GFR} = \frac{\text{No. of total live births in a year}}{\text{MYP of females of RAG of that region}} \times 1000$$

**Age-specific fertility rate:**

$$\text{ASFR} = \frac{\text{No. of TLB in a year in a sp age gp}}{\text{Females of that age gp of that region}} \times 1000$$

**Total fertility rate:** Sum of all age-specific fertility or total number of children per couple.

**Gross reproductive rate:** Number of female children born per women of reproductive age.

It can be assessed by a cross-section study via asking about female children of women cohort who have experienced their whole reproductive period.

$$\text{GRR} = \frac{\text{No. of female children born in a chohort of women}}{\text{No. of females in same cohort}}$$

**Net reproductive rate:** Number of female children born by a girl in her whole reproductive life if she experiences the present fertility and mortality pattern of that region.

It is assessed by a longitudinal study via following girls cohort for their whole reproductive period.

## COMPUTERS IN STATISTICS

### In calculation of 'Sample Size'

**Sample size** can directly be calculated online from different web sites.

### Steps to Calculate Sample Size online from Web Sites

- Open website to calculate 'sample size'.
- Select and click type of outcome analysis will be done.

- Some default values are given which are also changeable as per choice
- Give inputs asked
- Click calculate
- Sample size will be shown directly on window.

   **e.g. http://stat.ubc.ca/~rollin/stats/ssize/**
1. Open website to calculate 'sample size' following window will appear.

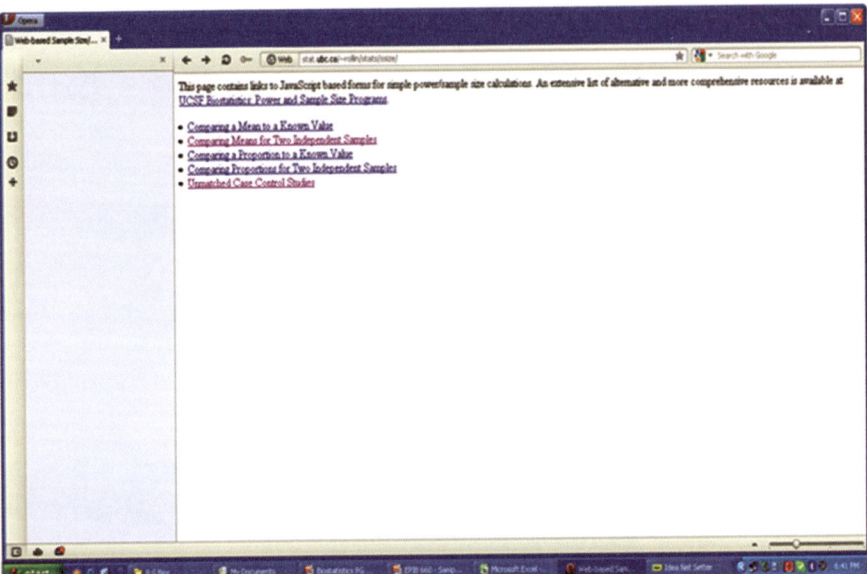

Select and click type of outcome analysis will be done.

For example, click type of outcome analysis comparing two independent samples. This window will appear.

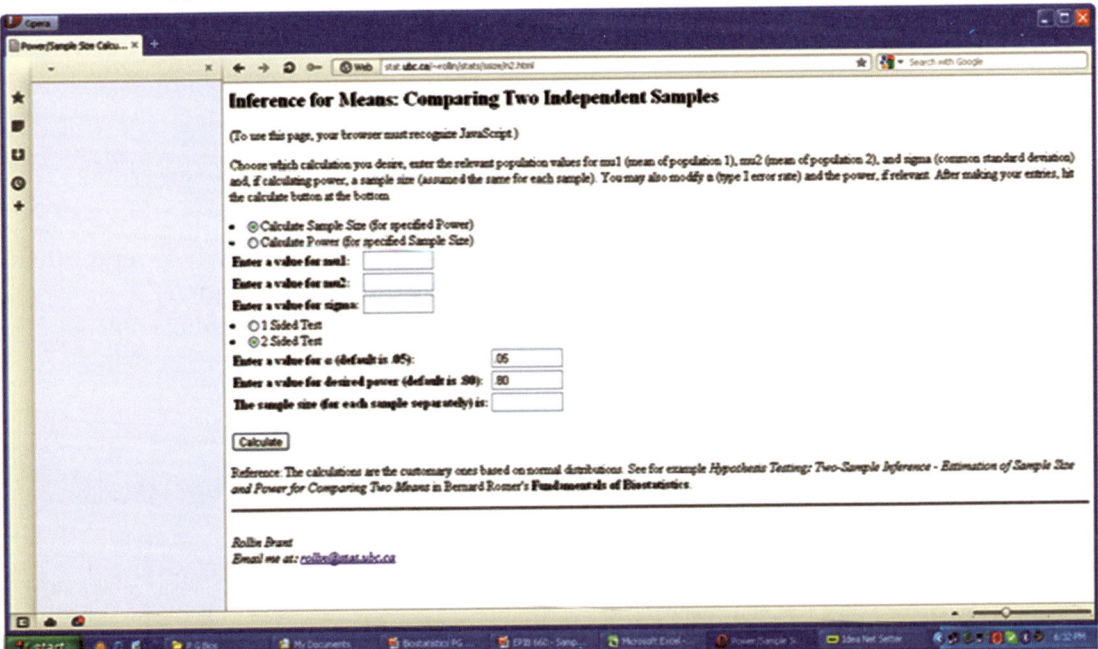

Some default values are given which are also changeable as per choice.

• Give inputs asked and click calculate.

For example, Mean 1 = 5, Mean 2 = 15 and SD = 14 inputting values.

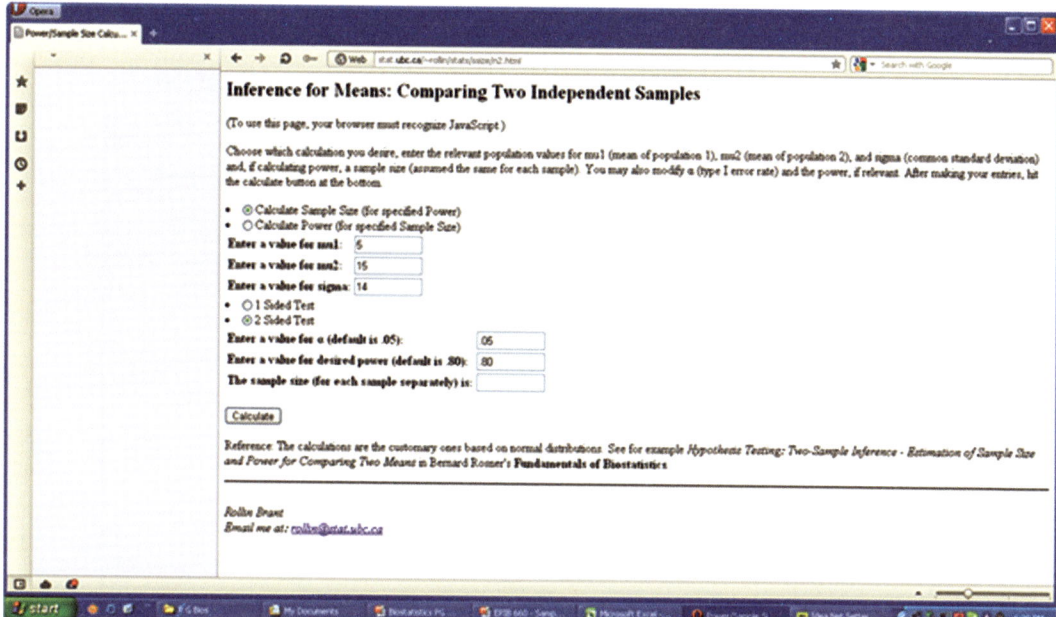

• Sample size will be shown directly on window.

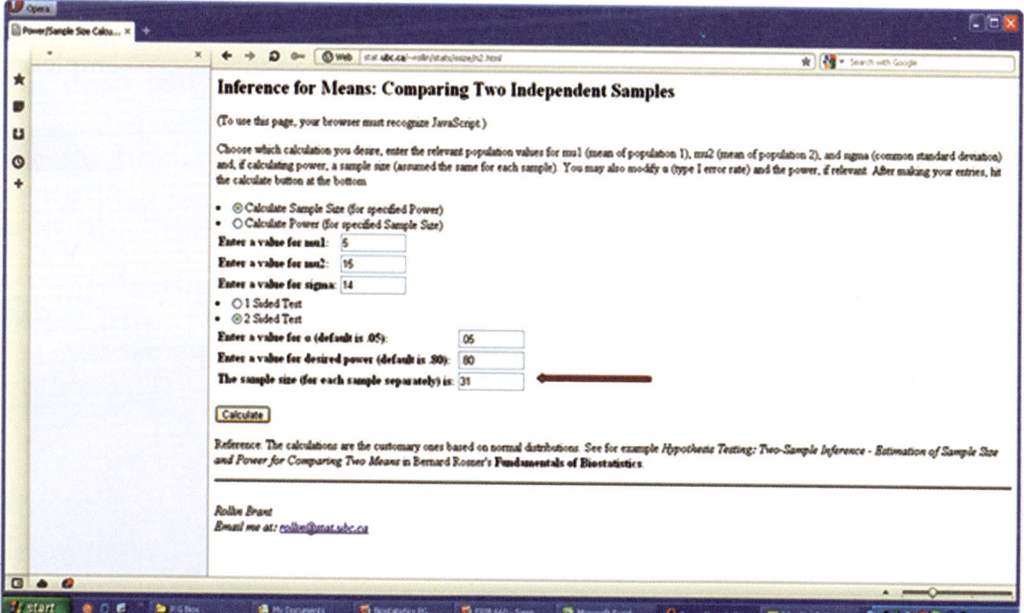

**Sample size** can directly be calculated from statistical softwares:

## Steps for Calculation from Statistical Software

1. Open software
2. Click 'Sample size'

3. Select and click type of outcome analysis.
4. Some default values are given which are also changeable as per choice.
5. Give inputs asked.
6. Click OK.
7. Sample size will be shown directly on window.
8. Some softwares also provide advisor to guide.

**Example: Primer** version 6

**Click advisor** to find out which test is required as per type of data

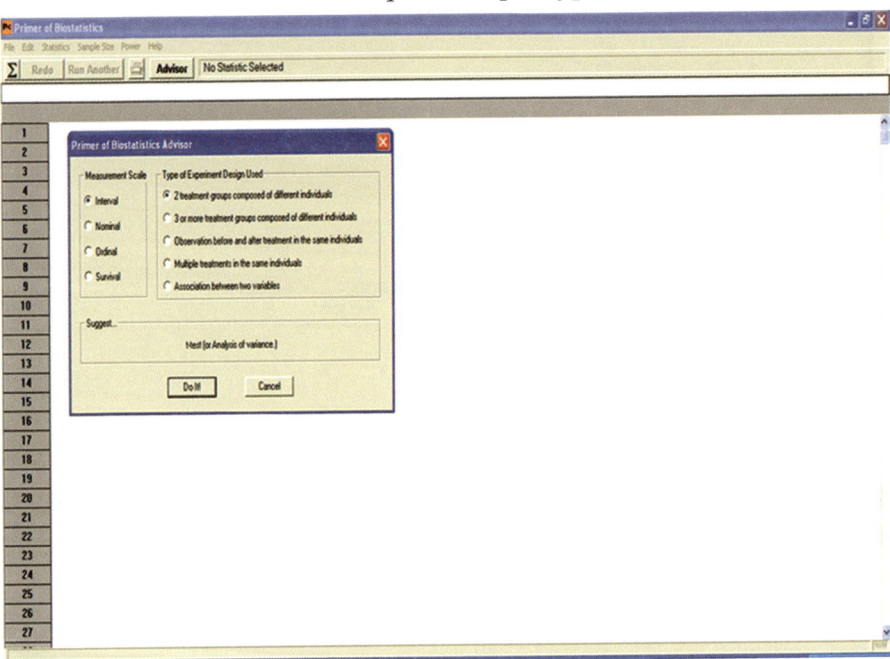

For example, if 2 different groups are compared of quantitative data, primer has suggested t-test.

**Click Sample Size**

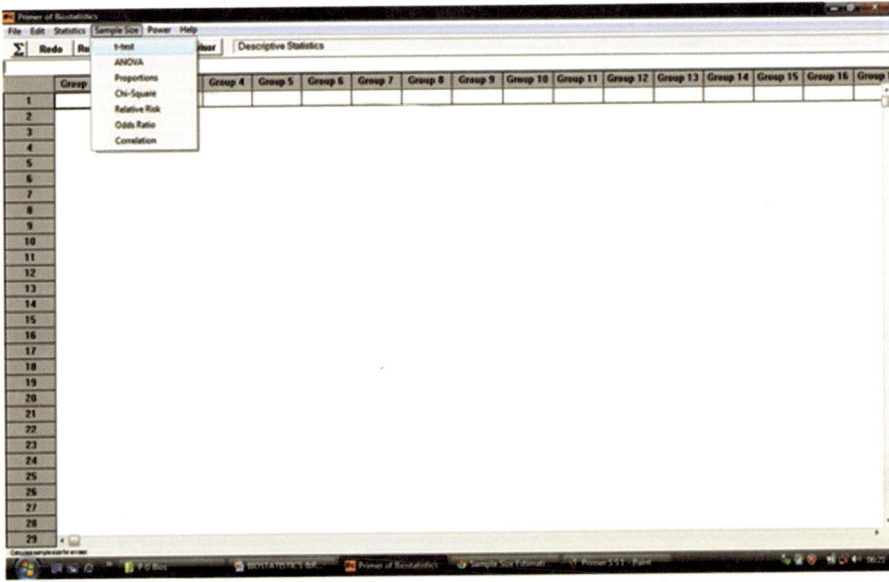

**Select and click t-test**

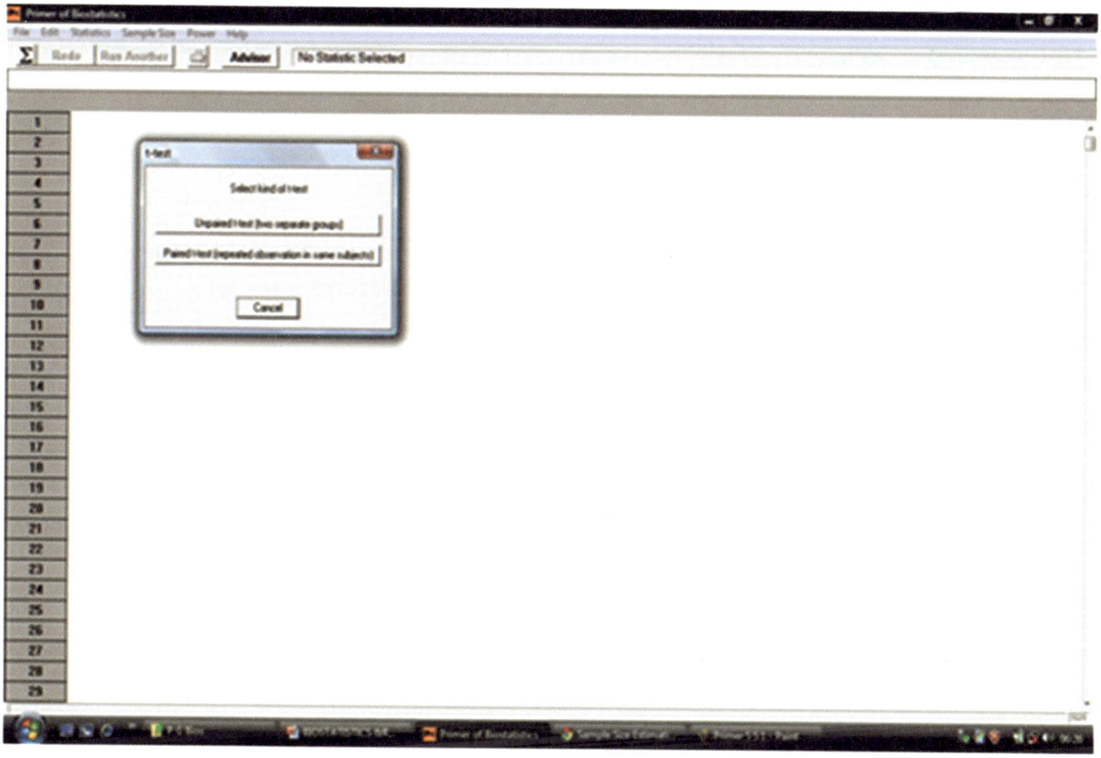

**Select and click unpaired,** this window will appear with by default 0.05 alpha error. **Give inputs** (alpha error may also be change, if one wants)

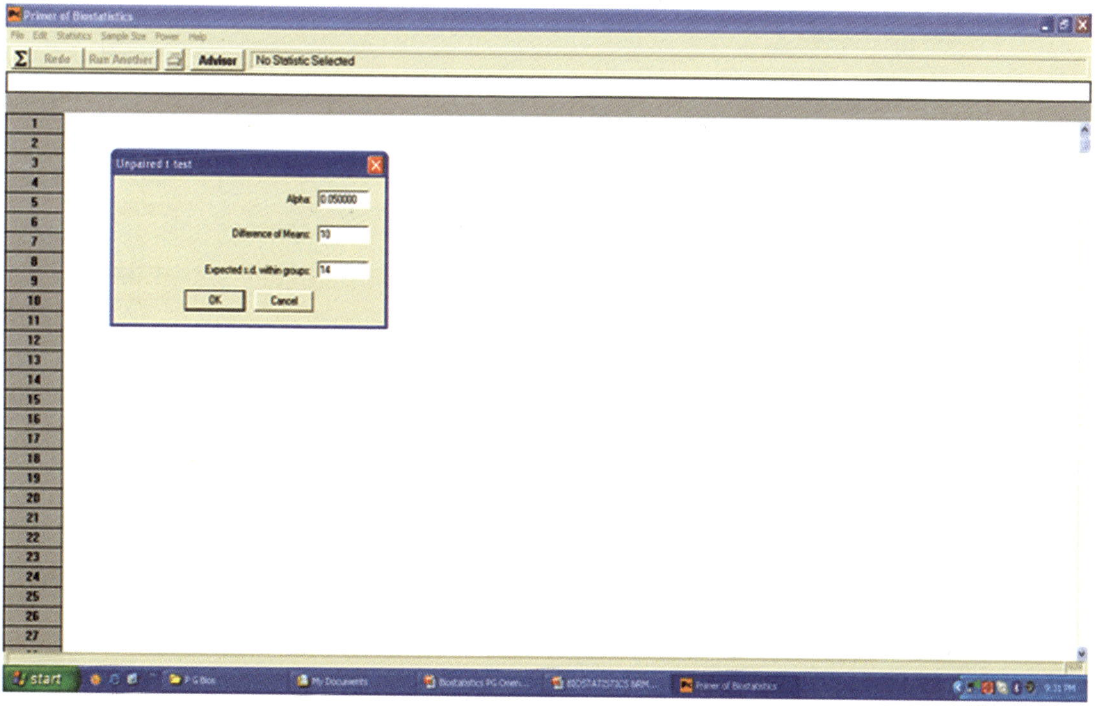

**Click OK, this window will appear asking about desired power.** By default it is given 80% but it may also be change as need.

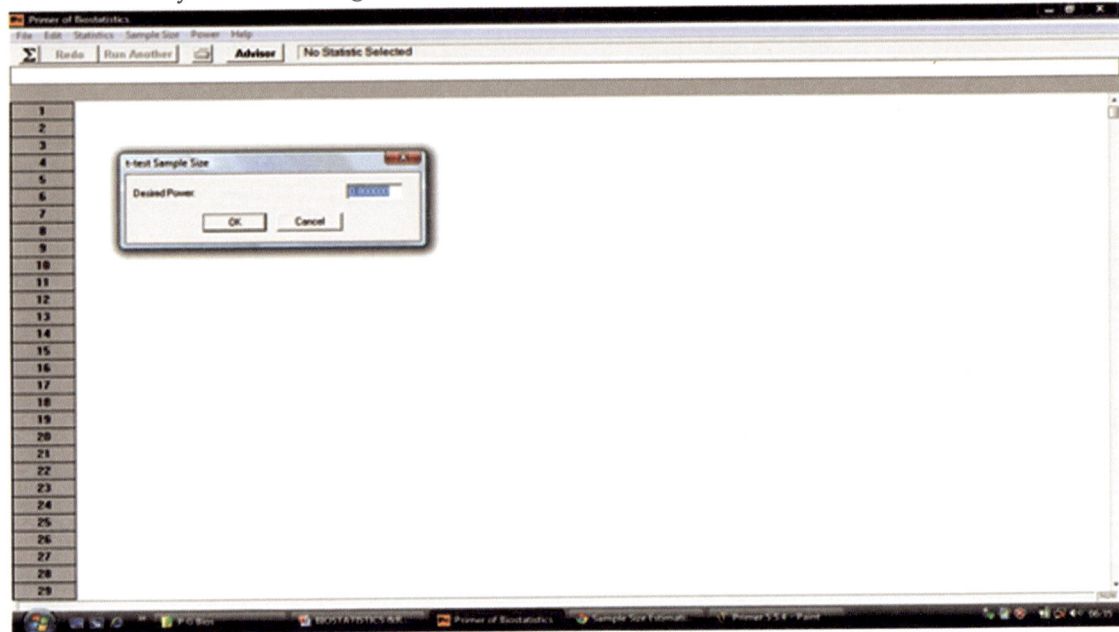

**Click OK**

Sample size window will appear showing sample size for each group at given alpha error, difference of means to be detected, expected SD within groups with desirable power.

**Sample size tables are also available online.**

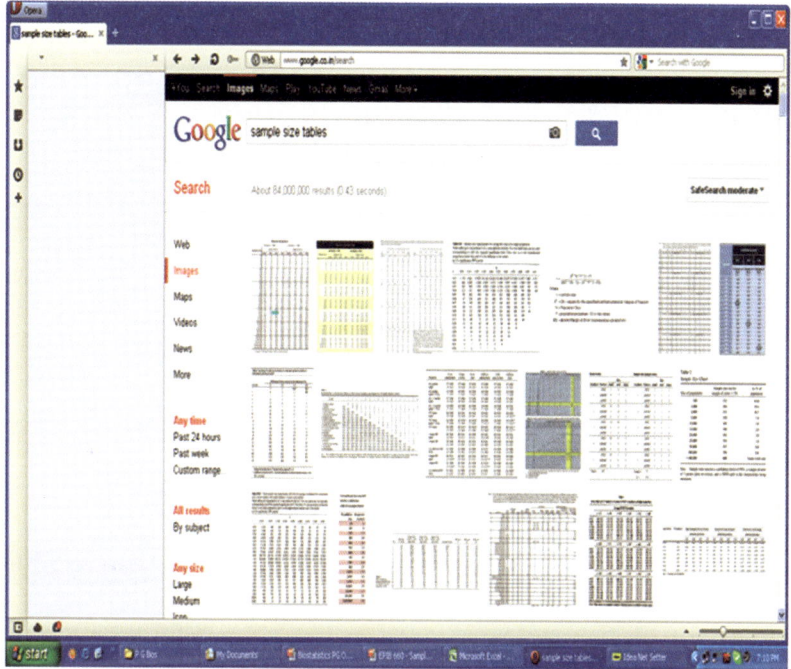

## Computer in Data Management and Analysis

**Entry of observation units in MS Excel:** Each row is for one observation unit (individual) and one column is for one variable.

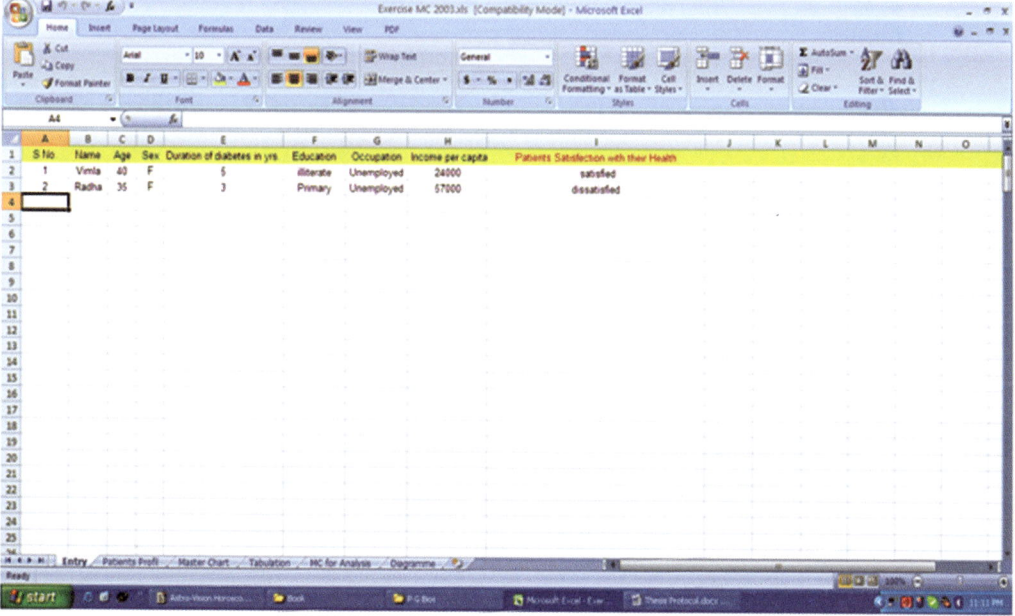

**If all observation units are entered with their variable, then it is known as 'Master Chart'.**

| S No | Name | Age | Sex | Duration of diabetes in yrs | Occupation | Education | Income per capita | Patients Satisfection with their Health |
|---|---|---|---|---|---|---|---|---|
| 1 | Vimla | 40 | F | 5 | Unemployed | illiterate | 24000 | satisfied |
| 2 | Radha | 35 | F | 3 | Unemployed | Primary | 57000 | dissatisfied |
| 3 | Anamika sharma | 55 | F | 5 | Unemployed | Graduate | 16666 | neither satisfied nor dissatisfied |
| 4 | Gulab devi | 48 | F | 5 | Unemployed | Middle | 15000 | neither satisfied nor dissatisfied |
| 5 | V K Gupta | 30 | M | 6 | Professional | PG | 300000 | neither satisfied nor dissatisfied |
| 6 | Rajendra Prasad | 28 | M | 2 | Semi-professional | Graduate | 60000 | satisfied |
| 7 | Meenal Singh | 23 | F | 5 | Unemployed | Graduate | 150000 | neither satisfied nor dissatisfied |
| 8 | Sheela Shrivastav | 35 | F | 2 | Unemployed | Graduate | 60000 | neither satisfied nor dissatisfied |
| 9 | Shashi Jain | 53 | F | 7 | Semi-professional | PG | 60000 | dissatisfied |
| 10 | Kaluram | 50 | M | 5 | Professional | Graduate | 60000 | satisfied |
| 11 | Rampyari devi | 50 | F | 10 | Unemployed | illiterate | 60000 | neither satisfied nor dissatisfied |
| 12 | Hukam Singh | 54 | M | 1 5 | Semi-skilled | Sec | 48000 | satisfied |
| 13 | Mohd Ali | 58 | M | 15 | Unskilled | Primary | 12000 | neither satisfied nor dissatisfied |
| 14 | Saroj | 49 | F | 20 | Unemployed | illiterate | 60000 | satisfied |
| 15 | Sameer | 55 | M | 5 | Professional | Graduate | 60000 | dissatisfied |
| 16 | Ram Prasad | 54 | M | 15 | Unskilled | Primary | 24000 | dissatisfied |
| 17 | Sitaram | 50 | M | 2 | Semi-professional | HSC | 60000 | neither satisfied nor dissatisfied |
| 18 | Sukhdeep | 35 | M | 5 | Professional | Graduate | 75000 | satisfied |
| 19 | Radha Devi | 35 | F | 10 | Unemployed | Middle | 80000 | neither satisfied nor dissatisfied |
| 20 | Rajkamal | 59 | M | 15 | Unemployed | Sec | 60000 | dissatisfied |
| 21 | Samundar Singh | 32 | M | 2 | Unskilled | Graduate | 40000 | neither satisfied nor dissatisfied |
| 22 | Kashuram | 45 | M | 2 | Semi-professional | illiterate | 40000 | satisfied |
| 23 | Kailash Rathi | 40 | M | 6 | Professional | PG | 84000 | neither satisfied nor dissatisfied |
| 24 | Sameera Khan | 25 | M | 4 | Unemployed | Graduate | 60000 | neither satisfied nor dissatisfied |

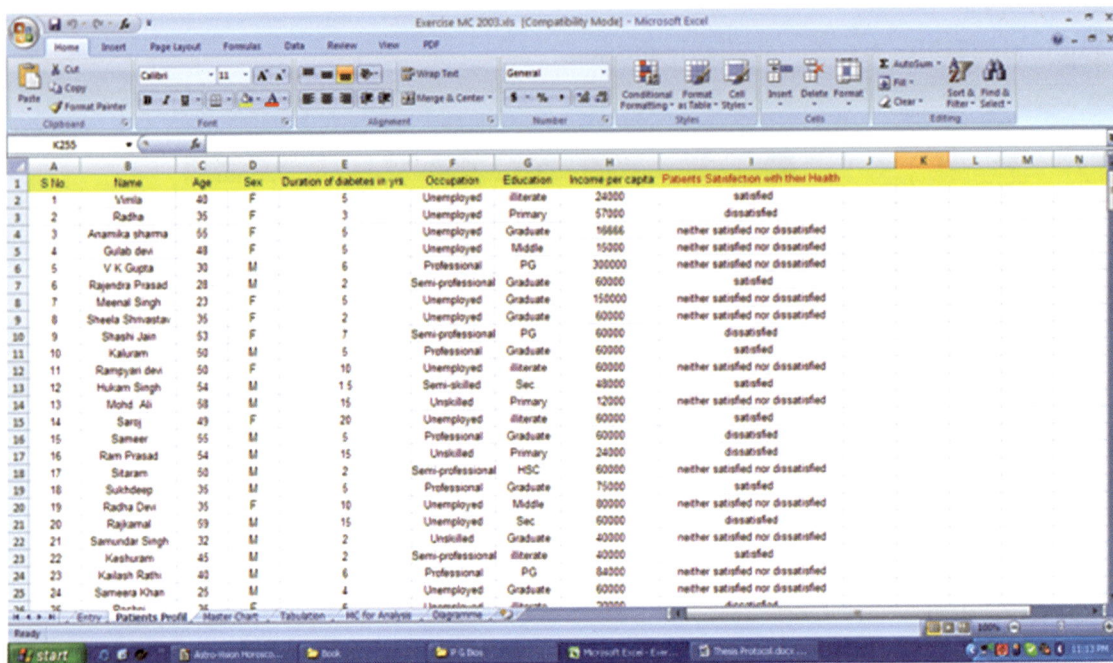

**After Master Chart, desired grouping of data will be done like this:**

Insert a column needing grouping

| S No | Name | Age | Age Groups | Sex | Duration of diabetes in yrs | Duration of DM Groups | Occupation | Education | Income per capita | SES | Patients Satisfection with their Health |
|---|---|---|---|---|---|---|---|---|---|---|---|
| 1 | Vimla | 40 | | F | 5 | | Unemployed | illiterate | 24000 | class II | satisfied |
| 2 | Radha | 35 | | F | 3 | | Unemployed | Primary | 57000 | class I | dissatisfied |
| 3 | Anamika sharma | 55 | | F | 5 | | Unemployed | Graduate | 16666 | class III | neither satisfied nor dissatisfied |
| 4 | Gulab devi | 48 | | F | 5 | | Unemployed | Middle | 15000 | class III | neither satisfied nor dissatisfied |
| 5 | V K Gupta | 30 | | M | 6 | | Professional | PG | 300000 | class I | neither satisfied nor dissatisfied |
| 6 | Rajendra Prasad | 28 | | M | 2 | | Semi-professional | Graduate | 60000 | class I | satisfied |
| 7 | Meenal Singh | 23 | | F | 5 | | Unemployed | Graduate | 150000 | class I | neither satisfied nor dissatisfied |
| 8 | Sheela Shrivastav | 35 | | F | 2 | | Unemployed | Graduate | 60000 | class I | neither satisfied nor dissatisfied |
| 9 | Shashi Jain | 53 | | F | 7 | | Semi-professional | PG | 60000 | class I | dissatisfied |
| 10 | Kaluram | 50 | | M | 5 | | Professional | Graduate | 60000 | class I | satisfied |
| 11 | Rampyari devi | 50 | | F | 10 | | Unemployed | illiterate | 60000 | class I | neither satisfied nor dissatisfied |
| 12 | Hukam Singh | 54 | | M | 1 5 | | Semi-skilled | Sec | 48000 | class I | satisfied |
| 13 | Mohd Ali | 58 | | M | 15 | | Unskilled | Primary | 12000 | class IV | neither satisfied nor dissatisfied |
| 14 | Saroj | 49 | | F | 20 | | Unemployed | illiterate | 60000 | class I | satisfied |
| 15 | Sameer | 55 | | M | 5 | | Professional | Graduate | 60000 | class I | dissatisfied |
| 16 | Ram Prasad | 54 | | M | 15 | | Unskilled | Primary | 24000 | class II | dissatisfied |
| 17 | Sitaram | 50 | | M | 2 | | Semi-professional | HSC | 60000 | class I | neither satisfied nor dissatisfied |
| 18 | Sukhdeep | 35 | | M | 5 | | Professional | Graduate | 75000 | class I | satisfied |
| 19 | Radha Devi | 35 | | F | 10 | | Unemployed | Middle | 80000 | class I | neither satisfied nor dissatisfied |
| 20 | Rajkamal | 59 | | M | 15 | | Unemployed | Sec | 60000 | class I | dissatisfied |
| 21 | Samundar Singh | 32 | | M | 2 | | Unskilled | Graduate | 40000 | class II | neither satisfied nor dissatisfied |
| 22 | Keshuram | 45 | | M | 2 | | Semi-professional | illiterate | 40000 | class II | satisfied |
| 23 | Kailash Rathi | 40 | | M | 6 | | Professional | PG | 84000 | class I | neither satisfied nor dissatisfied |
| 24 | Sameera Khan | 25 | | M | 4 | | Unemployed | Graduate | 60000 | class I | neither satisfied nor dissatisfied |

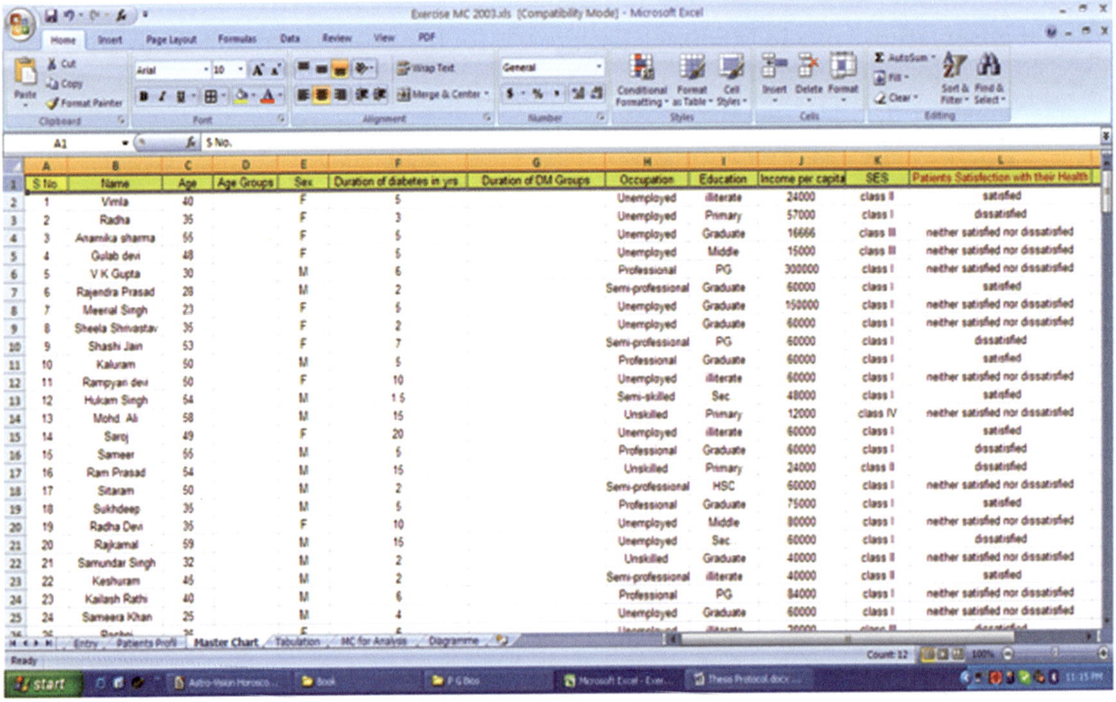

## Copy desired column

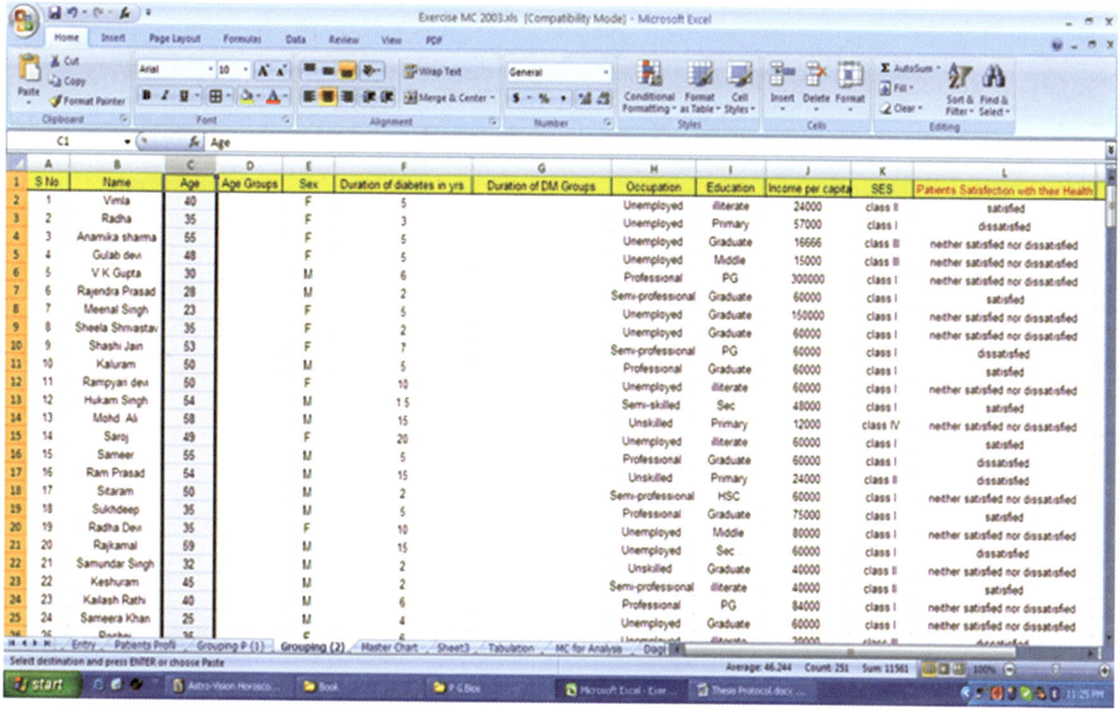

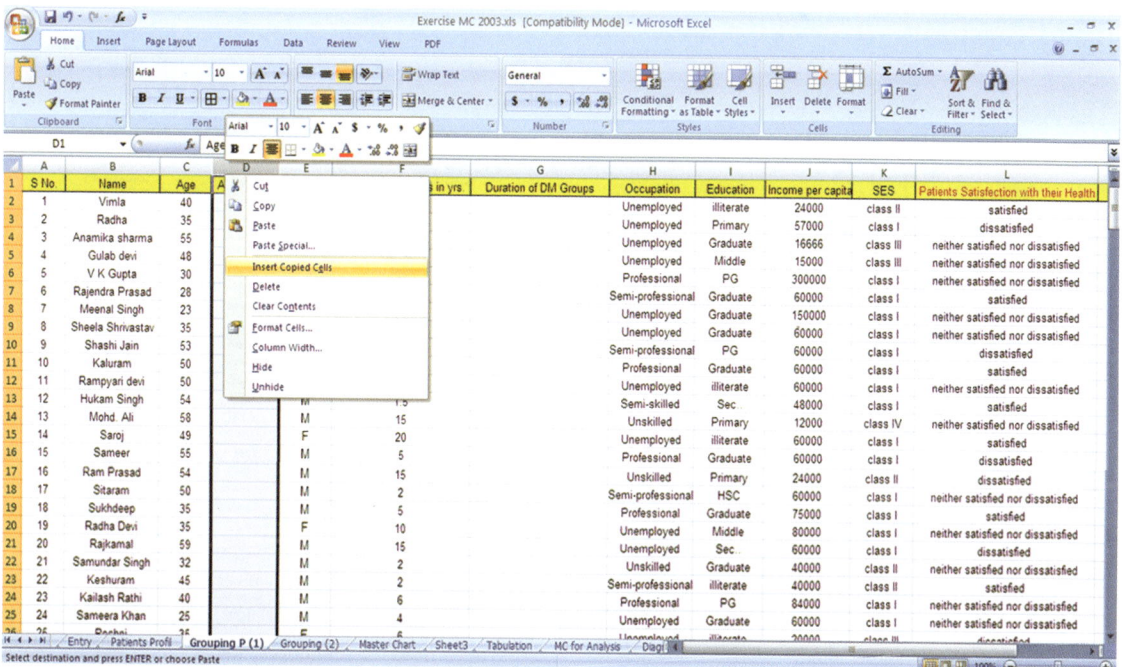

## Insert copied cells after copied variable column to be grouped

Click 'Filter' after selecting group column

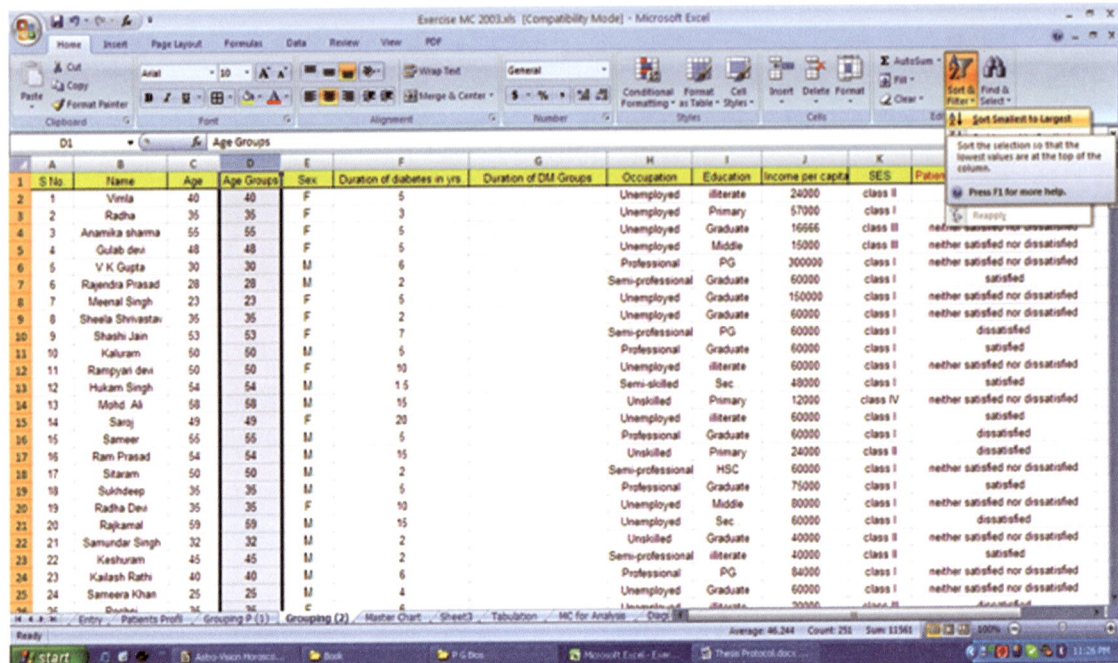

Always select expand selection, it will expand the selection for other variables also

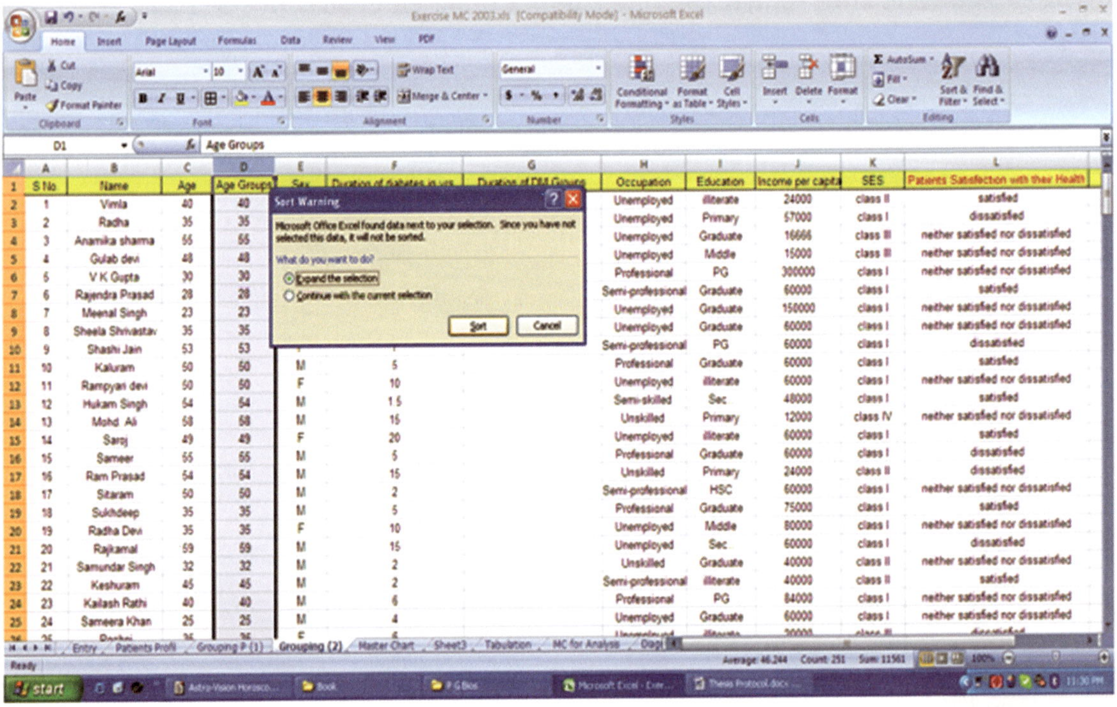

Click sort: This window will appear showing sorted column in ascending manner

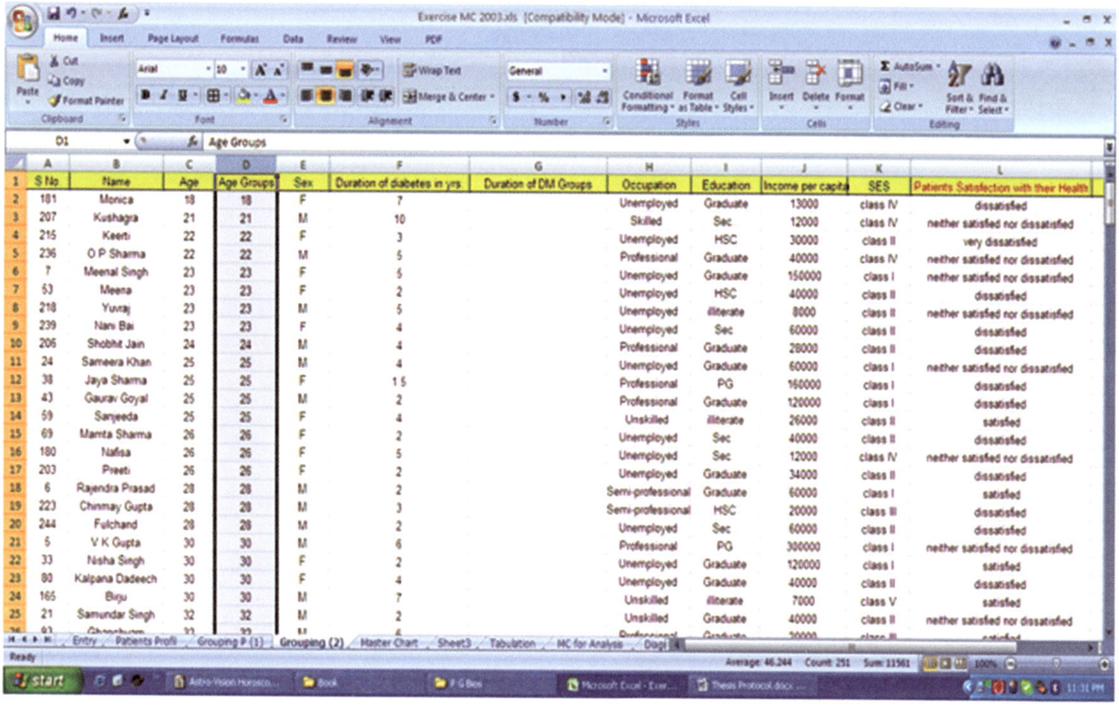

Click 'Filter' from title bar as shown here

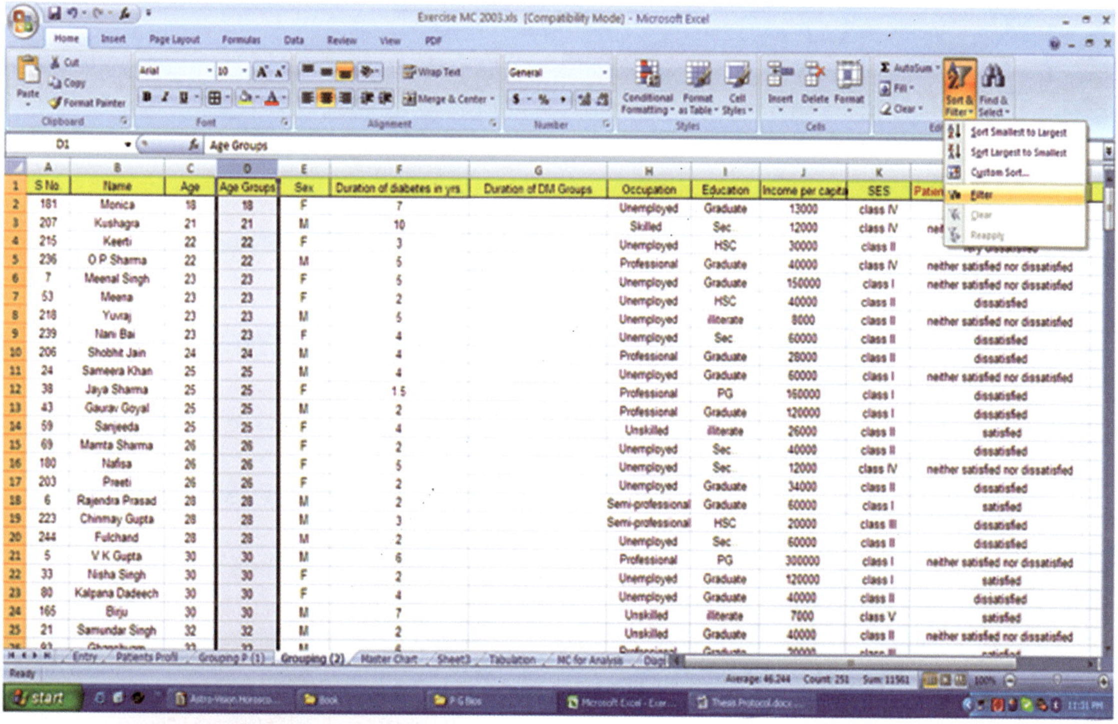

Sign of filter will appear on that column as shown here

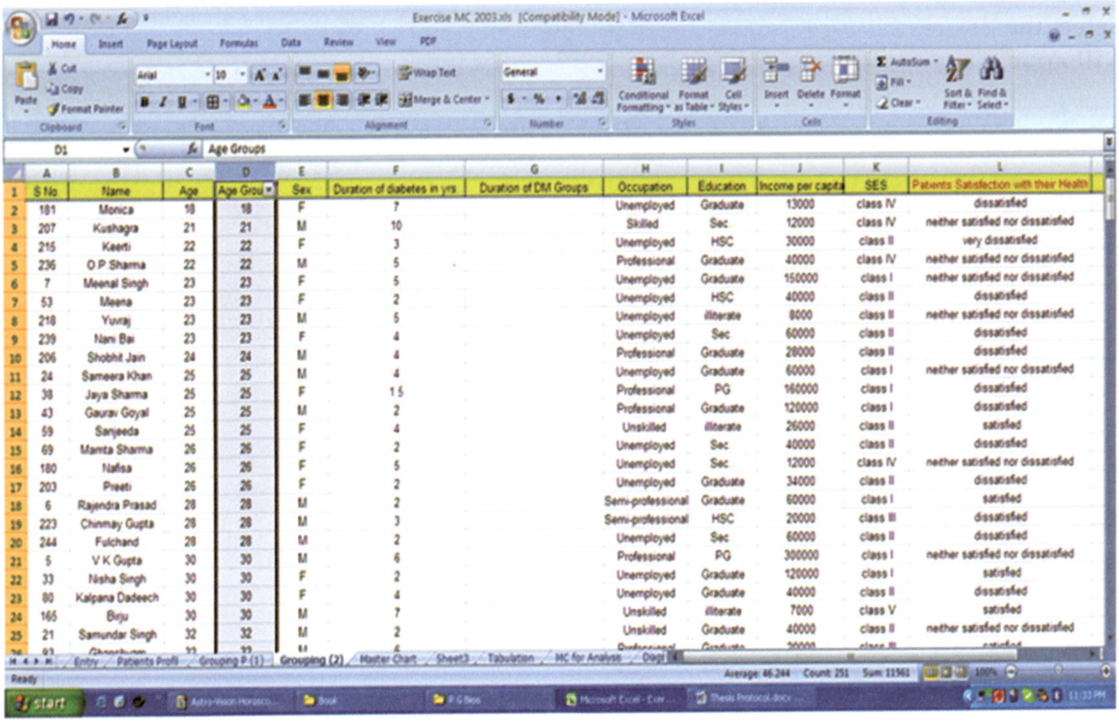

| S No | Name | Age | Age Group | Sex | Duration of diabetes in yrs | Duration of DM Groups | Occupation | Education | Income per capita | SES | Patients Satisfaction with their Health |
|---|---|---|---|---|---|---|---|---|---|---|---|
| 181 | Monica | 18 | 18 | F | 7 | | Unemployed | Graduate | 13000 | class IV | dissatisfied |
| 207 | Kushagra | 21 | 21 | M | 10 | | Skilled | Sec | 12000 | class IV | neither satisfied nor dissatisfied |
| 215 | Keerti | 22 | 22 | F | 3 | | Unemployed | HSC | 30000 | class II | very dissatisfied |
| 236 | O.P.Sharma | 22 | 22 | M | 5 | | Professional | Graduate | 40000 | class IV | neither satisfied nor dissatisfied |
| 7 | Meenal Singh | 23 | 23 | F | 5 | | Unemployed | Graduate | 150000 | class I | neither satisfied nor dissatisfied |
| 53 | Meena | 23 | 23 | F | 2 | | Unemployed | HSC | 40000 | class II | dissatisfied |
| 218 | Yuvraj | 23 | 23 | M | 5 | | Unemployed | illiterate | 8000 | class II | neither satisfied nor dissatisfied |
| 239 | Nani Bai | 23 | 23 | F | 4 | | Unemployed | Sec | 60000 | class II | dissatisfied |
| 206 | Shobhit Jain | 24 | 24 | M | 4 | | Professional | Graduate | 28000 | class II | dissatisfied |
| 24 | Sameera Khan | 25 | 25 | M | 4 | | Unemployed | Graduate | 60000 | class I | neither satisfied nor dissatisfied |
| 38 | Jaya Sharma | 25 | 25 | F | 15 | | Professional | PG | 160000 | class I | dissatisfied |
| 43 | Gaurav Goyal | 25 | 25 | M | 2 | | Professional | Graduate | 120000 | class II | dissatisfied |
| 59 | Sanjeeda | 25 | 25 | F | 4 | | Unskilled | illiterate | 26000 | class II | satisfied |
| 69 | Mamta Sharma | 26 | 26 | F | 2 | | Unemployed | Sec | 40000 | class II | dissatisfied |
| 180 | Nafisa | 26 | 26 | F | 5 | | Unemployed | Sec | 12000 | class IV | neither satisfied nor dissatisfied |
| 203 | Preeti | 26 | 26 | F | 2 | | Unemployed | Graduate | 34000 | class II | dissatisfied |
| 6 | Rajendra Prasad | 28 | 28 | M | 2 | | Semi-professional | Graduate | 60000 | class I | satisfied |
| 223 | Chinmay Gupta | 28 | 28 | M | 3 | | Semi-professional | HSC | 20000 | class III | dissatisfied |
| 244 | Fulchand | 28 | 28 | M | 2 | | Unemployed | Sec | 60000 | class II | dissatisfied |
| 5 | V K Gupta | 30 | 30 | M | 6 | | Professional | PG | 300000 | class I | neither satisfied nor dissatisfied |
| 33 | Nisha Singh | 30 | 30 | F | 2 | | Unemployed | Graduate | 120000 | class I | satisfied |
| 80 | Kalpana Dadeech | 30 | 30 | F | 4 | | Unemployed | Graduate | 40000 | class II | satisfied |
| 165 | Birju | 30 | 30 | M | 7 | | Unskilled | illiterate | 7000 | class V | satisfied |
| 21 | Samundar Singh | 32 | 32 | M | 2 | | Unskilled | Graduate | 40000 | class II | neither satisfied nor dissatisfied |

Click on sign of filter in group column or from title bar, filter options will be seen on window. Desired numbers for grouping may be selected as shown here

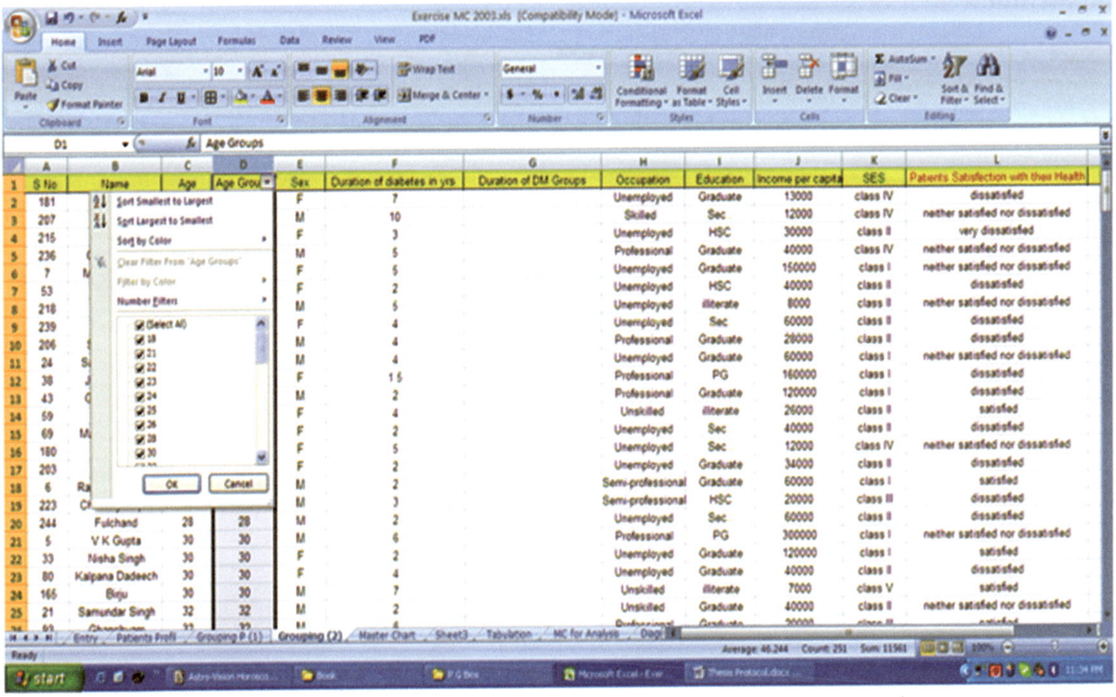

Select the desirable groups and then click OK. Window having only the desired numbers will appear as follows

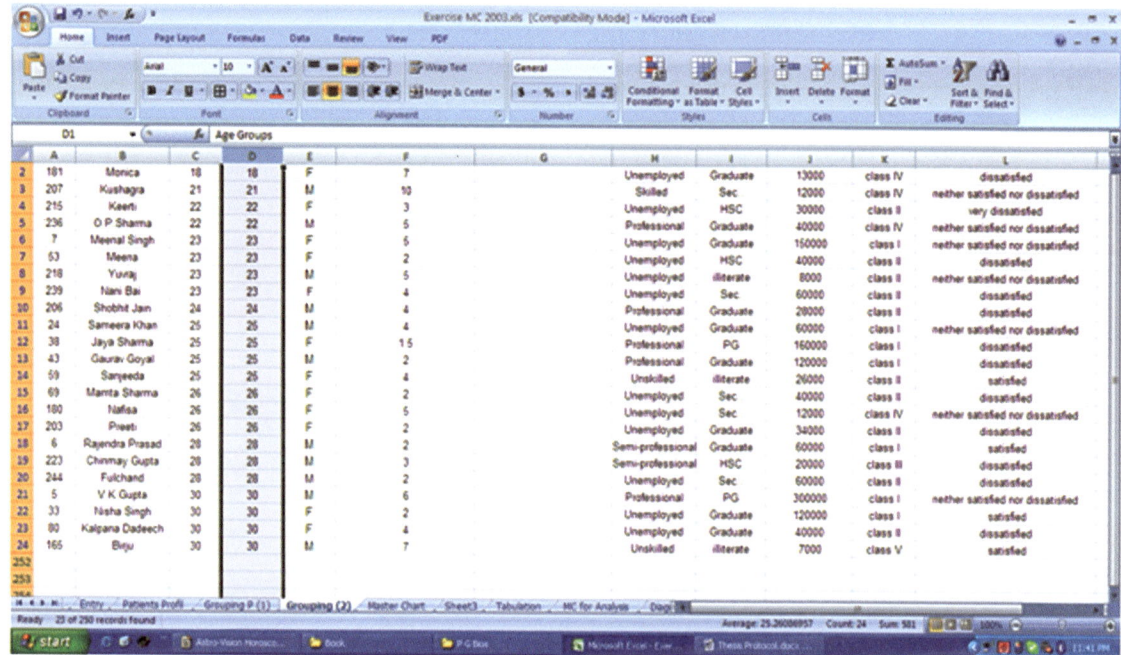

This window will be of desirable group, give it desired name as follows

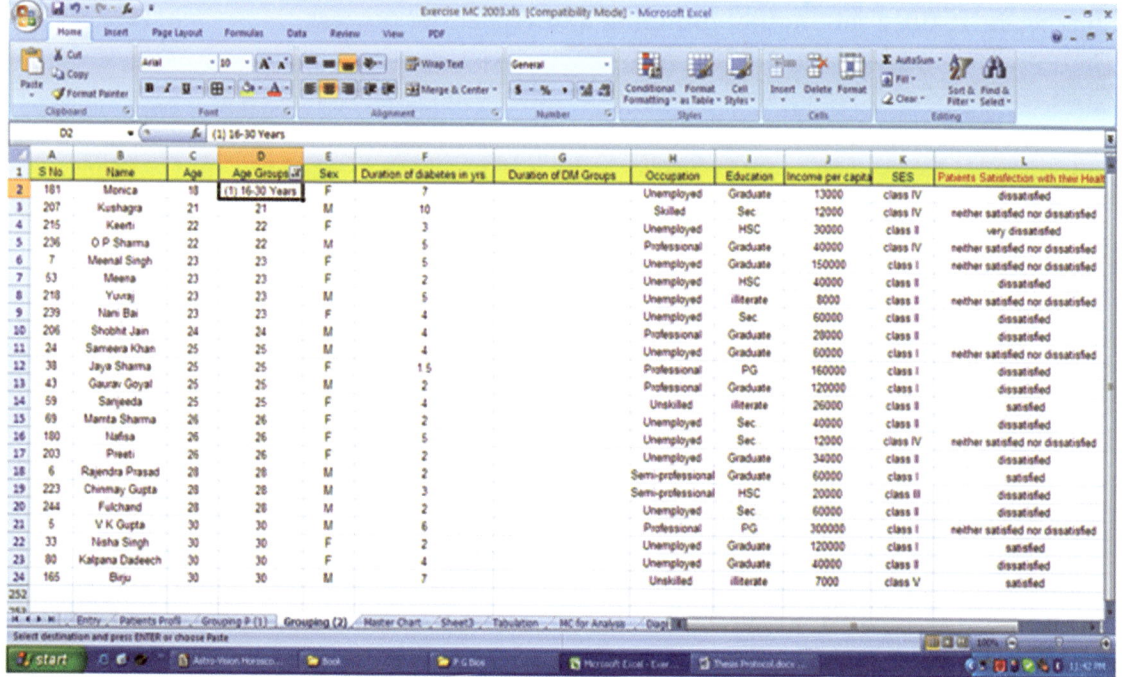

# Catch the cell when + sign appears and drag it till end of that group as follows

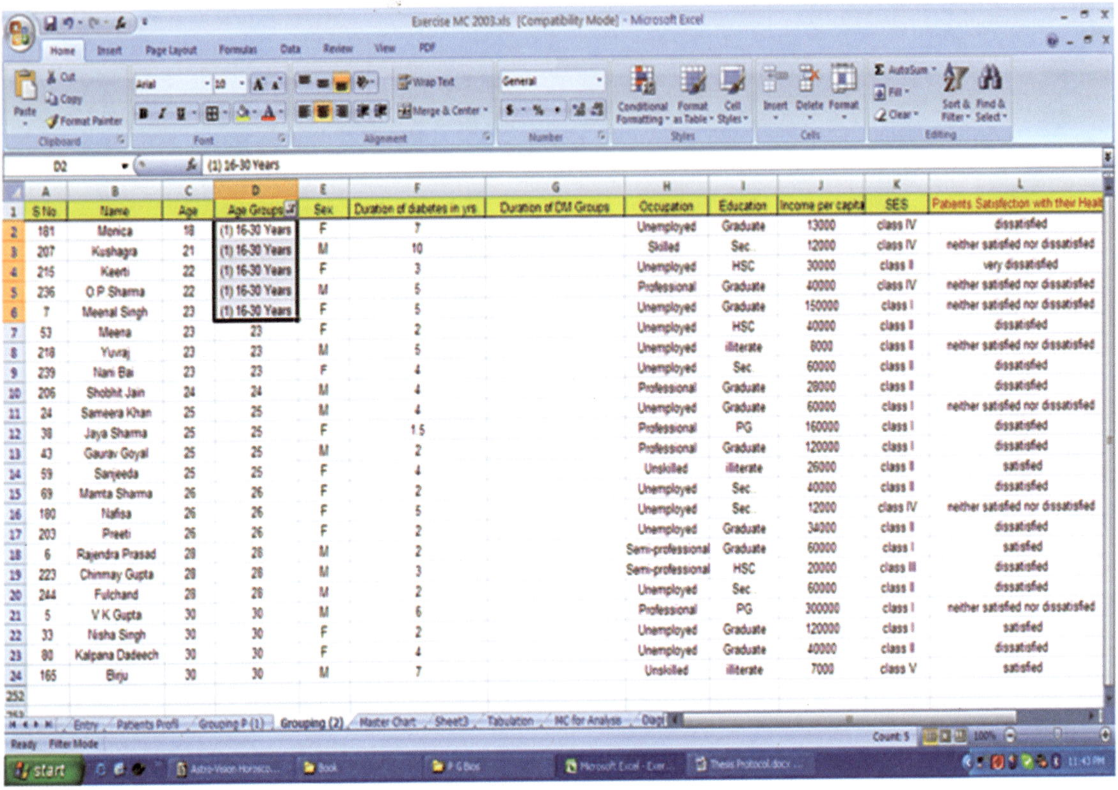

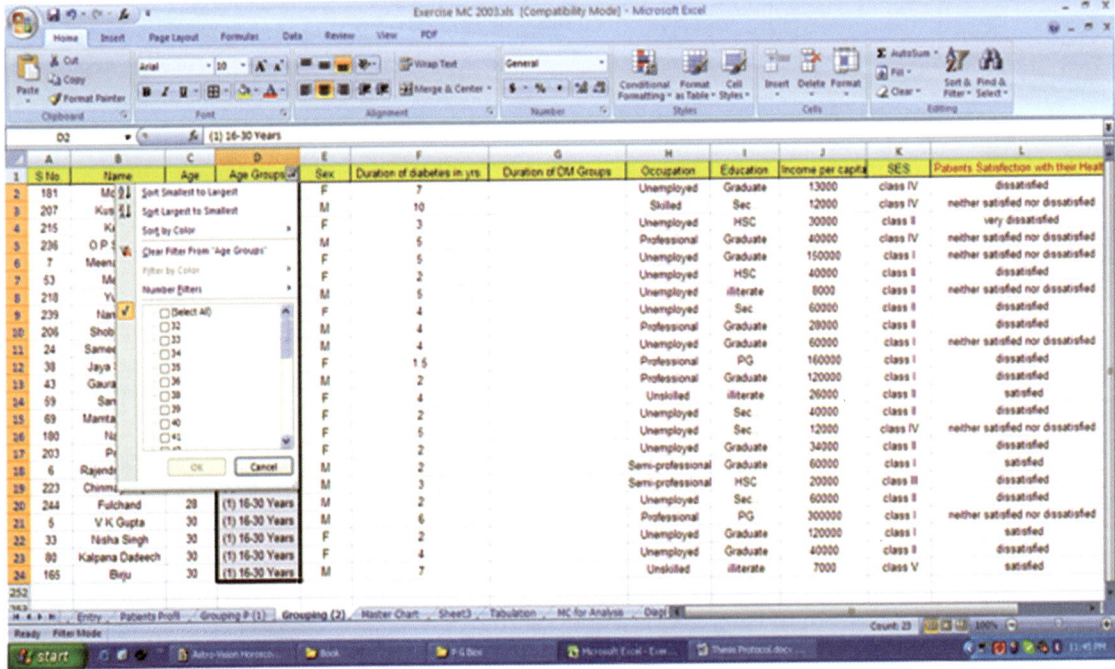

# Click again at filter for another grouping and repeat the process

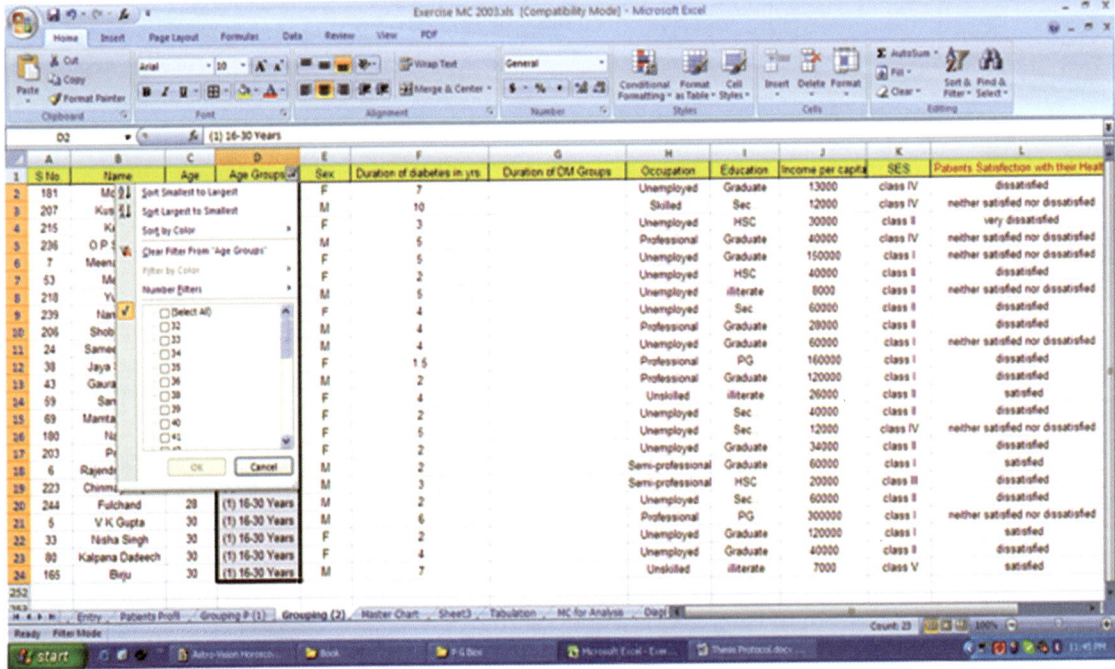

## By selecting another group

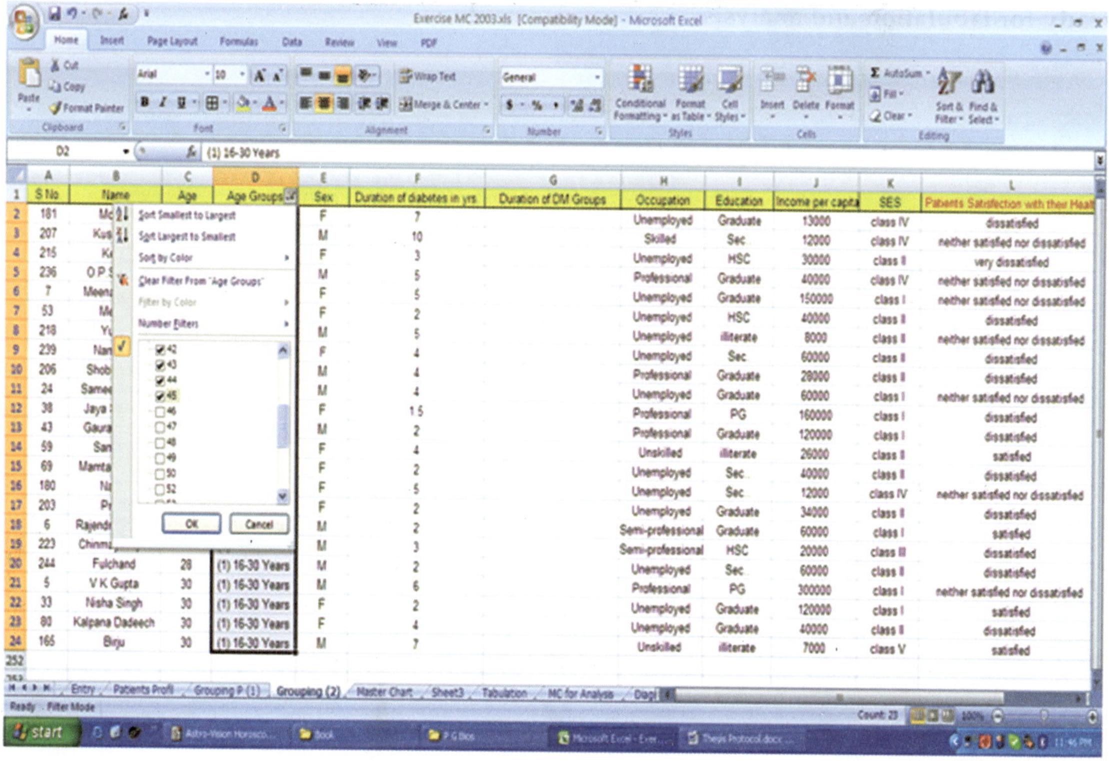

## Likewise grouping may be done for whole column. Start grouping for another variable.

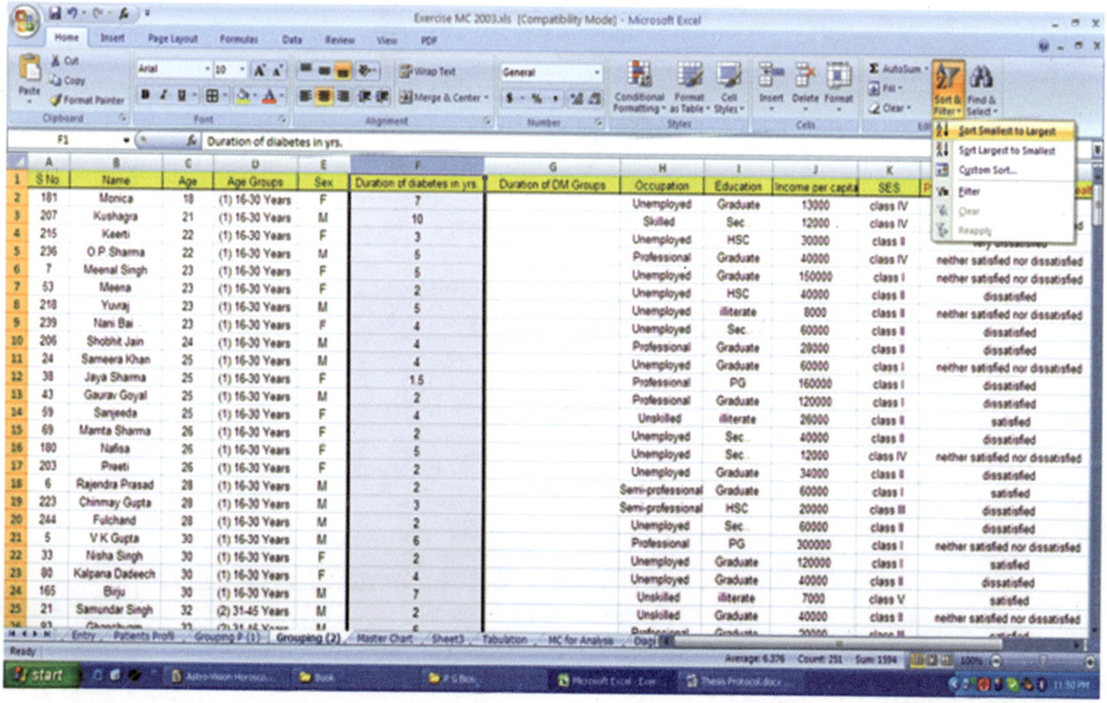

| S No | Name | Age | Age Groups | Sex | Duration of diabetes in yrs | Duration of DM Groups | Occupation | Education | Income per capita | SES | Patients Satisfaction with their Health |
|---|---|---|---|---|---|---|---|---|---|---|---|
| 181 | Monica | 18 | (1) 16-30 Years | F | 7 | | Unemployed | Graduate | 13000 | class IV | dissatisfied |
| 207 | Kushagra | 21 | (1) 16-30 Years | M | 10 | | Skilled | Sec. | 12000 | class IV | |
| 215 | Keerti | 22 | (1) 16-30 Years | F | 3 | | Unemployed | HSC | 30000 | class II | |
| 236 | O P Sharma | 22 | (1) 16-30 Years | M | 5 | | Professional | Graduate | 40000 | class IV | neither satisfied nor dissatisfied |
| 7 | Meenal Singh | 23 | (1) 16-30 Years | F | 5 | | Unemployed | Graduate | 150000 | class I | neither satisfied nor dissatisfied |
| 53 | Meena | 23 | (1) 16-30 Years | F | 2 | | Unemployed | HSC | 40000 | class II | dissatisfied |
| 218 | Yuvraj | 23 | (1) 16-30 Years | M | 5 | | Unemployed | illiterate | 8000 | class II | neither satisfied nor dissatisfied |
| 239 | Nani Bai | 23 | (1) 16-30 Years | F | 4 | | Unemployed | Sec. | 60000 | class II | dissatisfied |
| 206 | Shobhit Jain | 24 | (1) 16-30 Years | M | 4 | | Professional | Graduate | 28000 | class II | dissatisfied |
| 24 | Sameera Khan | 25 | (1) 16-30 Years | M | 4 | | Unemployed | Graduate | 60000 | class I | neither satisfied nor dissatisfied |
| 38 | Jaya Sharma | 25 | (1) 16-30 Years | F | 1.5 | | Professional | PG | 160000 | class I | dissatisfied |
| 43 | Gaurav Goyal | 25 | (1) 16-30 Years | M | 2 | | Professional | Graduate | 120000 | class I | dissatisfied |
| 59 | Sanjeeda | 25 | (1) 16-30 Years | F | 4 | | Unskilled | illiterate | 26000 | class II | satisfied |
| 69 | Mamta Sharma | 26 | (1) 16-30 Years | F | 2 | | Unemployed | Sec. | 40000 | class II | dissatisfied |
| 180 | Nafisa | 26 | (1) 16-30 Years | F | 5 | | Unemployed | Sec. | 12000 | class IV | neither satisfied nor dissatisfied |
| 203 | Preeti | 26 | (1) 16-30 Years | F | 2 | | Unemployed | Graduate | 34000 | class II | dissatisfied |
| 6 | Rajendra Prasad | 28 | (1) 16-30 Years | M | 2 | | Semi-professional | Graduate | 60000 | class I | satisfied |
| 223 | Chinmay Gupta | 28 | (1) 16-30 Years | M | 3 | | Semi-professional | HSC | 20000 | class III | dissatisfied |
| 244 | Fulchand | 28 | (1) 16-30 Years | M | 2 | | Unemployed | Sec. | 60000 | class II | dissatisfied |
| 5 | V K Gupta | 30 | (1) 16-30 Years | M | 6 | | Professional | PG | 300000 | class I | neither satisfied nor dissatisfied |
| 33 | Nisha Singh | 30 | (1) 16-30 Years | F | 2 | | Unemployed | Graduate | 120000 | class I | satisfied |
| 80 | Kalpana Dadeech | 30 | (1) 16-30 Years | F | 4 | | Unemployed | Graduate | 40000 | class II | dissatisfied |
| 165 | Birju | 30 | (1) 16-30 Years | M | 7 | | Unskilled | illiterate | 7000 | class V | satisfied |
| 21 | Samundar Singh | 32 | (2) 31-45 Years | M | 2 | | Unskilled | Graduate | 40000 | class II | neither satisfied nor dissatisfied |

**Repeat the process for other groups and other variable. Finally master chart is become ready for tabulation and analysis.**

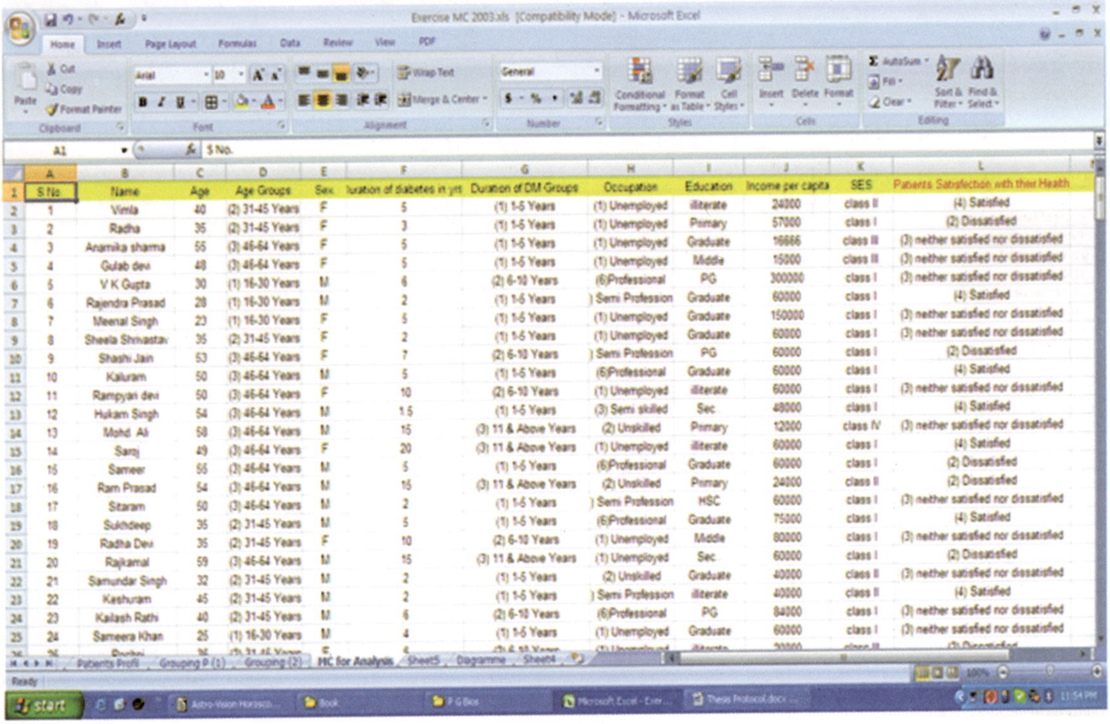

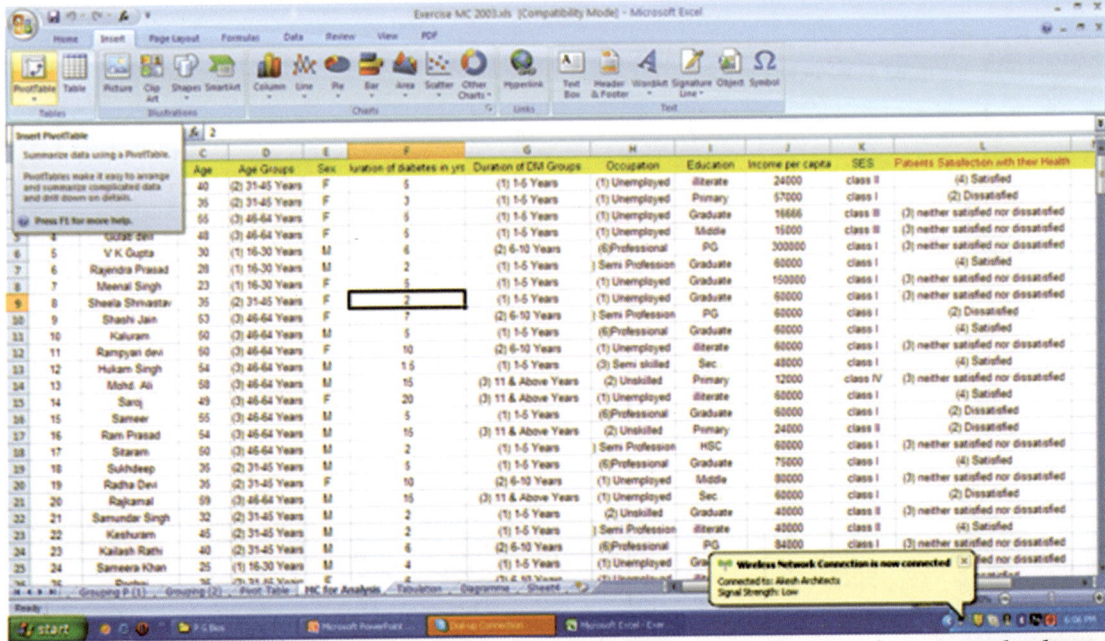

**For tabulation-click insert pivot table as follows**

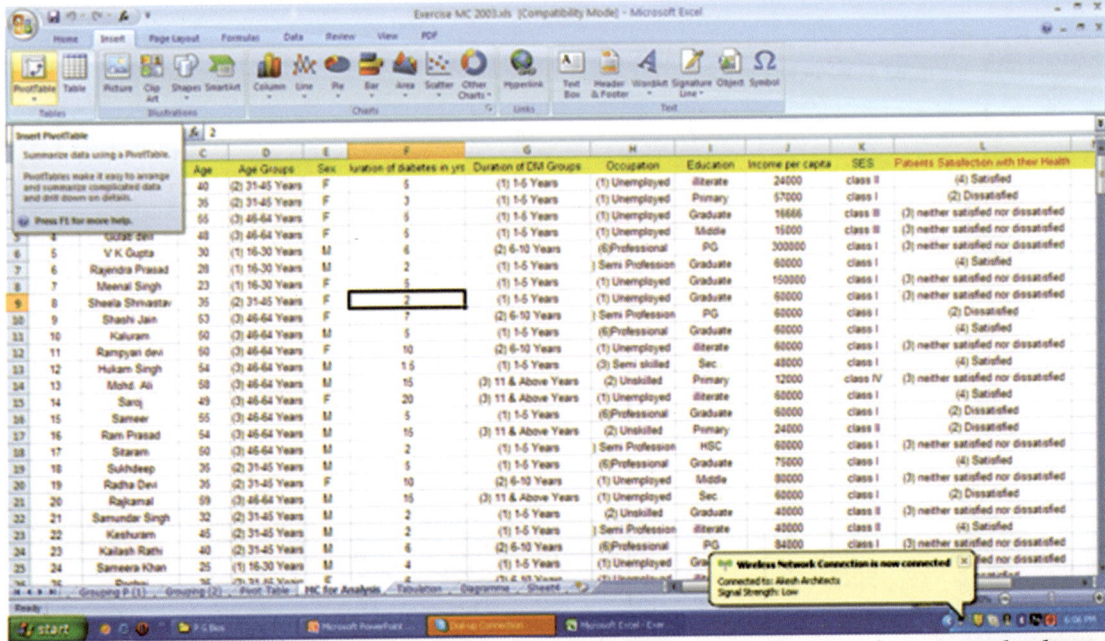

This window will appear showing table area and variable area with space for row and column. Select 'Row" and Column by dragging the cursor in window designed for it in right side of window. Simultaneously table will be shown on left side of window. Desired table will be framed by repeating the process with desirable variables.

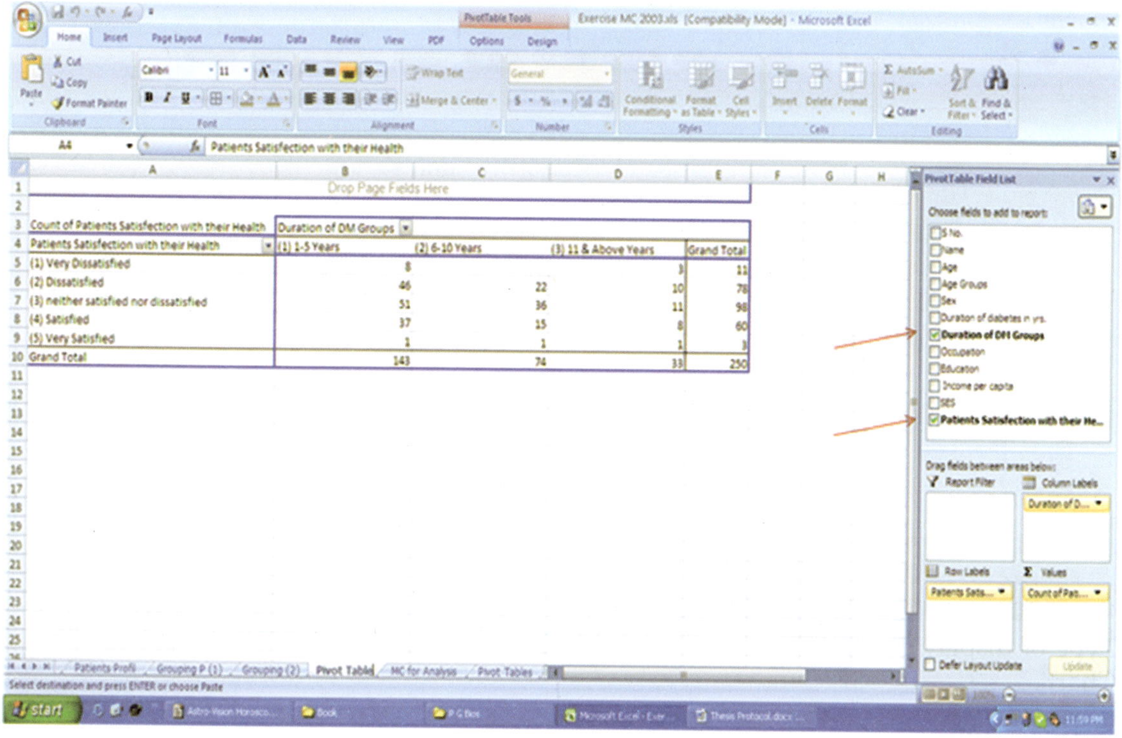

**For making chart – Insert 'Chart'**

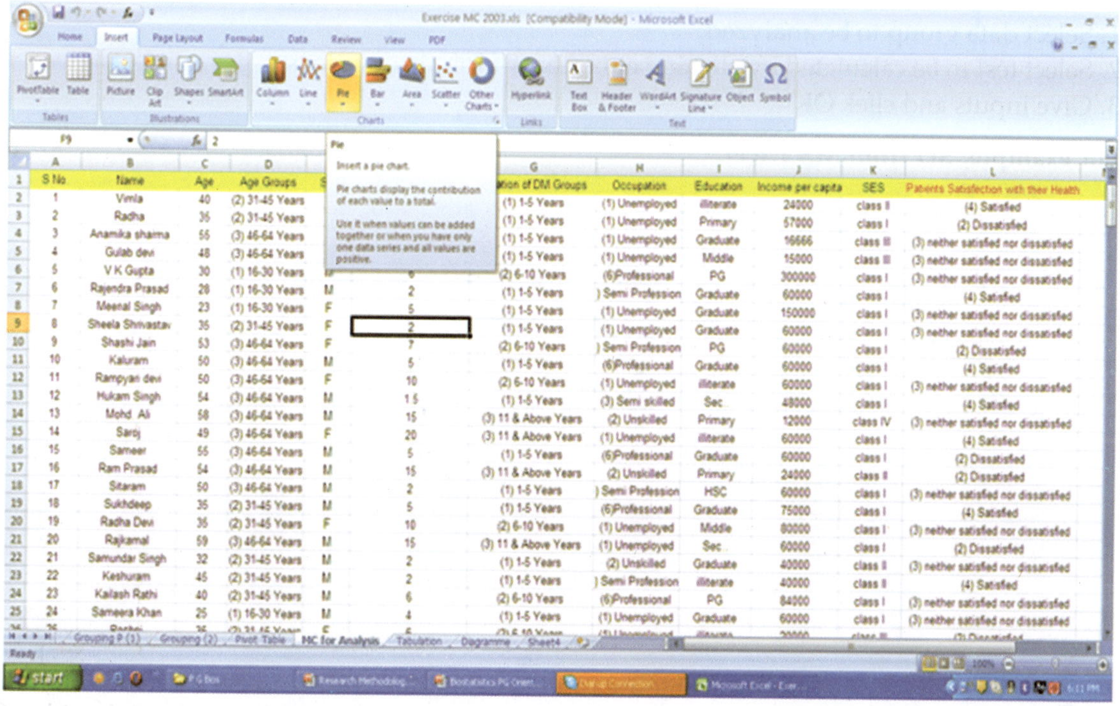

**Chart of selected table will appear on window.**

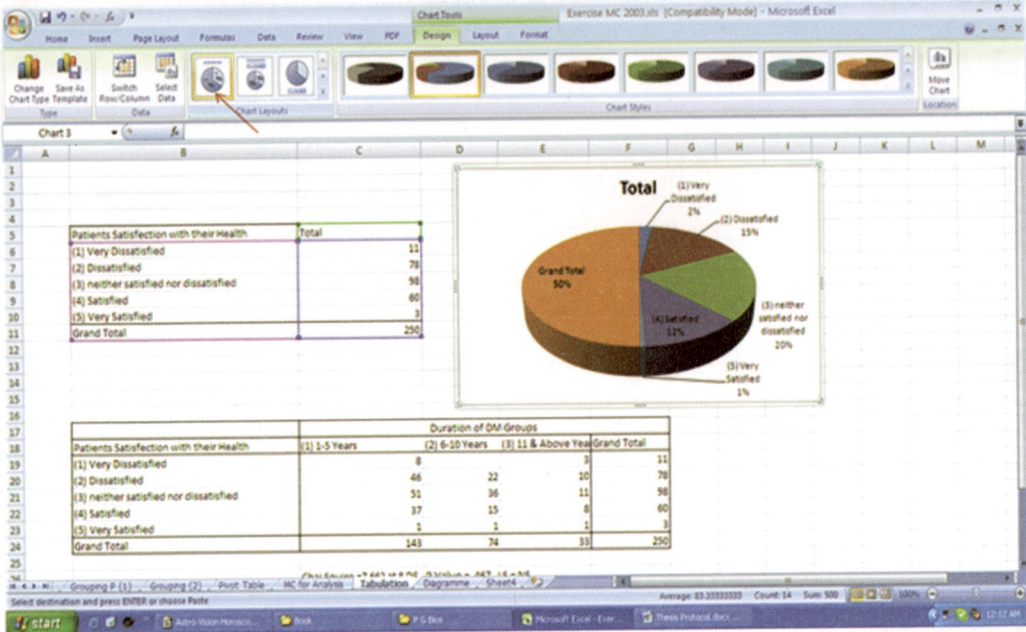

Type of display of chart can be selected. Charts type can be changed by clicking 'Change Chart'.

## Data Analysis

### Steps for Data Analysis

1. Select data group to be analyzed.
2. Select test to be calculated by clicking either fx or formula on title bar
3. Give inputs and click OK.

**For example, SD from MS Excel**

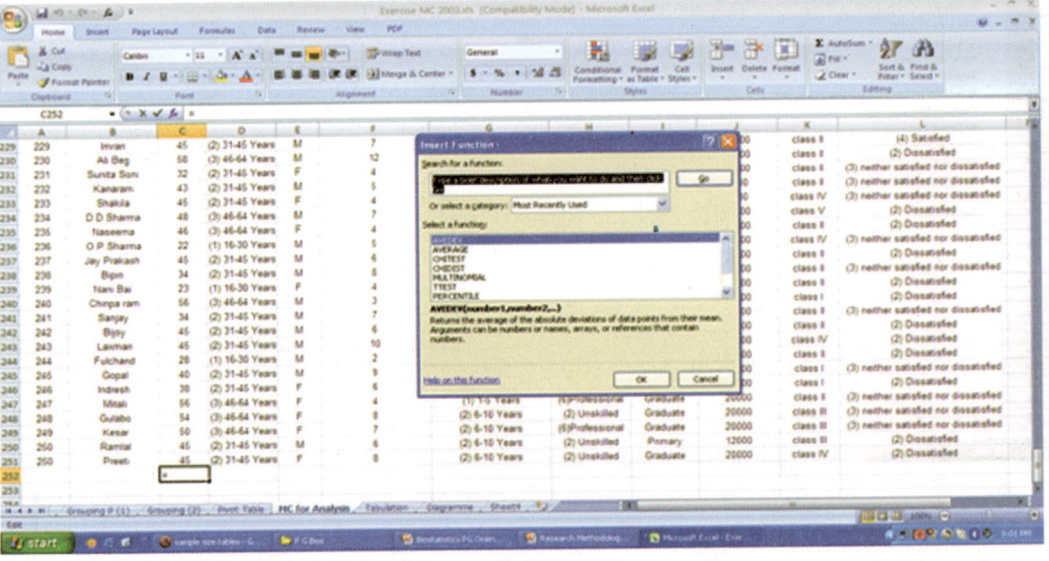

Following another window will appear asking cell range of data for calculation. Given input SD will be seen on window. If Ok is clicked, it will be on desired place on main window

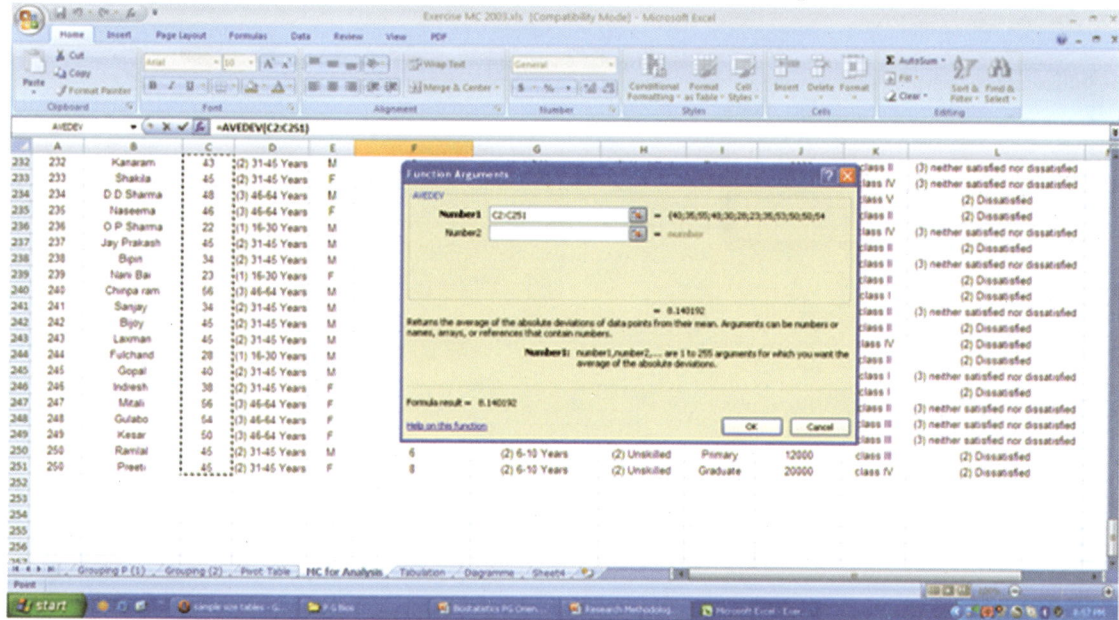

For further analysis, 'Primer' software can be downloaded free from net. (SPSS is more advanced software for this purpose but it is a licensed.) Primer is having advisor also to suggest type of test required as per type of data, e.g. **t-test from Primer.**

**Click Statistics and then click 't' test among all type of statistics**

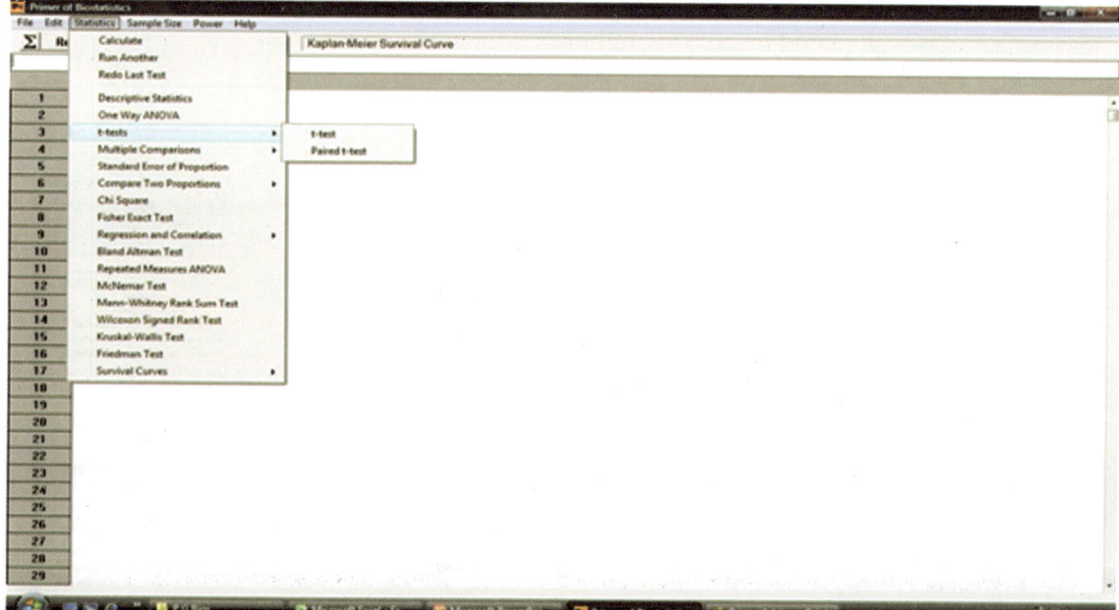

**Select type, e.g. t-test, following window will appear**

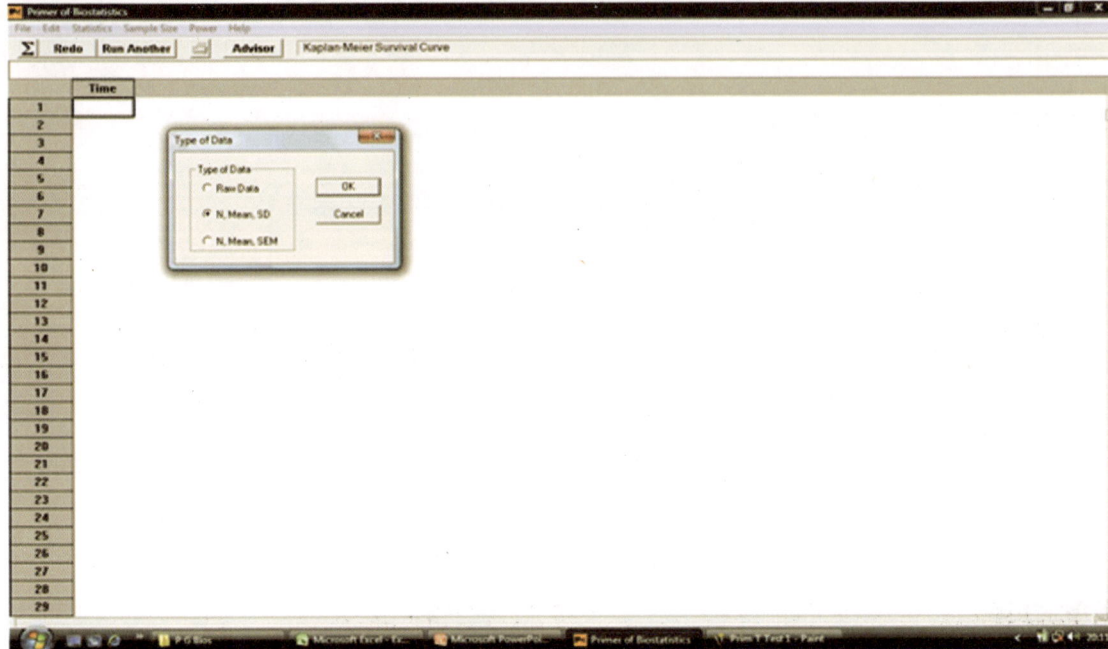

Select type of inputs for desired calculation then give inputs and click OK.

**'t' test window will appear. Give inputs and Click 'Σ'**

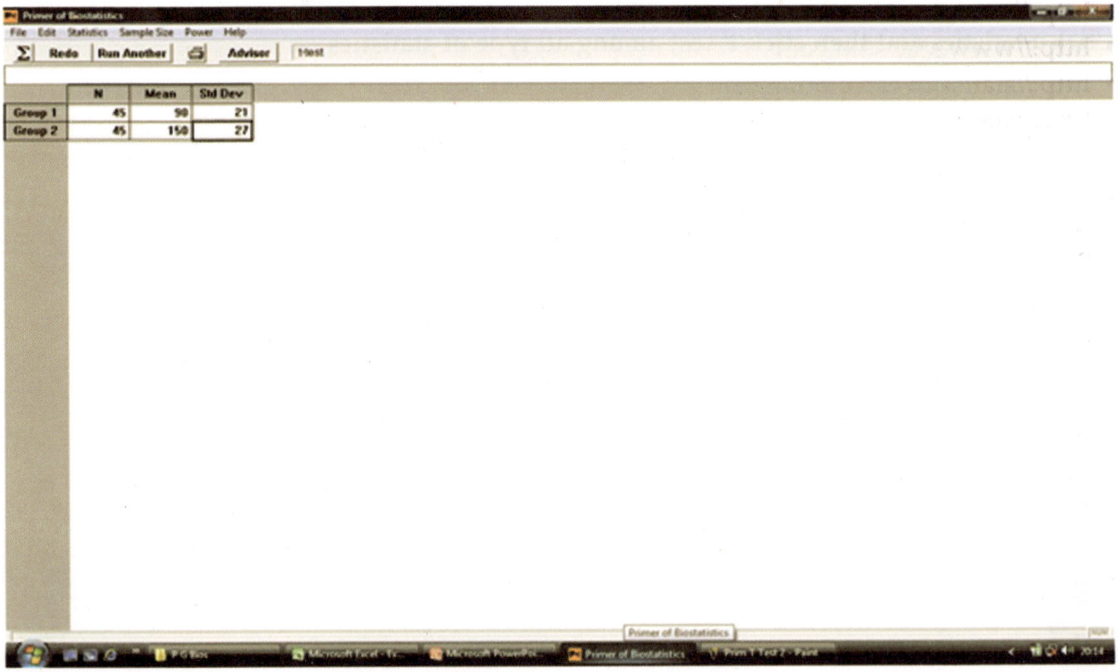

| | N | Mean | Std Dev |
|---|---|---|---|
| Group 1 | 45 | 90 | 21 |
| Group 2 | 45 | 150 | 27 |

**Result will be displayed with 'P' value.**

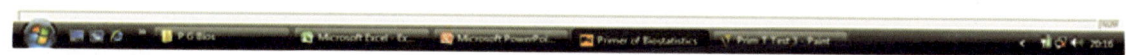

## Websites Related to Statistics

- **http://stattrek.com**
- **http://vassarstat.net**
- **http://www.scribd.com**
- **http://www.statistixl.com**
- **http://statistics calculators.com**
- **http://stat.ubc.ca/~rollin/stats/ssize/**

## Computer Softwares Related to Statistics

- Microsoft Excel
- SPSS
- Epi info
- Epi tab
- Mini tab
- Graph Pad
- Primer
- Medical

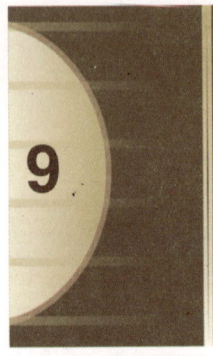

# Thesis Protocol

## Thesis Protocol (Plan for Thesis)

Thesis protocol is considered an official document submitted to the university before doing thesis work and it needs to resonance with the same. It is also said that better is the planning, the work will be better. So, to make their thesis work more towards perfection, majority of medical colleges have their research review boards to approve these protocols prior to submission to the university.

## Following are the Steps to Prapare a Thesis Protocol

1. Identify research problem: Problem is gap between ideal and present situation. Research problem refers to some difficulty a researcher experiences and wants to obtain a solution for the same, i.e. a question or issue to be examined.

2. Prioritize the problems in the view of internal and external criteria of selection

| Internal criteria | External criteria |
|---|---|
| • Researcher's interest | • Research ability of the problem |
| • Researcher's competence | • Importance and urgency |
| • Researcher's own resources: | • Novelty of the problem |
|   – Human resource | • Feasibility |
|   – Money | • Facilities |
|   – Material | • Social relevance |
|   – Time | • Public health importance |

3. Define the problem in the form of 'Title of the Research': Problem statement should be clear, precise, self-explanatory and include:
    i. What
    ii. How
    iii. When
    iv. Where

4. Make hypothesis: $H_0$ null hypothesis and $H_a$ alternative hypothesis (descriptive studies are to generate hypothesis, so there is no need to assume a hypothesis).

5. Define the research objectives: Research objectives are the statements of the questions that are to be investigated with the goal of answering the overall research problem.

    i. Research objectives should be clear and achievable.

    ii. Generally, they are written as statements, using the word "to"

        1. (For example, 'to discover ____', 'to determine ____', 'to establish ____', 'to find out ____', 'to assess ____', etc.)

    iii. Objectives should be achieved at the end of the study.

6. **Collect review of literature:** Literature review is the documentation of a published and unpublished work in the areas of specific interest to the researcher. It will help in:

    i. Knowing the work done before in the same field

    ii. Making researchable hypothesis

    iii. Getting the population parameters regarding the problem identified

    iv. Understanding the methodology of the research for problem identified

    v. Getting data for comparison with observations of the proposed research

7. Define study area
8. *Selection of study design
9. Define study universe with inclusion and exclusion criteria
10. *Calculate adequate sample size
11. *Select appropriate sampling technique
12. Prerequisites of study: Study tools, orientation trainings, consent of other department involved, etc.
13. *Planning for data collection, compilation, data entry and analysis
14. Ethical clearance: Consent from:

    i. Institutional Research Review Board

    ii. Ethical committee of the institute

    iii. Observational units

*With the help of chapter 'Research Methodology and Biostatistics' or discuss your study with statistician or epidemiologist.

**Recommended format of thesis-protocol** is as follows:

| Name of page/s | Content | Proposed pages |
| --- | --- | --- |
| **Title page** | Title, submitted to, submitted by, under guidance of | 1 |
| **Certificate from institution** | As per institutional format | 1 |
| **Introduction** | Importance and justification of research problem | 1–2 |
| **Review of literature** | Brief review of literature | 2–4 |
| **Purpose of study** | Public health importance | 1 |
| **Hypothesis** | Assumptions about study | 1 |
| **Aims and objectives** | Researchable statements | 1 |
| **Methodology** | Study area, study design, study period, study universe, study population including | 3–10 |

*Contd.*

*Contd.*

| Name of page/s | Content | Proposed pages |
|---|---|---|
| | inclusion and exclusion criteria, sample size, sampling technique, define variables, procedure outcome variables and outcome analysis | |
| Flow chart | Showing study design | 1 |
| Seed article | Almost similar study reference, of which data is used for calculation of sample size | |
| References | Almost similar study references (10–15) | 1–2 |
| Consent form | | 1 |
| Study tool | Proforma/schedule | 1–5 |

Total pages:15–30 + seed article

## Other Desirable Technicalities

1. *Four copies to be submitted to research review board
2. A4 size paper
3. Line spacing: Double space
4. Margins: At least 2.5 cm on both sides
5. Font: Times New Roman or Arial
6. Font size: 127
7. Pattern: Justified
8. As far as possible in active voice and in future tens

* After approval, 11 copies will be submitted to university.

Note: It is advisable that thesis topics of last five years should not be repeated.

## Structure of the Thesis Protocol

### Page No. 1

1. **Title page:** This page includes:
    i. Title of thesis (write in title case or capital letters)
    ii. Submitted to 'Name of the University'
    iii. Submitted for what? i.e. Degree (with discipline) for which the thesis is being submitted
    iv. Years of scheduled examination of candidate
    v. Submitted by 'Name of Candidate'
    vi. Under guidance of 'Name and Designation of Guide'

It is very important that it should perfectly match with final thesis report (Annexure 1).

### Page No. 2

2. **Letter to the university forwarded from guide and principal:** Letter to university should be attached taking permission from the university quoting about proposed study with personal details. This letter should be written through proper channel and duly forwarded and recommended by guide and principal of the institute (Annexure 2).

**Page No. 3 and 4**

3. **Introduction:** It is to establish the purpose of proposed research. This is accomplished by discussing the relevant available *literature (with references). It should answer following step-by-step:

   1. What is the research problem?
   2. Why is it an important problem?
   3. What had been done so far in this connection?
   4. Where is the lacuna which requires further explanation/research?
   5. How will this proposed study help in solving lacuna/problem?

   *Latest review articles or systematic reviews on the related topic are particularly useful because they summarize all the researches done on a subject over a brief period of time.

**Page No. 5**

4. **Purpose of study:** Here public health importance of the proposed study will be quoted, i.e. how this study will be beneficial to the population.

**Page No. 6**

5. **Hypothesis:** Research hypothesis is a predictive statement that relates an independent variable to a dependent variable.

   Hypothesis should be state in the form of:

   i. **Null hypothesis ($H_0$):** It is the default hypothesis that 'there is no significant difference in outcomes of both (or if > 2 groups then various) groups'.

   ii. **Alternate hypothesis ($H_a$):** It is hypothesis other than the default hypothesis that 'there is significant difference in outcomes of both (or if > 2 groups then various) groups'.

**Page No. 7**

6. **Aims and objectives:** What is to be found out from doing this proposed research should be narrated prior to precede for research.

   **Aim:** Overall goal of the proposed study.

   **Objectives:** Research objectives are the statement of the questions that are to be investigated with the goal of answering the overall research problem.

   If, e.g. a study is 'A Study on Utilization of Intranatal Services in field practice area of RHTC, Naila (Jaipur).

   **Aim:** To study the utilization of intranatal services in field practice area of RHTC, Naila.

   **Objectives:**

   1. To find out proportion of institutional deliveries among total deliveries in field practice area of RHTC, Naila.
   2. To determine the factors associated with institutional deliveries in field practice area of RHTC, Naila.
   3. To determine the factors associated with home deliveries in field practice area of RHTC, Naila.

## Page No. 8

### 7. Methodology:

i. **Study area:** Where the proposed study will be carried out. Whether in community, laboratory or in hospital; if it is in the community then geographically define the area and if it is in the hospital then which hospital, whether in wards or operation theater or OPD specify the exact location.

ii. **Study period:** When the proposed study will be carried out. Write down the proposed starting date to estimated date of completion.

iii. **Study design:** Write down the study design of proposed study. To find out the study design, following questions should be answered:

    a. Whether the study is community based or hospital based?

    b. What is the direction of study?

    c. What is the method of selection of subject? (Random or non-random: Preference is to given to random technique.)

    d. Whether control group is to be taken or not?

    e. Whether the effect of some intervention is to be studied or not?

    f. Whether there is comparison between groups or not?

(According to answers of these questions, study design is to be selected. With the help of chapter 'Research Methodology and Biostatistics' or with statistician.)

iv. **Study universe:** Population frame from where the study population will be selected. This target population of your study should be defined.

v. **Study population:** Study population is to be selected from study universe as per the inclusion and exclusion criteria.

    a. **Inclusion criteria:** Inclusion criteria will define the population/subjects to be included in the proposed study, e.g. to study the utilization of intranatal services females who have delivered child within a month period will be included in study on recall basis.

    b. **Exclusion criteria:** Exclusion criteria should also be well defined to exclude the subjects from above screened population, e.g. in above example; among females screened as per inclusion criteria, females seriously ill, not able to recall and do not want to participate in the proposed study will be excluded.

    **Selection of control:** It is recommended in analytical and experimental studies. Control population should also be defined taking into consideration of confounding factors.

vi. **Sample size:** Adequate sample size should be calculated to get the result applicable to universe with minimum resources. Calculation of sample size will be done as per followings:

    a. Allowable beta error (conventionally 0.2) or Power = 1-beta error = 0.8

    b. Allowable alpha error (conventionally 0.05)

    c. Type of study design selected

    d. Population parameters available

    e. Type of outcomes

    f. Type of analysis will be done

*Finally to estimate the total number of subjects to be included in the study, non-response rate, dropout rate should also be taken into consideration.

vii. **\*Sampling technique:** Appropriate sampling technique should be chosen to avoid selection bias. Appropriate sampling technique should be random via giving every subject equal chance to appear in the study population and none of them should have zero probability. There are the different types of random sampling techniques which may be selected as per the type of study. It should be cleared how the randomization will be done in study.

**Blinding:** Blinding is being unknown about the group to which individual belongs to while assessing the outcome. It can further reduce personal biases and is strongly recommended in interventional studies.

viii. **Working definition:** Variables to be assessed should be well defined to make understand the meaning of variable and its grouping. It becomes more necessary to make study variables uniform, if more than one investigator is there; in such a case orientation training may be organized prior to data collection to keep uniformity of observations.

ix. **Procedures involved:** Various procedures involved in the study should also be detailed prior to study, e.g. procedure for intervention, procedure for withdrawal, procedure for randomization, procedure for blinding, procedure for data collection (study tool), procedure for outcome measurement (measurement tools), outcome analysis procedure, etc.

x. **Outcome variables:** Outcome variables are the variables (value of which vary with individual) that are selected to know the outcome of the study. These variables should be valid, i.e. should measure the outcome it is supposed to measure. For exemple:

- To measure the utilization of intranatal services 'proportion of institution delivery' is a valid indicator.
- To find out the effect of Yoga on hypertension 'mean blood pressure' before and after the yoga is a valid indicator.
- To compare the effect of two medicines on diabetes 'serum blood sugar level' in both the group is a valid outcome variable, etc.

**Outcome** may be primary and secondary.

**Primary outcomes** are in main thirst areas on which the hypothesis and objectives are decided. Sample size is calculated on the basis of these primary.

**Secondary outcomes** are other possible outcome of interest.

xi. **\*Outcome analysis:** Outcome analysis is done to get the inferences. It should be done in such a way that answer to the objectives should be obtained out of this analysis. It is done with the help of appropriate test of significance.

For inferences, level of significance should also be pre-defined (conventionally 0.05). This analysis depends on type of data, type of outcome variables and type of inference (as per aims and objectives) needed. So help of statistician or statistical software may be required.

* With the help of chapter 'Research Methodology and Biostatistics' or with statistician.

8. **Flow chart:** Whole procedure of study (study design) is shown in schematic flow chart for better understanding at a glance.

9. **Seed article:** Reference almost similar to proposed study. Outcome data of seed article is used for calculation of sample size.

10. **References:** References, referred in the proposed study should be written in order of preference as it appears in the text. Standard method should be choosen to write down references like:

    Simkhada B, Teijlingen E, Porter M, Simkhada P. Factors affecting the utilization of antenatal care in developing countries: systematic review of the literature. J Adv Nurs. 2007;61:244 – 260.

    USAID 2007. Focused antenatal care: providing integrated, individualized care during pregnancy. http://www.accesstohealth.org/toolres/pdfs/ACCESStechbrief_FANC.pdf

11. **Consent form:** Consent should be 'Informed Consent Form' and it should be in local language or in language study subjects can understand. It should be signed by every subject (observation unit) taking part in the study after giving consent to be included in study. Before presenting it to the subject for sign, it should be conformed that consent form has information about:

    - Study design
    - Population parameter available
    - Types of outcomes
    - Title of the research
    - Investigator's name and designation
    - Procedure of the research
    - Expected duration of the subject's participation
    - Benefits that might be expected to the subject or to others
    - Any foreseeable risk or discomfort to the subject resulting from participation in the study
    - Any compensation/reimbursement/insurance cover for participation or risk involved.
    - Contact number of person responsible in case of emergency
    - Extent to which confidentiality of records could be maintained
    - Freedom of the individual to participate or to withdraw from research any time without penalty or loss of benefits.

12. **Schedule/proforma:** It is data collection tool. It should have following parts:

    **Introductory schedule:** In this schedule, general information about the subject should be written including address and mobile number.

    **Specific schedule:** In this schedule, specific information as per pre-decided aims and objectives about the subject should be written. It should have reasonable and analyzable data information. If study is intervention study, then more than one specific schedule is required, i.e. pre-intervention specific schedule and post-intervention schedule.

13. **Annexure:** Some additional information may be given in the form of annexure.

## Thesis Report

Thesis is also an official document submitted to the university before appearing in university examination of MD/MS. It should be in resonance with the thesis protocol previously submitted to the university.

**Following are steps before writing a thesis:**

- After Institutional Research Review Board and ethical clearance, study should be conducted with proper consent of subjects.
- Data should be collected as per previously planned in protocol.
- Data should be entered in Microsoft Excel worksheet/SPSS worksheet in the form of master chart.
- *Data thus collected in the form of master chart should be grouped or classified as per aims and objectives.
- *These collected data then should be analyzed to get inferences with the help of computer and statistical software as and when required.

**Structure of the thesis and other technicalities**: Structure is same as in thesis protocol except:

- Thesis should be written in past tense.
- Explanatory approach should be used.
- Observations, discussions, conclusions and recommendations are also added to it.

***Observations:** Observations will take following steps:

- After collection of data in the form of master chart, grouping and classification of data will be done as per aims and objectives.
- Observation will be drawn from master chart ready for analysis.
- Observation will be drawn in the form of tables, graphs and charts as describe elsewhere.
- Inferences drawn from tables and charts are also included in observations.

* "with the help of computer application in thesis".

**Discussion:** It is discussing of the observations of the present study with national/state norms and with findings of other authors in detail.

**Conclusions:** Final conclusion drawn from the observations and discussion is summarized here.

**Recommendations**: Recommend desirable actions as per observations and conclusions.

**Recommended format of thesis** is as follows:

| Name of page/s | Contents | Proposed pages |
|---|---|---|
| **Title page** | Title, submitted to, submitted by, under guidance of | 1 |
| **Certificate from institution** | As per institutional format | 1 |
| **Introduction** | Importance and justification of research problem | 5–10 |
| **Review of literature** | Brief review of literature | 15–35 |
| **Purpose of study** | Public health importance | 1 |
| **Hypothesis** | Assumptions about study | 1 |
| **Aims and objectives** | Researchable statements | 1 |
| **Methodology** | Study area, study design, study period, study universe, study population including inclusion and exclusion criteria, sample size, sampling technique, define variables, procedure outcome variables and outcome analysis | 10–25 |
| **Flow chart** | Showing study design | 1 |
| **Observations** | Tables, charts and graphs with their inferences | 15–35 |
| **Discussion** | Comparison of observations of present study with observations of other studies | 15–35 |
| **Conclusions** | Finally concluded from observations and discussion | 3–7 |
| **Recommendations** | Recommendations as per observations and conclusions | 5–10 |
| **References** | Almost similar study reference (50–100) | 6–12 |
| **Annexure** | Certificates from RRB of institute | 1 |
| | Certificates from ethical committee | 1 |
| | Consent form | 1 |
| | Study tool-proforma/schedule | 1–5 |
| | Master chart | |

Total Pages: 80–180

## Annexure of Thesis Protocol/Report

1. Title page
2. Letter to university
3. Flow chart
4. Inform consent

## PLAN OF DISSERTATION

### COMPARATIVE STUDY OF DYNAMIC HIP SCREW AND DYNAMIC HELICAL HIP SYSTEM IN STABLE INTERTROCHANTERIC FRACTURES OF FEMUR IN ELDERLY PATIENTS

Submitted to the

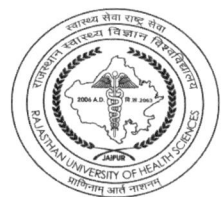

## RAJASTHAN UNIVERSITY OF HEALTH SCIENCES

### Jaipur (Rajasthan)

For the degree of

### M.S. (Orthopaedic), 2014

Submitted by

### Dr. Prerna Gupt

Under the supervision and guidance of:
### Dr. Mahesh Sharma

Associate Professor, Department of Orthopaedic

S.M.S. Medical College and Attached Hospitals

Jaipur (Rajasthan)

To

The Registrar

Rajasthan University of Health Sciences

Jaipur.

**THROUGH PROPER CHANNEL**

Subject : Submission of plan of dissertation entitled **"Comparative Study of Dynamic Hip Screw and Dynamic Helical Hip System in Stable Intertrochanteric Fractures of Femur in Elderly Patients"**

Respected sir,

I am enclosing herewith eleven copies of my plan of dissertation on the subject cited above for M.S. (**Orthopaedic**) Examination, 2014. My particulars are as follows:

Name: **Dr. Prerna Gupt**

Post-Graduate Student in Orthopaedic

S.M.S Medical college and Attached Hospitals, Jaipur

University Registration: 214/11

Enrolment Number: 57/11

Date of Admission: 25.7.2011

Name of guide: **Dr. MAHESH SHARMA**

Associate Professor, Department of **Orthopaedic**

I shall be highly obliged if you kindly convey the approval of the plan of dissertation at the earliest.

Thanking you

Yours faithfully

**Dr. Prerna Gupt**

Recommended and forwarded

**Dr. Mahesh Sharma**

Associate Professor, Department of **Orthopaedic**

S.M.S. Medical College and Attached Hospitals

Jaipur  (Rajasthan)

## Flow Chart

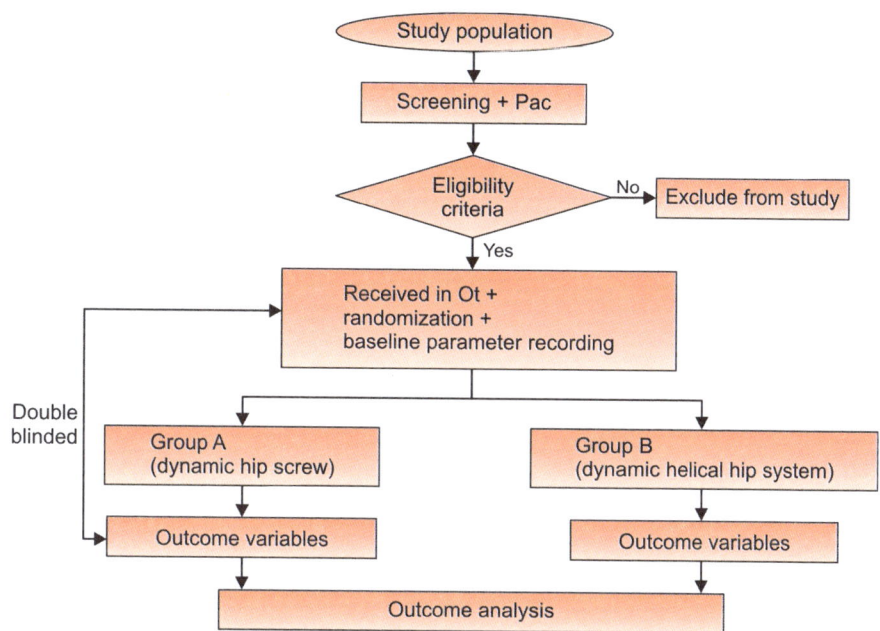

## सूचित सहमति पत्र

अध्ययन का नाम ...................................................................................................

अध्ययन दिनांक ...................................................................अध्ययन नम्बर .......................

सहभागी का पूरा नाम ...............................................................................................

जन्मतिथि / उम्र .....................................................................................................

पता .................................................................................................................

1. मुझे अध्ययन अन्वेषक ने विस्तार से सब तथ्यों को समझा दिया है तथा मुझे प्रश्न पूछने का अवसर प्रदान किया। मुझे पूर्णतः से शोध में होने वाली प्रक्रिया की जानकारी प्रदान कर दी गई है।

2. मैनें समझ लिया है कि इस अध्ययन में मेरी सहभागिता स्वैच्छिक है, तथा यह कि मैं बिना कोई कारण बताए किसी भी समय अपनी चिकित्सीय देखभाल या कानूनी अधिकारों पर प्रभाव पड़े बिना हट जाने के लिये स्वतंत्र हूं।

3. मैनें समझ लिया है वि, चिकित्सीय प्रयोजक की ओर से काम करने वाले अन्य नैतिकता समिति तथा विनियामक अधिकारियों का चालू अध्ययन तथा इससे सम्बंधित हो सकने वाले किसी अनुसंधान से सम्बंधित मेरे स्वास्थ्य व अभिलेखों को देखने के लिए मेरी अनुमति की आवश्यकता नही होगी भले ही मैं इस परीक्षण से हट ही क्यों न जांऊ। तथापि मैनें समझ लिया है कि तृतीय पक्ष को दी गई या कारित की गई किसी जानकारी में मेरी पहचान को उजागर नही किया जाएगा।

4. उपर्युक्त अध्ययन में भाग लेने के लिये मैं सहमत हूं।

हस्ताक्षर साक्षी                                          हस्ताक्षर मरीज

पता :                                                       पता :

                                                              रजिस्ट्रेशन नं:

# Investigation and Management of an Epidemic

## Investigation and Management of an Epidemic

**Cluster of cases:** Aggregation of cases locally is known as clustering of cases.

**Outbreak:**  Unusual occurrence of the disease/cases in excess of its normal expectation, i.e. two standard deviation from the endemic frequency but limited to localised increase.

**Epidemic:** Unusual occurrence of the disease/cases in excess of its normal expectation, i.e. two standard errors from the endemic frequency over a larger geographic area.

## Benefits of Epidemic Investigation
- To determine the magnitude and distribution of disease (time, place, person )
- To control ongoing/current outbreak
- To determine factors responsible (source and mode of transmission)
- To evaluate the effectiveness of existing  surveillance activities at local level
- To evaluate the effectiveness of preventive measures
- To respond to public, political and legal concerns
- To prevent occurrence of future outbreaks
- To provide research opportunity

## Early Warning Symptoms of Outbreak
- Clustering of cases
- Increase in cases or deaths
- Acute illness of an unknown aetiology
- Shifting in age distribution of cases
- High vector density
- Natural disasters

## Source of Information about Outbreak/Epidemic
- Rumour register: To be kept in standardized format at each institution
- Community informants: Private and public sector
- Media: Important source of information
- Review of routine data: Through 'Triggers'

## Levels of Response to different Triggers

| Trigger | Significance | Level of response |
|---------|--------------|-------------------|
| 1. | Suspected outbreak | Local response to health workers and medical officers |
| 2. | Outbreak | Local and district response by district surveillance officer and rapid response team |
| 3. | Confirmed outbreak | Local, district and state level |
| 4. | Epidemic | Local, district and state level |
| 5. | Natural disaster | Local, district, state and central level |

## Deciding Factors for Investigation

- Severity of illness
- Number of cases
- Availability of preventive and control measures
- Availability of resources
- Public, political and legal concerns
- Research opportunity

## Balance of investigation and control while responding to an outbreak

| | | Source of disease | |
|---|---|---|---|
| | | Known | Unknown |
| **Aetiology** | Known | Control +++ <br> Investigate + | Control + <br> Investigate +++ |
| | Unknown | Control +++ <br> Investigate +++ | Control + <br> Investigate +++ |

## Steps in investigation and management of outbreak/epidemic:

1. Preparation for field
2. Verify disease and establish existence of epidemic
3. Make provisional diagnosis and develop working case definition
4. Case finding and case management (rapid house-to-house survey and line listing of cases)
5. Laboratory investigation
6. Entomological and environmental investigations
7. Data analysis and descriptive epidemiology
8. Generate hypothesis
9. Test hypothesis
10. Implement preventive/control measures
11. Initiate and maintain surveillance
12. Communicate findings (interim report and final report)
13. Follow up of outbreak
14. Evaluation of outbreak management
15. Documentation and sharing of lessons learnt

## Step1. Preparation for Field

1. **Rapid respond team (RRT)** is formed on urgent basis whenever there is doubt of epidemic.
    a. Composition:
        i. Epidemiologist, clinician and microbiologist.
        ii. Entomologist when vector-borne disease is suspected.
        iii. Animal health specialist/veterinary surgeon when zoonotic disease is suspected.
    b. Gathered on ad hoc basis when needed
    c. Role: Confirm and investigate outbreaks
    d. Responsibility:
        i. Assist in the investigation and response
        ii. Primary responsibility rests with local health staff
2. Scientific and investigative issues for addressing the team has to have:
    a. Appropriate scientific knowledge
    b. Supplies and equipments
    c. A plan of action
3. Management and operational issues:
    a. A good epidemiologist must be a good manager, collaborator and a good co-ordinator
    b. Selection of team members
    c. Contact with local staff
    d. Involved local agencies
    e. Communication with clinical community
    f. Operational and logistic details

## Step: 2. Verify Disease and Established Existence of Epidemic

1. Properly identify the disease:
    a. Clinical findings
    b. Laboratory findings
    c. Review the clinical findings with lab results
    d. Summarize clinical features using frequency distributions.
2. Observe the number of cases with more or less same symptoms and findings with short time period.
3. Establish existence of epidemic:
    a. **Observed cases are compared with expected number of cases:** Observed cases should be two standard deviation excess of expected number of cases.
    b. **Expected number of cases:** Expected number of cases may be received from record of previous few years.

## Step: 3. Make Provisional Diagnosis and Develop Working Definition of Disease

- Make provisional diagnosis of disease.
- Develop working definition of disease for survey.
    - Standard set of criteria for deciding, if an individual should be classified as having the

health condition/disease under investigation.
- Clinical criteria, restrictions of place, person and time.
- Clinical criteria should be based on simple and objective measures.

## Step 4. Case Finding and Case Management

Define population at risk through:

1. **Passive surveillance:** Find out cases among similar cases reporting to the health centre.
2. **Active surveillance:** Find out cases through **rapid household/community survey.**
3. **By studying line:** Line listing cases, i.e. finding out the serial of cases occurring in that area. It may be found out through proper recording details of each case.

   **By studying line listing of cases:**
   - Name, age, sex, address
   - Date of onset of illness
   - Signs/symptoms
   - Investigation reports
   - Treatment taken
   - Outcome
4. Management of cases

## Step 5. Laboratory Investigation

After finding out cases, they should be confirmed though laboratory investigation. So followings should be pre-decided:
- Appropriate clinical specimens
- Time of sample collection
- Method of collection
- Selection of transport media
- Labelling
- Storage and transportation of samples
- Selection of lab

## Step 6. Environmental, Entomological and Zoonotic Surveys

Environmental, entomological and zoonotic surveys are also done with the help of concerned persons to find out the possible aetiology of the disease.
- Entomological survey (density of vectors, indices)
- Study of zoonotic reservoir (if required)
- Study of environmental conditions: Collect data on:
  - Rainfall
  - Humidity
  - Temperature
  - Drinking water supply
  - Environmental sanitation

– Man made situations—developmental, irrigation projects
– Any health activity taken up in recent past.

## Step 7. Data Analysis and Descriptive Epidemiology

- **Time distribution:** When is the disease occurring?
- **Place distribution:** Where is it occurring?
- **Person distribution:** Who is getting the disease?

**Time distribution:** Number of cases occurring with time should be found out, it will say about:

1. Magnitude
2. Distinguish epidemic from endemic
3. Pattern of spread
4. Where we are in course of epidemic
5. Deduce probable time of exposure

## Time Distribution

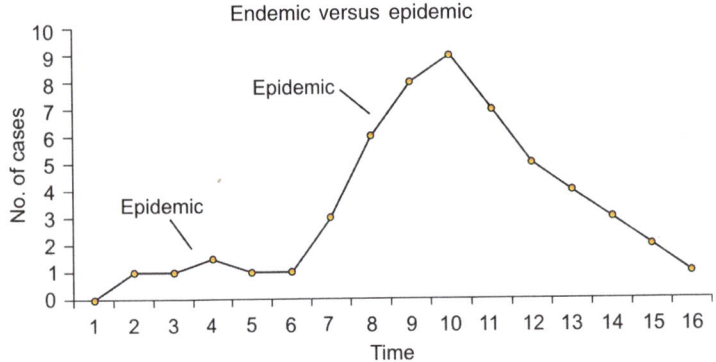

Endemic versus epidemic

**Endemic:** Constant presence of a disease or infectious agent at a usual level, *without importation* from outside, within a geographically defined area.

**Epidemic:** Unusual occurrence of the disease/event/specific health-related behaviour clearly in excess of its normal expectation.

## The Types of Epidemic Curves

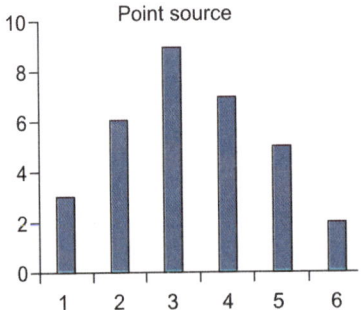

Point source

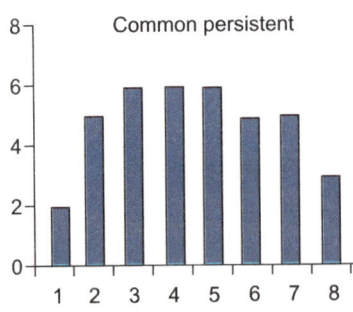

Common persistent

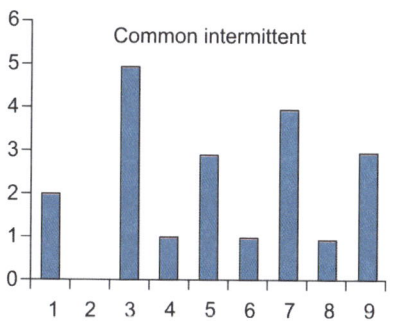

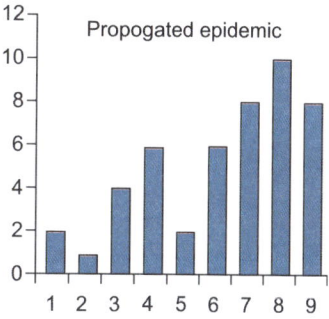

**Person distribution:** Specialties of affected persons like age, sex, occupation, marital status, behaviour, history of migration, etc.

**Place distribution**

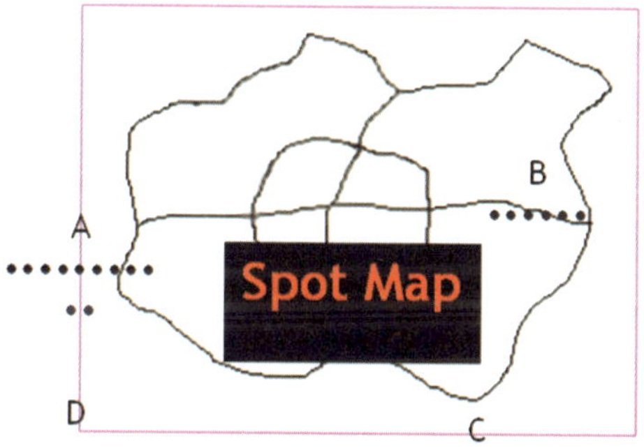

**Clustering of cases through spot map**

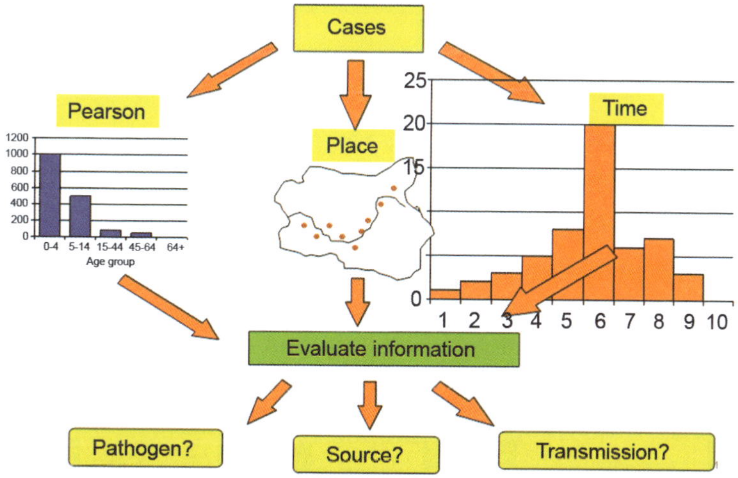

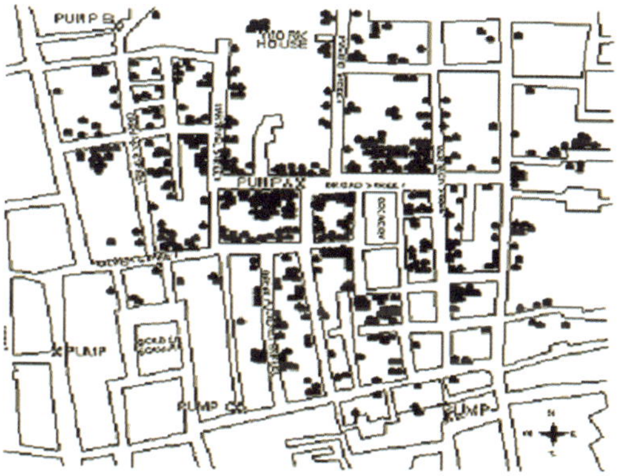

### Step 8. Generate Hypothesis

Hypothesis is generated from data analysis and interpretation about:

1. Characteristics of the population
2. Specific cause (source, agent)
3. Environmental factors

4. Expected outcome
5. Dose response relationship of medicine
6. Time response relationship of medicine

## Step 9. Test Hypothesis

Use of analytical epidemiology to test the hypothesis: It is done by:

**Odds ratio (cross product ratio):** Odds ratio is used in case control study, case control study is suitable for outbreaks without a well-defined population. It measures the strength of association between exposure and outcome.

|  | Cases | Control |
|---|---|---|
| Exposed | a | b |
| Not exposed | c | d |

$$\text{Odds ratio} = \frac{ad}{bc}$$

**Risk ratio/relative risk:** It is calculated in cohort studies, a cohort study is suitable for an outbreak in a well-defined population.

|  | Diseased | Non-diseased | Total |
|---|---|---|---|
| Exposed | a | b | $a + b = H_1$ |
| Not exposed | c | d | $c + d = H_0$ |
| Total | $a + c = V_1$ | $b + d = V_2$ | $a + b + c + d = T$ |

$$\text{Risk ratio} = \frac{\text{Attack rate in exposed group}}{\text{Attack rate in unexposed group}} = \frac{\left(\dfrac{a}{a+b}\right) \times 100}{\left(\dfrac{c}{c+d}\right) \times 100}$$

Larger the relative risk, the stronger the association between exposure and disease.

**Attributable risk:** It indicates to what extent the disease under study can be attributed to the exposure.

$$\text{Attibuted risk} = \frac{(\text{Incidence among exposed} - \text{Incidence among unexposed}) \times 100}{\text{Incidence among exposed}}$$

**Statistical significance :** It measures probability of study results occurring by chance.

$$\text{Chi-square test value} = \frac{T\,(ad - bc)^2}{H_1\, H_0\, V_1\, V_2}$$

Find out P value from Chi-square table, if it is >0.05 accept null hypothesis otherwise accept alternate hypothesis.

**Compare and reconcile with laboratory and environmental studies.**

## Step 10. Implement Control Measures

**General measures:** Till source and route of transmission identified general measures should be taken like isolation, counsel to change behaviours, decontamination, control vector population, etc.

**Specific measures:** Based upon the results of the investigation:

1. **Agent:** Removing the source
2. **Environment:** Interrupting transmission
3. **Host:**
    a. Personnel protection:
        i. Personnel protective measures
        ii. Immunization
        iii. Chemoprophylaxis
    b. Case management

### Step 11. Initiate and Maintain Surveillance

1. To monitor control and preventive measures.
2. For active surveillance to find out new cases. It can provide information about
    - New cases
    - Changing trends of the disease
    - Feedback to modify the policies and the system to redefine the objectives.

### Step 12. Communicate Findings

**Interim report:** Written report to higher authourities and oral briefing to local authorities to describe

What we did? …. Procedure of investigation and management of an outbreak/epidemic

What we found?.... Observations/results of investigation of an outbreak/epidemic

What we think should be done about it?... Recommendations based on observations

Written report in scientific format.

### Final Report of Investigation of an Outbreak/Epidemic

### Executive Summary

- Structure with subheadings
- < one page or < 300 words

### Background

- Geographic location
- Climatic conditions
- Demographic status
- Socioeconomic situation
- Organization of health services
- Normal disease prevalence

### Methods Used for the Investigation

- **Epidemiological methods:**
    - Case definition
    - Case search methods

   – Data collection method

   – Analytical studies, if any

   – Data analysis

- **Laboratory methods:**
  - Appropriate clinical specimens
  - Method of collection
  - Selection of transport media
  - Storage and transportation of samples
  - Selection of lab
- **Environmental investigations:**
  - Rainfall
  - Humidity
  - Temperature
  - Drinking water supply
  - Environmental sanitation
  - Man made situations—developmental, irrigation projects
  - Any health activity taken up in recent past

## Major Observations/Results

- Epidemiological results (descriptive and analytic epidemiology of disease identified)
- Current status of transmission, control measures adopted/initiated

**Conclusion: Genesis of outbreak** (diagnosis, source, vehicles)

**Recommendations:** Suggestion for prevention of such outbreak

### Step 13. Follow-up of Outbreak/Epidemic

Follow-up should be done to:

- Detect last case
- Detect and treat late complications
- Complete the documentation of the outbreak

### Step14. Evaluate Outbreak/Epidemic Management

Evaluate the overall management of outbreak/epidemic for:

- Genesis of the outbreak
- Early or late detection of outbreak
- Preparedness for the outbreak
- Management of the outbreak
- Control measures undertaken and their impact

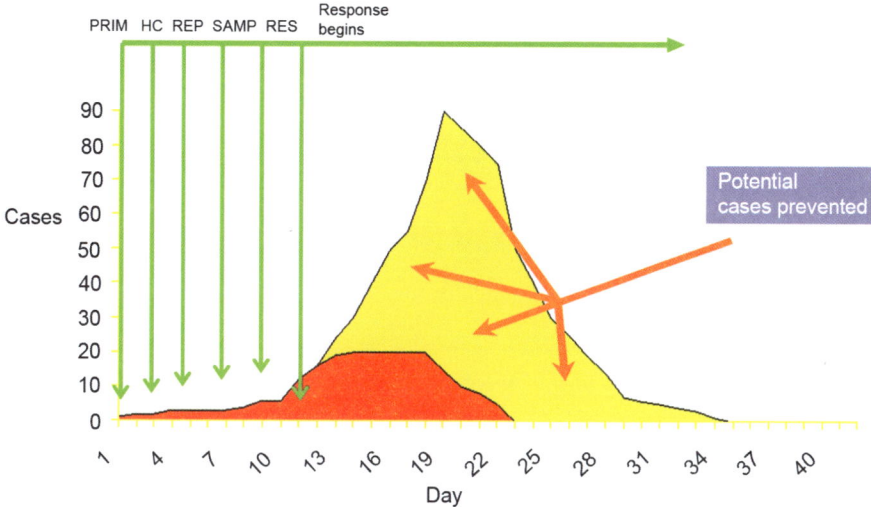

## Step 15. Documentation and Sharing of Lessons Learnt

Documentation and sharing of lessons learnt through:
- Organize post-outbreak seminar
- Provide feedback to state and district RRTs
- Develop case studies on selected outbreaks for training RRT members
- Publish the study for public circulation.

# 11

# Exercises

## Exercises

1. Match the following:

| Research question | Study design |
|---|---|
| 1. Prevalence | Cohort |
| 2. Incidence | RCT |
| 3. Risk ratio | Cross-sectional |
| 4. Relative risk | RCT (before and after) |
| 5. Effect of medicine | Cohort |
| 6. Comparison of effect of 2 medicines | Case-control |

2. Calculate sample size at 95% confidence limit for case series type of study, if prevalence of diseases to be studied is 15% in the defined population.

3. Calculate sample size at 95% confidence limit for case series type of study assuming standard deviation 20 with allowable error 5.

4. Find out sample size for comparing two proportions assuming α error 0.05 and power 80%, if a previous study shows 15% and 45% proportion in both groups of defined population.

5. Find out sample size for comparing two means assuming α error 0.05 and power 80%, if a previous study shows respective means 5 and 15 in both groups with SD within groups 10 in defined population.

6. Find out sample size for case-control study assuming α error 0.05 and power 80%, if a previous study shows OR 5.

7. Find out sample size for analytical study assuming α error 0.05 and power 80%, if a previous study shows correlation 0.6.

8. Find out sample size for comparing effect of two medicines assuming α error 0.05 and power 80%, if a previous study shows treated patient 15% with one and 45% with other medicine.

9. Find out sample size to identify the effect of a haematinic medicine assuming α error 0.05 and power 80%, if a previous study shows proportion of anaemic population 75% before the intervention and 15% after intervention.

10. Find out sample size to identify the effect of a haematinic medicine assuming α error 0.05 and power 80%, if a previous study shows mean haemoglobin of population 8 ± 3 before the intervention and 11 ± 4 after intervention.

11. Find out sample size for comparing effect of two tests assuming $\alpha$ error 0.05 and power 80%, if a previous study shows sensitivity 95% with one and 65% with other test.

12. Find out sample size to identify the agreement of association between two tests assuming $\alpha$ error 0.05 and power 80%, if a previous study shows agreement of association between two tests 0.6.

13. If sample size calculated was 450 under five children estimate working sample size for a 30 cluster sampling technique assuming non-response rate 10%.

14. Find the arithmetic mean and SD of the marks obtained by 10 students of a class in Mathematics in a certain examination. The marks obtained are:

$$55, 40, 61, 75, 47, 20, 65, 57, 67, 45$$

15. Find the arithmetic mean and SD from the following frequency table.

| Marks | 52 | 58 | 60 | 65 | 68 | 70 | 75 |
|---|---|---|---|---|---|---|---|
| No. of students | 7 | 5 | 4 | 6 | 3 | 3 | 2 |

16. Birth weights (in kg) of 60 children born in a village in year 2012 are as follows:

| | | | | | | | | | | | |
|---|---|---|---|---|---|---|---|---|---|---|---|
| 3.63 | 3.79 | 3.46 | 2.82 | 3.36 | 4.17 | 3.54 | 3.57 | 2.70 | 3.52 | 3.42 | 3.52 |
| 3.15 | 3.44 | 3.12 | 3.27 | 4.14 | 3.93 | 3.90 | 2.58 | 3.82 | 3.04 | 4.02 | 3.41 |
| 4.29 | 4.23 | 3.75 | 4.36 | 3.89 | 3.49 | 4.06 | 4.76 | 3.54 | 3.70 | 3.60 | 2.64 |
| 2.91 | 3.09 | 3.34 | 3.74 | 3.46 | 5.02 | 3.36 | 3.65 | 3.00 | 3.19 | 4.50 | 2.52 |
| 3.38 | 3.23 | 4.44 | 2.36 | 4.09 | 3.85 | 2.22 | 3.97 | 1.91 | 4.26 | 3.50 | 3.54 |

Calculate the mean, median, and standard deviation of these results and draw histogram. Describe and comment on this data set.

17. The following results are of plasma digoxin levels (in ng/ml) for 16 patients currently receiving a daily digoxin dose of 0.25 mg.

| | | | | | | | |
|---|---|---|---|---|---|---|---|
| 1.65 | 0.60 | 0.75 | 0.95 | 0.85 | 0.55 | 0.65 | 1.30 |
| 0.70 | 0.80 | 0.90 | .080 | .095 | 1.10 | 0.85 | 0.60 |

Describe and comment on this data set.

18. The following data are weight (in lbs) and cholesterol (in mg/dl) measurements collected from 14 adult males for a CAD study. Determine if there is any evidence of a relationship between the two variables.

| Weight | Cholesterol | Weight | Cholesterol |
|---|---|---|---|
| 168 | 135 | 262 | 269 |
| 175 | 403 | 181 | 311 |
| 173 | 294 | 143 | 286 |
| 158 | 312 | 140 | 403 |
| 154 | 311 | 187 | 244 |
| 214 | 222 | 163 | 353 |
| 176 | 302 | 164 | 252 |

19. In an initial trial of a newly developed anaesthetic, the time from administration of the anaesthetic until induction of anaesthesia was recorded for 10 patients, and the effective dosage rate used (in mg/kg) was calculated from the patients' weight. Describe and test the relationship between induction time and dosage rate.

| Dose (mg/kg) | Induction time (min) | Dose (mg/kg) | Induction time (min) |
|---|---|---|---|
| 1.3 | 25 | 1.3 | 21 |
| 1.9 | 13 | 2.1 | 11 |
| 1.5 | 19 | 0.7 | 31 |
| 1.1 | 23 | 1.6 | 14 |
| 1.0 | 26 | 0.9 | 24 |

20. In a study of the effect of age on the duration of anaesthesia, 10 patients ranging in age from 22 to 80 years were given an epidural anaesthetic agent. Blood samples were collected at intervals after administration, and the rate of total plasma clearance (expressed in ml/min) was calculated for each patients.

| Plasma clearance (ml/min) | Age | Plasma clearance (ml/min) | Age |
|---|---|---|---|
| 610 | 22 | 300 | 58 |
| 510 | 25 | 370 | 60 |
| 400 | 31 | 405 | 64 |
| 450 | 43 | 280 | 70 |
| 420 | 52 | 320 | 80 |

Describe and test the relationship between plasma clearance and age, fit 95% confidence limits to the predicted plasma clearance rates at age 25 and at age 55.

21. Match the following:

| *Research question* | *Test of significance* |
|---|---|
| 1. Effect of medicine | Correlation |
| 2. Comparison of effect of 2 medicines | Regression |
| 3. Comparison of 2 proportions | Kappa |
| 4. Agreement of association between two tests | Chi-squre |
| 5. Correlation | Paired 'T' test |
| 6. Change of 1 unit in X change how much in Y | Unpired 'T' test |

22. Following data gives you reporting of high blood pressure among users of OCPs and other methods of contraception tests that proportion of hypertensive among users of oral contraceptive pills differ significantly at 5% level of significance from user of other contraceptive methods. Prove or disprove it.

|  | Hypertensive | Normotensive | Total |
|---|---|---|---|
| OCP user | 16 | 64 | 80 |
| Others | 30 | 90 | 120 |

23. A study conducted to find out association of exposure to environmental tobacco smoke and occurrence of asthma revealed following data:

|        | Exposed | Not exposed | Total |
|--------|---------|-------------|-------|
| Asthma | 45      | 15          | 60    |
| Normal | 105     | 135         | 240   |
| Total  | 150     | 150         | 300   |

Find out the Chi-square value and test the hypothesis about exposure to ETS and its association with occurrence of asthma.

24. Following is result of a test BCPE

|                 | Breast Cancer (D+) | No Breast Cancer (D −) | Totals |
|-----------------|--------------------|------------------------|--------|
| BCPF test (T+)  | 570                | 150                    | 720    |
| BCPF t est (T−) | 30                 | 850                    | 880    |
| Total           | 600                | 1000                   | 1600   |

Infer about its sensitivity, specificity, PPV and NPV.

25. Figure below shows the result of a cohort study of cancer breast found in a block having population 10800; followed for one and half years, i.e. started since 1st January 2011 to 30 June 1012.

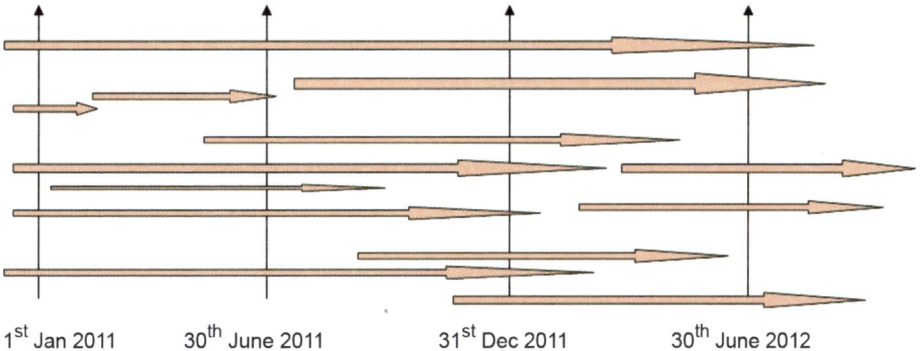

| 1$^{st}$ Jan 2011 | 30$^{th}$ June 2011 | 31$^{st}$ Dec 2011 | 30$^{th}$ June 2012 |

**Calculate the values of the following measures:**

1. Prevalence of breast cancer on:
   a. 1st Jan. 2011
   b. 30th June 2011
   c. 31st Dec. 2011
   d. 30th June 2012

2. Incidence rate of breast cancer in:
   a. Year 2011
   b. Mid-year 2011 to mid-year 2012

3. Mortality rate of breast cancer

4. Estimate probability of dying in 6 months on assuming the constant rate model.

5. Find out one year survival of breast cancer case assuming the constant rate model.

26. Complete the following life table:

| Year (t) | N | D | L | N1/2L | P(F) | P(S) | S(t) |
|---|---|---|---|---|---|---|---|
| 1 | 234 | 24 | 3 | | | | |
| 2 | 207 | 27 | 11 | | | | |
| 3 | 169 | 31 | 9 | | | | |
| 4 | 129 | 17 | 7 | | | | |
| 5 | 105 | 7 | 13 | | | | |
| 6 | 85 | 6 | 6 | | | | |
| 7 | 73 | 5 | 6 | | | | |
| 8 | 62 | 3 | 10 | | | | |
| 9 | 49 | 2 | 13 | | | | |
| 10 | 34 | 4 | | | | | |

27. In the following table, population of a community is given with cases and deaths of disease 'A' and disease 'B'.

| Year | 2006 | 2007 | 2008 | 2009 | 2010 |
|---|---|---|---|---|---|
| Population | 320 | 350 | 390 | 430 | 480 |
| Cases of 'A' | 23 | 31 | 33 | 29 | 50 |
| Deaths due to 'A' | 5 | 8 | 9 | 2 | 14 |
| Cases of 'B' | 43 | 31 | 24 | 19 | 8 |
| Deaths due to 'B' | 12 | 11 | 9 | 9 | 4 |
| Total deaths | 45 | 54 | 32 | 44 | 34 |

1. Find out incidence rates of disease 'A' in this population for different years.
2. Find out incidence rates of disease 'B' in this population for different years.
3. Calculate all possible mortality and morbidity statistics with above data available.
4. What would you conclude about the disease 'A'?
5. What would you conclude about the disease 'B'?
6. Compare and comment on disease 'A' and disease 'B'.

28. In a study out of 250 cases of breast cancer, 134 cases were having children whereas out of 250 matched controls 246 were having children.
   1. What type of study is this?
   2. What is the risk ratio of breast cancer, in nullipara?
   3. Discuss the results.

29. 1000 smokers and same number of matched non-smokers were followed for 15 years. Lung cancer was developed in 58 among smokers group and 24 in non-smokers group.
   1. What type of study is this?
   2. Calculate absolute risk, relative risk and attributed risk of lung cancer in smokers.
   3. Discuss the results.

30. The following results were obtained for treatment of type I diabetes with Insulin 50/50 and Insulin 30/70.

| | | Blood sugar level | |
|---|---|---|---|
| | | Controlled | Uncontrolled |
| Treatment group | Insulin 50/50 | 236 | 14 |
| of cases | Insulin 30/70 | 188 | 62 |

1. What type of study is this?
2. Calculate success management rate of type I diabetes with Insulin 50/50
3. Calculate success management rate of type I diabetes with Insulin 30/70.
4. Whether Insulin 50/50 is more effective than Insulin 30/70 ?

31. The following results were obtained for cancer of the prostate after an average follow-up time of 6 years:

| | | Cases | |
|---|---|---|---|
| | | *Number* | *Incidence rate* |
| Treatment group | Vitamin E supplementation | 99000 | 11.6 |
| of cases | No supplementation | 151000 | 17.8 |

1. Calculate the person-years at risk in the two study groups separately.
2. Estimate the "relative risk" and "attributed risk" measuring the effect of daily supplementation with vitamin E on the risk prostate cancer.
3. Estimate either the excess fraction or preventive fraction, whichever is more appropriate.
4. Describe the proportional impact of vitamin E supplementation.
5. Discuss the results. What can be concluded from these estimates?

# Appendix

## India's Demography

| | |
|---|---|
| Capital | New Delhi at 28°36.82N 77°12.52E |
| Largest city | Mumbai |
| Official language(s) | Hindi, English |
| Government | Federal parliamentary |

## Legislature Parliament of India

- Upper house     Rajya Sabha
- Lower house     Lok Sabha

## Independence from the United Kingdom

- Dominion     15 August 1947
- Republic     26 January 1950

| | |
|---|---|
| Area | Total 3,287,263 km$^2$ |
| Water (%) | 9.56 |
| Population | 1,210,193,422 (2011 Census) |
| Density | 370.4/km$^2$ (2011 Census) |
| GDP (nominal) | 2011 estimate |
| • Total | 1.848 trillion[7] (10th) |
| • Per capita | 1,388[6] (140th) |
| HDI (2011) | 0.547[9] (medium) (134th) |
| Currency | Indian rupee (INR) |
| Time zone | IST (UTC + 05:30) |
| Date formats | dd-mm-yyyy (AD) |
| Drives on the | left |
| ISO 3166 code | IN |
| Internet TLD | .in |
| Calling code | 91 |

## States of India

| | | |
|---|---|---|
| 1. Andhra Pradesh | 2. Arunachal Pradesh | 3. Assam |
| 4. Bihar | 5. Chhattisgarh | 6. Goa |
| 7. Gujarat | 8. Haryana | 9. Himachal Pradesh |
| 10. Jammu and Kashmir | 11. Jharkhand | 12. Karnataka |
| 13. Kerala | 14. Madhya Pradesh | 15. Maharashtra |
| 16. Manipur | 17. Meghalaya | 18. Mizoram |

| | | |
|---|---|---|
| 19. Nagaland | 20. Orissa | 21. Punjab |
| 22. Rajasthan | 23. Sikkim | 24. Tamil Nadu |
| 25. Tripura | 26. Uttar Pradesh | 27. Uttarakhand |
| 28. West Bengal | | |

## Union Territories

| | | |
|---|---|---|
| 1. Andaman and Nicobar Islands | 2. Chandigarh | 3. Dadra and Nagar Haveli |
| 4. Daman and Diu | 5. Lakshadweep | |
| 6. National Capital Territory of Delhi | 7. Pondicherry | |

## National Symbols

| | |
|---|---|
| Flag | Tricolour |
| Emblem | Sarnath Lion Capital |
| Anthem | Jana Gana Mana |
| Song | Vande Mataram |
| Calendar | Saka |
| Flower | Lotus |
| Fruit | Mango |
| Tree | Banyan |
| Bird | Indian Peafowl |
| Land animal | Royal Bengal Tiger |
| River | Ganga |

## IMPORTANT DAYS

### January

**Month activity:** Alzheimer Awareness Month
**Week activity:** January 15 to January 21—National Non-Smoking Week

### Single day events:

- 10th January: World Laughter Day
- 12th January: National Youth Day
- 15th January: Army Day
- 26th January: India's Republic Day and International Customs Day
- 26th January: International Customs Day
- 30th January: Martyrs' Day
- 30th January: Anti-Leprosy Day

### February

**Month activity:** Heart Month

### Week activity:

- February 5 to February 11: Eating Disorders Awareness Week
- February 5 to February 11: White Cane Week

## Single day events:

- 4th February: World Cancer Day
- 6th February: International Day of Zero Tolerance to Female Genital Mutilation
- 12th February: Sexual and Reproductive Health Awareness Day
- 24th February: Central Excise Day
- 28th February: National Science Day

## March

### Month activity:

- "Help Fight Liver Disease" Month
- National Colorectal Cancer Awareness Month
- National Kidney Month
- National Nutrition Month
- National Social Work Month
- Red Cross Month

### Week activity:

- March 4 to March 10: Pharmacist Awareness Week
- March 11 to March 17: Canadian Agricultural Safety Week
- March 11 to March 17: World Glaucoma Week
- March 12 to March 18: Brain Awareness Week
- March 18 to March 24: Poison Prevention Week

### Single day events

- 8th March: International Women's Day
- 15th March: World Disabled Day
- 15th March: World Consumer Right Day
- 16th March: Measles Vaccination Day
- 21st March: World Forestry Day
- 21st March: International Day for the Elimination of Racial Discrimination.
- 22nd March: World Water Day
- 23rd March: World Meteorological Day
- 24th March: World TB Day
- 26th March: Purple Day—The Global Day of Epilepsy Awareness

## April

### Month activity:

- Daffodil Days: Cancer Awareness
- Irritable Bowel Syndrome (IBS) Awareness Month
- Oral Health Month
- Parkinson's Awareness Month

**Week activity:**
- April 8 to April 14: National Dental Hygienists Week
- April 21 to April 28: National Immunization Awareness Week
- April 22 to April 28: National Organ and Tissue Donor Awareness Week

**Single day events:**
- 2nd April: World Autism Awareness Day
- 5th April: National Maritime Day
- 7th April: World Health Day
- 17th April: World Haemophilia Day
- 18th April: World Heritage Day
- 22nd April: World Earth Day
- 23rd April: World Bank and Copyright Day
- 25th April: World Malaria Day

## May

**Month activity:**
- Cystic Fibrosis Month
- Foot Health Awareness Month
- Hepatitis Awareness Month
- Huntington's Disease Awareness Month
- Multiple Sclerosis Awareness Month
- National Physiotherapy Month
- Speech and Hearing Awareness Month

**Week activity:**
- May 1 to May 7: National Summer Safety Week
- May 6 to May 12: Emergency Preparedness Week
- May 6 to May 12: National Hospice Palliative Care Week
- May 6 to May 12: North American Occupational Safety and Health Week
- May 7 to May 13: National Mental Health Week
- May 7 to May 13: National Nursing Week
- May 28 to June 1: Spine Week

**Single day events:**
- 1st May: International Labor Day
- 1st May: World Asthma Day
- 3rd May: Press Freedom Day
- 5th May: Save Lives: Clean Your Hands
- 6th May: Annual Hike for Hospice Palliative Care
- May (2nd Sunday): Mother's Day

- 8th May: World Red Cross Day
- 11th May: National Technology Day
- 12th May: International Nursing Day
- 15th May: International Day of the Family
- 17th May: World Telecommunication Day
- 17th May: International Day Against Homophobia
- 20th May: World Autoimmune Arthritis Day
- 24th May: Commonwealth Day
- 28th May: National Multiple Births Awareness Day
- 31st May: Anti-Tobacco Day

## June

### Month activity:

- Spina Bifida and Hydrocephalus Awareness Month
- Stroke Awareness Month

**Week activity:** June 4 to June 10: National Sun Awareness Week

### Single day events:

- 3rd June: National Cancer Survivors Day
- 4th June: International Day of Innocent Children Victims of Aggression.
- 5th June: World Environment Day
- 6th June: Clean Air Day
- 14th June: World Blood Donor Day
- June (3rd Sunday): Fathers Day
- 26th June: International Day Against Drug Abuse and Illicit Trafficking
- 27th June: World Diabetes Day

## July

**Week activity:** 17th July to 23rd July: Anti-Fly Week

### Single day events:

- 1st July: International Joke Day
- 6th July: World Zoonoses Day
- 11th July: World Population Day
- 28th July: World Hepatitis Day

## August

**Week activity:** August 1st to August 7th: World Breastfeeding Week

### Single day events:

- 3rd August: International Friendship Day
- 6th August: Hiroshima Day
- 9th August: Quit India Day and Nagasaki Day

- 15th August: Independence Day in India.
- 19th August: World Humanitarian Day
- 29th August: National Sports Day.

## September
### Month activity:

- Breakfast for Learning Month
- Childhood Cancer Awareness Month
- Men's Cancer Health Awareness Month
- National Arthritis Month
- Ovarian Cancer Awareness Month

**Multi-days activity:** September 15 to September 23: AIDS Walk for Life

### Single day events:

- 5th September: World Teachers' Day
- 8th September: World Literacy Day
- 9th September: Fetal Alcohol Spectrum Disorder (FASD) Awareness Day
- 10th September: World Suicide Prevention Day
- 16th September: World Ozone Day
- 21st September: World Alzheimer's Day
- 26th September: Day of the Deaf
- 27th September: World Tourism Day
- 28th September: World Rabies Day
- 29th September: World Heart Day

## October
### Month activity:

- Autism Awareness Month
- Breast Cancer Awareness Month
- Eye Health Month
- Healthy Workplace Month
- International Walk to School Month
- Learning Disabilities Awareness Month
- National Occupational Therapy Month
- Psoriasis Awareness Month
- SIDS (Sudden Infant Death Syndrome) awareness Month
- The Flu Shot: Influenza Immunization Awareness Month

### Week activity:

- September 30 to October 6: Mental Illness Awareness Week
- October 7 to October 13: Fire Prevention Week
- October 15 to October 19: National Infection Control Week
- October 17 to October 23: National School Safety Week

## Single day events

- 1st October: International day of the Elderly
- 1st October: Blood Donation Day
- 2nd October: Cleanliness Day
- 2nd October: Leprosy Day
- 2nd October: T.B. Seal Campaign Day
- 3rd October: World Habitat Day
- 4th October: World Animal Welfare Day
- 7th October: World Habitation Day
- 8th October: Indian Air Force Day
- 9th October: World Post Office Day
- 10th October: National Postal Day
- 10th October: World Mental Health Day
- 12th October: World Sight Day
- 13th October: International Day for Disaster Reduction
- 13th October: World Sight Day
- 13th October: UN International Day for National Disaster Reduction
- 14th October: World Standards Day
- 15th October: World White Cane Day (guiding the Blind).
- 16th October: World Food Day
- 22nd October: International Stuttering Awareness Day
- 24th October: UN Day, World Development Information Day
- 30th October: World Thrift Day

## November

### Month activity:

- Crohn's and Colitis Awareness Month
- Cardipulmonary Resuscitation (C.P.R.) Awareness Month
- Diabetes Month
- Lung Cancer Awareness Month
- Canada: Prostate Cancer Awareness Month
- Osteoporosis Month
- Pancreatic Cancer Awareness Month

### Week activity:

- November 6 to November 12: National Pain Awareness Week
- November 6 to November 12: National Seniors Safety Week
- November 24 to November 30: National Home Fire Safety Week

### Single day events:

- 12th November: World Pneumonia Day
- 14th November: World Diabetes Day
- 12th November: Children's Day (in India)
- 16th November: World COPD (Chronic Obstructive Pulmonary Disease) Day

- 20th November: National Child Day
- 25th November: International Day for the Elimination of Violence Against Women
- 29th November: International Day of Solidarity with Palestinian People

## December

**Month activity:** The Lung Association's Christmas Seal Campaign

### Single day events

- 1st December: World AIDS Day
- 3rd December: International Day of Disabled Persons
- 4th December: Navy Day
- 7th December: Armed Forces Flag Day
- 10th December: Human Right Day
- 10th December: International Day for Broadcasting
- 18th December: Minorities Right Day
- 23rd December: Kisan Divas (Farmer's Day)

### WORLD HEALTH DAY THEMES

- 1950: Know own health services.
- 1951: Health for your child and the world's children.
- 1952: Healthy surroundings make healthy people.
- 1953: Health is wealth.
- 1954: The nurse: Pioneer of health.
- 1955: Clean water means better health.
- 1956: Destroy disease-carrying insects.
- 1957: Food and health.
- 1958: Ten years of health progress.
- 1959: Mental illness and mental health in the world today.
- 1960: Malaria eradication—a world challenge.
- 1961: Accidents need not happen.
- 1962: Preserve sight—prevent blindness.
- 1963: Hunger: Disease of millions.
- 1964: No trace of tuberculosis.
- 1965: Smallpox—constant alert.
- 1966: Man and his cities.
- 1967: Partners in health.
- 1968: Health in the world of tomorrow.
- 1969: Health, labour and productivity.
- 1970: Early detection of cancer saves lives.
- 1971: A full life despite diabetes.
- 1972: Your heart is your health.

- 1973: Health begins at home.
- 1974: Better food for a healthier world.
- 1975: Smallpox—point of no return.
- 1976: Foresight prevents blindness.
- 1977: Immunize and protect your child.
- 1978: Down with high blood pressure.
- 1979: A healthy child—a sure future.
- 1980: Smoking or health: The choice is yours.
- 1981: Health for all by the year 2000.
- 1982: Add life to years.
- 1983: Health for all by 2000 AD: The count down has began.
- 1984: Children's health: Tomorrow's wealth.
- 1985: Healthy youth: Our best resource.
- 1986: Healthy living: Every one a winner.
- 1987: Immunization: A chance for every child.
- 1988: Health for All: All for health.
- 1989: Let's talk health.
- 1990: Our planet our health—think globally—act locally.
- 1991: Should disaster strike—be prepared.
- 1992: Heart beat: The rhythm of health.
- 1993: Handle life with care: Prevent violence and negligence.
- 1994: Oral health for healthy life.
- 1995: Target 2000—"World without polio.
- 1996: Healthy cities for better life.
- 1997: Emerging infectious diseases: Global response—global alert.
- 1998: Safe motherhood (pregnancy is special—let's make it safe).
- 1999: Active aging makes the difference.
- 2000: Safe blood starts with me: Blood saves life.
- 2001: Mental Health: New understanding, new hope.
- 2002: Reducing risks, promoting healthy life.
- 2003: Shape the future of life.
- 2004: Road safety.
- 2005: Make every mother and child count.
- 2006: Working together for health.
- 2007: Invest in health, build a safer future.
- 2008: Protect health from climate change.
- 2009: Save life, make hospitals safe in emergencies.
- 2010: Urbanization and health.
- 2011: Antimicrobial resistance: No action today no cure tomorrow.
- 2012: Good health adds life to years.

## Chi-square Table

| Degree of freedom (df) | At P value | | |
|---|---|---|---|
| | P = 0.05 | P = 0.01 | P = 0.001 |
| 1 | 3.84 | 6.64 | 10.83 |
| 2 | 5.99 | 9.21 | 13.82 |
| 3 | 7.82 | 11.35 | 16.27 |
| 4 | 9.49 | 13.28 | 18.47 |
| 5 | 11.07 | 15.09 | 20.52 |
| 6 | 12.59 | 16.81 | 22.46 |
| 7 | 14.07 | 18.48 | 24.32 |
| 8 | 15.51 | 20.09 | 26.13 |
| 9 | 16.92 | 21.67 | 27.88 |
| 10 | 18.31 | 23.21 | 29.59 |
| 11 | 19.68 | 24.73 | 31.26 |
| 12 | 21.03 | 26.22 | 32.91 |
| 13 | 22.36 | 27.69 | 34.53 |
| 14 | 23.69 | 29.14 | 36.12 |
| 15 | 25.00 | 30.58 | 37.70 |
| 16 | 26.30 | 32.00 | 39.25 |
| 17 | 27.59 | 33.41 | 40.79 |
| 18 | 28.87 | 34.81 | 42.31 |
| 19 | 30.14 | 36.19 | 43.82 |
| 20 | 31.41 | 37.57 | 45.32 |
| 21 | 32.67 | 38.93 | 46.80 |
| 22 | 33.92 | 40.29 | 48.27 |
| 23 | 35.17 | 41.64 | 49.73 |
| 24 | 36.42 | 42.98 | 51.18 |
| 25 | 37.65 | 44.31 | 52.62 |
| 26 | 38.89 | 45.64 | 54.05 |
| 27 | 40.11 | 46.96 | 55.48 |
| 28 | 41.34 | 48.28 | 56.89 |
| 29 | 42.56 | 49.59 | 58.30 |
| 30 | 43.77 | 50.89 | 59.70 |

Table gives the highest value of Chi-square at particular degree of freedom.

## 'Z' Score Test

| 'Z' | At positive 'Z' score with P value | | | | | At negative' Z' score with P value | | | | |
|---|---|---|---|---|---|---|---|---|---|---|
| Score | < 0.001 | 0.01 | 0.02 | 0.05 | 0.09 | <0.001 | 0.01 | 0.02 | 0.05 | 0.09 |
| 0.0 | 0.5000 | 0.5040 | 0.5080 | 0.5199 | 0.5359 | 0.5000 | 0.4960 | 0.4920 | 0.4801 | 0.4641 |
| 0.1 | 0.5398 | 0.5438 | 0.5478 | 0.5596 | 0.5753 | 0.4602 | 0.4562 | 0.4522 | 0.4404 | 0.4247 |
| 0.2 | 0.5793 | 0.5832 | 0.5871 | 0.5987 | 0.6141 | 0.4207 | 0.4168 | 0.4129 | 0.4013 | 0.3829 |
| 0.3 | 0.6179 | 0.6217 | 0.6255 | 0.6368 | 0.6517 | 0.3821 | 0.3783 | 0.3745 | 0.3632 | 0.3483 |
| 0.4 | 0.6554 | 0.6591 | 0.6628 | 0.6736 | 0.6879 | 0.3446 | 0.3409 | 0.3372 | 0.3300 | 0.3121 |
| 0.5 | 0.6915 | 0.6950 | 0.6985 | 0.7088 | 0.7224 | 0.3085 | 0.3050 | 0.3015 | 0.2912 | 0.2776 |
| 0.6 | 0.7257 | 0.7291 | 0.7324 | 0.7422 | 0.7549 | 0.2743 | 0.2709 | 0.2676 | 0.2578 | 0.2451 |
| 0.7 | 0.7580 | 0.7611 | 0.7642 | 0.7734 | 0.7852 | 0.2420 | 0.2389 | 0.2358 | 0.2266 | 0.2148 |
| 0.8 | 0.7881 | 0.7910 | 0.7939 | 0.8023 | 0.8133 | 0.2119 | 0.2090 | 0.2061 | 0.1977 | 0.1867 |
| 0.9 | 0.8159 | 0.8186 | 0.8212 | 0.8289 | 0.8389 | 0.1841 | 0.1814 | 0.1788 | 0.1711 | 0.1611 |
| 1.0 | 0.8413 | 0.8438 | 0.8461 | 0.8531 | 0.8621 | 0.1587 | 0.1562 | 0.1539 | 0.1469 | 0.1379 |
| 1.1 | 0.8643 | 0.8665 | 0.8686 | 0.8749 | 0.8830 | 0.1357 | 0.1335 | 0.1314 | 0.1251 | 0.1170 |
| 1.2 | 0.8849 | 0.8869 | 0.8888 | 0.8944 | 0.9015 | 0.1151 | 0.1131 | 0.1112 | 0.1056 | 0.0985 |
| 1.3 | 0.9032 | 0.9049 | 0.9066 | 0.9115 | 0.9177 | 0.0968 | 0.0951 | 0.0934 | 0.0885 | 0.0823 |
| 1.4 | 0.9192 | 0.9207 | 0.9222 | 0.9265 | 0.9319 | 0.0808 | 0.0793 | 0.0778 | 0.0735 | 0.0681 |
| 1.5 | 0.9332 | 0.9345 | 0.9357 | 0.9394 | 0.9441 | 0.0668 | 0.0655 | 0.0643 | 0.0606 | 0.0559 |
| 1.6 | 0.9452 | 0.9463 | 0.9474 | 0.9505 | 0.9545 | 0.0548 | 0.0537 | 0.0526 | 0.0495 | 0.0455 |
| 1.7 | 0.9554 | 0.9564 | 0.9573 | 0.9599 | 0.9633 | 0.0446 | 0.0436 | 0.0427 | 0.0401 | 0.0367 |
| 1.8 | 0.9641 | 0.9649 | 0.9656 | 0.9678 | 0.9706 | 0.0359 | 0.0351 | 0.0344 | 0.0322 | 0.0294 |
| 1.9 | 0.9713 | 0.9719 | 0.9726 | 0.9744 | 0.9767 | 0.0287 | 0.0281 | 0.0274 | 0.0257 | 0.0233 |
| 2.0 | 0.9772 | 0.9778 | 0.9783 | 0.9798 | 0.9817 | 0.0228 | 0.0222 | 0.0217 | 0.0202 | 0.0183 |
| 2.1 | 0.9821 | 0.9826 | 0.9830 | 0.9842 | 0.9857 | 0.0179 | 0.0174 | 0.0170 | 0.0158 | 0.0143 |
| 2.2 | 0.9861 | 0.9864 | 0.9868 | 0.9878 | 0.9890 | 0.0139 | 0.0136 | 0.0132 | 0.0122 | 0.0110 |
| 2.3 | 0.9893 | 0.9896 | 0.9898 | 0.9906 | 0.9916 | 0.0107 | 0.0104 | 0.0102 | 0.0094 | 0.0084 |
| 2.4 | 0.9918 | 0.9920 | 0.9922 | 0.9929 | 0.9936 | 0.0082 | 0.0080 | 0.0078 | 0.0071 | 0.0064 |
| 2.5 | 0.9938 | 0.9940 | 0.9941 | 0.9946 | 0.9952 | 0.0062 | 0.0060 | 0.0059 | 0.0054 | 0.0048 |
| 2.6 | 0.9953 | 0.9955 | 0.9956 | 0.9960 | 0.9964 | 0.0047 | 0.0045 | 0.0044 | 0.0040 | 0.0036 |
| 2.7 | 0.9965 | 0.9966 | 0.9967 | 0.9970 | 0.9974 | 0.0035 | 0.0034 | 0.0033 | 0.0030 | 0.0027 |
| 2.8 | 0.9974 | 0.9975 | 0.9976 | 0.9978 | 0.9981 | 0.0026 | 0.0025 | 0.0024 | 0.0022 | 0.0019 |
| 2.9 | 0.9981 | 0.9982 | 0.9982 | 0.9984 | 0.9986 | 0.0019 | 0.0018 | 0.0018 | 0.0016 | 0.0014 |
| 3.0 | 0.9987 | 0.9987 | 0.9987 | 0.9989 | 0.9990 | 0.0013 | 0.0013 | 0.0013 | 0.0012 | 0.0010 |
| 3.1 | 0.9990 | 0.9991 | 0.9991 | 0.9992 | 0.9993 | 0.0010 | 0.0009 | 0.0009 | 0.0008 | 0.0007 |
| 3.2 | 0.9993 | 0.9993 | 0.9994 | 0.9994 | 0.9995 | 0.0007 | 0.0007 | 0.0006 | 0.0006 | 0.0005 |
| 3.3 | 0.9995 | 0.9995 | 0.9995 | 0.9996 | 0.9997 | 0.0005 | 0.0005 | 0.0005 | 0.0004 | 0.0003 |
| 3.4 | 0.9997 | 0.9997 | 0.9997 | 0.9997 | 0.9998 | 0.0003 | 0.0003 | 0.0003 | 0.0003 | 0.0002 |
| z | < 0.001 | 0.01 | 0.02 | 0.05 | 0.09 | <0.001 | 0.01 | 0.02 | 0.05 | 0.09 |

## Table for 't' Test

| Degree of freedom | At P value | | | |
|---|---|---|---|---|
| | 0.1 | P = 0.05 | P = 0.01 | P = 0.001 |
| 1 | 6.31 | 12.71 | 63.66 | 636.62 |
| 2 | 2.92 | 4.30 | 9.93 | 31.60 |
| 3 | 2.35 | 3.18 | 5.84 | 12.92 |
| 4 | 2.13 | 2.78 | 4.60 | 8.61 |
| 5 | 2.02 | 2.57 | 4.03 | 6.87 |
| 6 | 1.94 | 2.45 | 3.71 | 5.96 |
| 7 | 1.89 | 2.37 | 3.50 | 5.41 |
| 8 | 1.86 | 2.31 | 3.36 | 5.04 |
| 9 | 1.83 | 2.26 | 3.25 | 4.78 |
| 10 | 1.81 | 2.23 | 3.17 | 4.59 |
| 11 | 1.80 | 2.20 | 3.11 | 4.44 |
| 12 | 1.78 | 2.18 | 3.06 | 4.32 |
| 13 | 1.77 | 2.16 | 3.01 | 4.22 |
| 14 | 1.76 | 2.14 | 2.98 | 4.14 |
| 15 | 1.75 | 2.13 | 2.95 | 4.07 |
| 16 | 1.75 | 2.12 | 2.92 | 4.02 |
| 17 | 1.74 | 2.11 | 2.90 | 3.97 |
| 18 | 1.73 | 2.10 | 2.88 | 3.92 |
| 19 | 1.73 | 2.09 | 2.86 | 3.88 |
| 20 | 1.72 | 2.09 | 2.85 | 3.85 |
| 21 | 1.72 | 2.08 | 2.83 | 3.82 |
| 22 | 1.72 | 2.07 | 2.82 | 3.79 |
| 23 | 1.71 | 2.07 | 2.82 | 3.77 |
| 24 | 1.71 | 2.06 | 2.80 | 3.75 |
| 25 | 1.71 | 2.06 | 2.79 | 3.73 |
| 26 | 1.71 | 2.06 | 2.78 | 3.71 |
| 27 | 1.70 | 2.05 | 2.77 | 3.69 |
| 28 | 1.70 | 2.05 | 2.76 | 3.67 |
| 29 | 1.70 | 2.05 | 2.76 | 3.66 |
| 30 | 1.70 | 2.04 | 2.75 | 3.65 |
| 40 | 1.68 | 2.02 | 2.70 | 3.55 |
| 60 | 1.67 | 2.00 | 2.66 | 3.46 |
| 120 | 1.66 | 1.98 | 2.62 | 3.37 |
| Infinity | 1.65 | 1.96 | 2.58 | 3.29 |

Table gives the highest value of 't' test at particular degree of freedom.

## Random Number Table

| | | | | | | | | | |
|---|---|---|---|---|---|---|---|---|---|
| 13962 | 70992 | 65172 | 28053 | 02190 | 83634 | 66012 | 70305 | 66761 | 88344 |
| 43905 | 46941 | 72300 | 11641 | 43548 | 30455 | 07686 | 31840 | 03261 | 89139 |
| 00504 | 48658 | 38051 | 59408 | 16508 | 82979 | 92002 | 63606 | 41078 | 86326 |
| 61274 | 57238 | 47267 | 35303 | 29066 | 02140 | 60867 | 39847 | 50968 | 96719 |
| 43753 | 21159 | 16239 | 50595 | 62509 | 61207 | 86816 | 29902 | 23395 | 72640 |
| 83503 | 51662 | 21636 | 68192 | 84294 | 38754 | 84755 | 34053 | 94582 | 29215 |
| 36807 | 71420 | 35804 | 44862 | 23577 | 79551 | 42003 | 58684 | 09271 | 68396 |
| 19110 | 55680 | 18792 | 41487 | 16614 | 83053 | 00812 | 16749 | 45347 | 88199 |
| 82615 | 86984 | 93290 | 87971 | 60022 | 35415 | 20852 | 02909 | 99476 | 45568 |
| 05621 | 26584 | 36493 | 63013 | 68181 | 57702 | 49510 | 75304 | 38724 | 15712 |
| 06936 | 37293 | 55875 | 71213 | 83025 | 46063 | 74665 | 12178 | 10741 | 58362 |
| 84981 | 60458 | 16194 | 92403 | 80951 | 80068 | 47076 | 23310 | 74899 | 87929 |
| 66354 | 88441 | 96191 | 04794 | 14714 | 64749 | 43097 | 83976 | 83281 | 72038 |
| 49602 | 94109 | 36460 | 62353 | 00721 | 66980 | 82554 | 90270 | 12312 | 56299 |
| 78430 | 72391 | 96973 | 70437 | 97803 | 78683 | 04670 | 70667 | 58912 | 21883 |
| 33331 | 51803 | 15934 | 75807 | 46561 | 80188 | 78984 | 29317 | 27971 | 16440 |
| 62843 | 84445 | 56652 | 91797 | 45284 | 25842 | 96246 | 73504 | 21631 | 81223 |
| 19528 | 15445 | 77764 | 33446 | 41204 | 70067 | 33354 | 70680 | 66664 | 75486 |
| 16737 | 01887 | 50934 | 43306 | 75190 | 86997 | 56561 | 79018 | 34273 | 25196 |
| 99389 | 06685 | 45945 | 62000 | 76228 | 60645 | 87750 | 46329 | 46544 | 95665 |
| 36160 | 38196 | 77705 | 28891 | 12106 | 56281 | 86222 | 66116 | 39626 | 06080 |
| 05505 | 45420 | 44016 | 79662 | 92069 | 27628 | 50002 | 32540 | 19848 | 27319 |

## Hospital Waste Categories

| Category no. | Type of waste |
|---|---|
| 1 | Human anatomical waste |
| 2 | Animal and slaughter house waste |
| 3 | Microbiology and biotechnology waste |
| 4 | Waste sharps |
| 5 | Discarded medicines and cytotoxic medicines |
| 6 | Soiled solid waste (other than plastic) |
| 7 | Solid (plastic) disposables |
| 8 | Liquid waste |
| 9 | Incineration waste |
| 10 | Municipal waste |

Hospital waste segregation, transportation and disposal as per category of waste.

## FINAL TREATMENT AND DISPOSAL

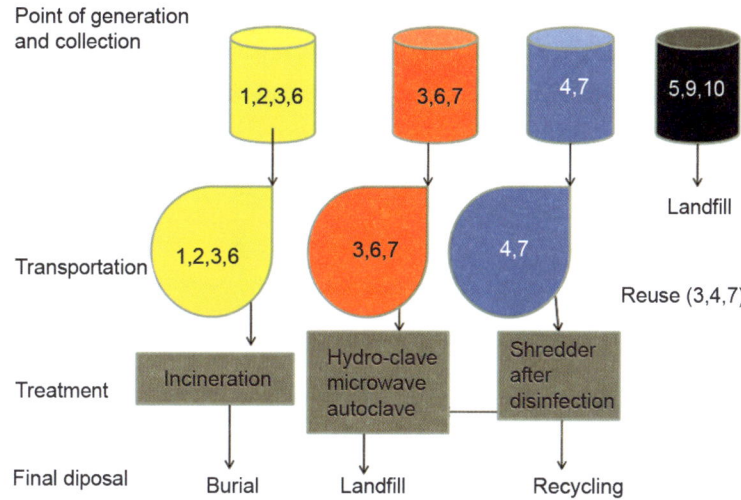

### Dos and Don'ts for Vaccine Refrigerators

### Dos

- Keep it in a cool room away from sunlight and at least 10 cm away from sunlight.
- Fix the plug permanently.
- Keep the ref levelled.
- Keep voltage stabilizer.
- Keep the vaccines at desired places with some space in between.
- Keep ice and icepacks in freezer and bottled filled with water in door always, to maintain temperature in case of emergency.
- Stick a paper nearby to note temperature at least for two times, i.e. one when session starts and other when session last.
- Mobile number of the person to whom should be contacted in emergency must be written on the above paper.

### Don'ts

- Do not open the door frequently.
- Do not use this refregarator for eatables.
- Do not keep vaccines in the door.
- Do not keep more than one month stock of vaccines.
- Do not keep expired vaccines.

# Index

**A**

Aflatoxin 81
Aganwadi centre 139
AICPI 33
Alum 99
Antenatal case 12, 37
Arthropods 84
At risk children 35
At risk mothers 35
Autoclave 154

**B**

BCG 109, 112, 119
Bed bug 91
Bitot's spot 119
Bleaching powder 50, 57, 99
Blood sampling 174
BMI 35
BMR units 41

**C**

Calcium hardness 52
Caries 120
Cereals 61
CHC 146
Child health record 14
Chlorine demand 50
Coffee 79
Cold boxes 116
Coliform test 168
Community survey 7
Condoms 102
Cyclops 91

**D**

DDT 96
Dettol 98
Diet and nutritional status 10
Differential diagnosis 5, 20
District hospital visit 149
DPT 109, 112
DT 110

**E**

Education 26
Environmental status 8
Epidemic dropsy 82

**F**

Family 25
Family schedule 9
Fluorosis 120
Food sampling 185
Fruits 70

**G**

Gaur's SES scale 30
General examination 4, 19
Goiter 120
Gram's staining 44

**H**

Hanging drop preparation 46
Harmonal contraceptive methods 104
Herpes 120
Horrock's apparatus 50
House fly 90
Housing conditions 7, 32
Hydroclave 155

**I**

Ice packs 115
ICTC visit 152
ILR 117, 118
Immunization card 128
Incinerator 156
Individual health record 21
IUDs 103

**K**

Kishori card 127
Kuppuswami SES scale 28
Kwashiorkor 119

**L**

Lathyrism 80
Lime 99
Living status 32
Louse 91

**M**

Magnesium (Mg) hardness 54
Malaria test kit 131
Mamta card 121
Management of family 26
Marasmum child 119
Measles 109, 112, 119
Microwave 155
Milk and milk product 75
Mosquitoes 85

**N**

Nasal swab 179
Nasopharyngeal swab 180
Non-vegetarian food 73
Nutritional status schedule 10
Nuts 77

**O**

Obstetric history 3
Occupation 27
OPV 109
ORS packets 125

**P**

P. Prasad's SES scale 28
Parboiling 63
Paris green 97
Partograph 126
Pellegra 120
Personal history 4
Personal hygiene 4, 19, 23
PHC 143
PNC record 13
Potassium permanganate 99
Pregnancy preparedness 38
Problem family 25
Pulses 63
Pyrethrum 97

**R**

Rat flea 91
RDA 39

Rectal swab 183
Religion 26
RHTC 137
Rickets 120
Road to health card 125
Roots and tubers 70

**S**

Safe water 161
Sand fly 90
Savlone 98
Sewage treatment plant 159
Social problem 12
Socioeconomic status 27
Sodium hypochlorite 99
Sputum sampling 177
Stool sampling 182
Subcentre 141
Sugar reaction of bacteria 46
Sulphate hardness 56
Systemic examination 5, 20

**T**

Tea 79
Tetanus 118
Thermocole boxes 116
Throat swab 179
Total hardness 51
TT vaccine 111

**U**

Udai Pareek SES scale 29
UHTC 135
Unmet need 11
Urine sampling 181

**V**

Vaccination 36, 111
Vaccine carrier 115, 116
Vegetables 66
Vitamin A 111

**W**

Water filtration plant 157
Water quality standard 171
Water sampling 163
Water sources 162
Wholesale price index 33
Whooping cough 119

# Reader's Note

**Reader's Note**